Clinical Cases in Implant Dentistry

Clinical Cases in Implant Dentistry

Edited by Preston Bailey

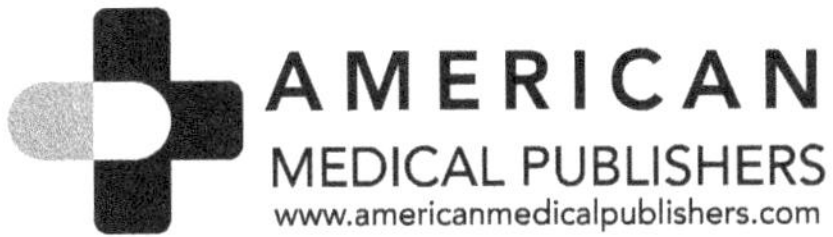

American Medical Publishers,
41 Flatbush Avenue,
1st Floor, New York,
NY 11217, USA

Visit us on the World Wide Web at:
www.americanmedicalpublishers.com

ISBN: 978-1-63927-052-1

Cataloging-in-Publication Data

Clinical cases in implant dentistry / edited by Preston Bailey.
p. cm.
Includes bibliographical references and index.
ISBN 978-1-63927-052-1
1. Dental implants. 2. Dentistry. I. Bailey, Preston.
RK667.I45 M63 2022
617.693--dc23

Table of Contents

Preface

A surgical process that supports a dental prosthesis such as bridge, crown and denture, by interfacing with the bone of jaw and skull is known as implant dentistry. The most common procedure in implant dentistry is osseointegration. In this process, the materials such as titanium are used to make an intimate bond to the bone. The complications related to the dental implants occur during the process of surgery such as bleeding and nerve injury. Complications such as infection and failure to osseointegrate, can also occur after the surgery. For the success of osseointegration, sufficient amount of healing time is necessary before the dental prosthetic is attached to the implant. This book outlines the processes and applications of modern implant dentistry in detail. It is a valuable compilation of topics, ranging from the basic to the most complex advancements in this field. With state-of-the-art inputs by acclaimed experts of this field, this book targets students and professionals.

After months of intensive research and writing, this book is the end result of all who devoted their time and efforts in the initiation and progress of this book. It will surely be a source of reference in enhancing the required knowledge of the new developments in the area. During the course of developing this book, certain measures such as accuracy, authenticity and research focused analytical studies were given preference in order to produce a comprehensive book in the area of study.

This book would not have been possible without the efforts of the authors and the publisher. I extend my sincere thanks to them. Secondly, I express my gratitude to my family and well-wishers. And most importantly, I thank my students for constantly expressing their willingness and curiosity in enhancing their knowledge in the field, which encourages me to take up further research projects for the advancement of the area.

Editor

1

Do we need CBCTs for sufficient diagnostics? - dentist-related factors

Josipa Radic[1], Raphael Patcas[2], Bernd Stadlinger[1], Daniel Wiedemeier[3], Martin Rücker[1] and Barbara Giacomelli-Hiestand[1*]

Abstract

Background: The aim of this study was to assess the diagnostic accuracy of various dentoalveolar pathologies based on panoramic radiography (OPG), cone beam computed tomography (CBCT) and printed 3D models in consecutive order; and to evaluate the impact of specialisation of residents in oral surgery (OS) versus residents in orthodontics (ORTH).

Methods: Fourteen residents were recruited to evaluate nine selected cases with different dentoalveolar pathologies. The residents were given for each case an OPG, a CBCT and a printed 3D model. For each case and imaging modality, the residents were asked several questions relating to (i) diagnosis, and (ii) the request for consecutive imaging in order to enable treatment. Further, aspects like impact of specialisation (OS versus ORTH), gender and years of experience were analysed.

Results: In this study, diagnostic accuracy (i) improved for OS from OPG to CBCT (OPG 66.3%, CBCT 83.4%) and likewise for ORTH (OPG 63.7%, CBCT 78.0%). 3D models generally did not seem more useful than CBCTs. For treatment planning (ii), residents in orthodontics considered OPGs significantly more often as sufficient compared to residents in oral surgery (OR 6.3, $p < 0.001$). Further, the odds to request a CBCT after OPG for treatment planning is influenced by dentist-related factors: female dentists (OR 3.8) or residents with limited professional experience as dentists (OR 3.0) asked more frequently for a CBCT.

Conclusions: Overall diagnostic accuracy is decent with OPG and can be improved with CBCT. Specialisation seems to have a moderate impact on diagnostic accuracy, but influences whether a CBCT was requested for treatment planning. Based on these findings, future studies shall analyse the diagnostic accuracy of specific pathologies in higher number in order to substantiate the present findings with regard to specific pathologies.

Keywords: Anatomy, CBCT, OPT, Oral surgery, Orthodontics

Background

Along with the clinical examination, radiological imaging is essential for a complete diagnosis in dental medicine [1, 2]. Orthopantomography (OPG), a two-dimensional panoramic radiograph, is widely used across all dental disciplines including oral surgery and orthodontics [3–5] to address basic diagnostic queries. An OPG contains an abundance of information on the teeth, mandible, maxilla, including the sinuses and the nasal cavity, and the temporomandibular joints. At the same time, OPG images suffer from important limitations [4, 6], such as being limited to two dimensions, distortion and blurring. In some cases, the broad coverage of the OPG will therefore still be insufficient to obtain an accurate diagnosis or enable the dentist to perform a treatment plan. According to most prevailing guidelines [7–9], three-dimensional imaging is recommended for patients who will benefit from cone beam computed tomography (CBCT) because the diagnosis would otherwise remain uncertain or the treatment plan unclear. CBCT scans of a region of interest have particularly been advocated by these guidelines for the assessment of bony structures and teeth, trauma, various pathologies or the assessment of topographical anatomy prior to surgical or orthodontic procedures.

* Correspondence: barbara.giacomelli@zzm.uzh.ch
[1]Clinic of Cranio-Maxillofacial and Oral Surgery, Centre of Dental Medicine, University of Zurich, Plattenstrasse 11, 8032 Zurich, Switzerland
Full list of author information is available at the end of the article

While the guidelines are hardly disputed, it must be noted that diagnostic accuracy and the effect on patient management (such as setting a treatment plan) are two different facets of imaging efficacy and have historically always been viewed in a hierarchical order [10, 11]. Moreover, an intrinsic difference between diagnostic accuracy and patient management must be respected. While diagnosis of a pathology should clearly remain unaffected by the dental specialisations, the treatment plan may ultimately differ between disciplines. The evaluation of a CBCT scan should therefore preferably include the impact on diagnostic accuracy as well as treatment approach.

With the introduction of commercial 3D-printing in dentistry, another diagnostic tool became available. The printing of CBCT DICOM-based surface reconstructed files with a semi-opaque material enables to obtain a "see-through" physical model of the scan. Yet, the diagnostic value of such printed models has to our knowledge not been researched.

Finally, the request for a CBCT should always be guided by the pursuit of improved diagnostic accuracy and the prospect of an enhanced treatment plan. Preferably, the indications for a CBCT should be based entirely on case-related factors. Yet, dentist-related factors might influence the request for a CBCT as well.

The aim of this study was therefore (i) to assess whether pathologies are accurately diagnosed in three different imaging modalities (OPG, CBCT, 3D model) of the same case, and (ii) whether the case is classified as treatable on the basis of the present imaging modality. Further, aspects like the impact of specialisation (oral surgery versus orthodontics), gender and years as a dentist were analysed.

Methods

Fourteen residents were recruited for this survey [7 residents in oral surgery (OS) and 7 residents in orthodontics (ORTH), respectively; $m = 6$, $f = 8$]. Their characteristics are listed in Table 1. Every resident assessed individually nine separate patient cases, each containing a distinct dentoalveolar pathology, as defined in the study planning process (Table 2).

For each patient case, an OPG, a CBCT and a printed 3D model were shown in sequential order to each resident. Each resident assessed each patient case and each type of imaging modality (OPG, CBCT, 3D model) on the basis of a questionnaire customised for this study. The questionnaire comprised diagnostic items and questions relating to diagnosis and patient management (treatability). The correct diagnosis of each case was determined by two independent and experienced senior consultants prior to the residents' assessment.

Medical records of the Clinic of Cranio-Maxillofacial and Oral Surgery and the Clinic of Orthodontics and Paediatric Dentistry of the University of Zurich, Switzerland were searched for patient cases with the following inclusion criteria:

- Treatment indication due to supernumerary, displaced or retained teeth, bone or teeth resorptions, or odontomas
- Availability of an OPG and a CBCT (Accuitomo 170)
- Patient age between 6 and 30 years
- Time lapse between OPG and CBCT no more than 6 months, no dental treatment performed between the imaging

Table 1 Characteristics of residents in oral surgery and orthodontics

Resident	Age (years)	Sex	Specialisation	Experience as a dentist (years)
1	31	m	OS	3 to 4
2	29	m	ORTH	3 to 4
3	34	m	ORTH	5 to 9
4	30	m	ORTH	5 to 9
5	29	f	OS	3 to 4
6	30	f	ORTH	3 to 4
7	34	m	ORTH	5 to 9
8	27	f	OS	1 to 2
9	28	f	ORTH	3 to 4
10	28	f	ORTH	1 to 2
11	29	f	OS	3 to 4
12	29	f	OS	1 to 2
13	28	f	OS	1 to 2
14	31	m	OS	3 to 4

m, male; *f*, female; *OS*, oral surgery; *ORTH*, orthodontics

Table 2 Description of the cases assessed

Case	Age (years)	Sex	Pathology	Time between OPG and CBCT
1	28	m	Tooth resorption	0 Mt
2	11	f	Retained tooth	3 Mt
3	14	m	Retained tooth	5 Mt
4	13	m	Mesiodens	1 Mt
5	18	f	Retained tooth	1 Mt
6	12	m	Tooth resorption	2 Mt
7	13	f	Retained tooth	1 Mt
8	17	m	Odontoma	0 Mt
9	13	f	Retained tooth	0 Mt

m, male; *f*, female; *Mt*, months

- Informed consent for further use of patient data for clinical research given by the patient and wherever necessary by the parents/legal guardians

Every resident assessed the cases separately in the presence of the same supervisor, in order to ascertain identical settings and equal instructions to the viewer software (Morita I-Dixel). Uncertainties were clarified prior to completing the questionnaires. Patient cases were anonymised and presented to every resident in the same order.

The residents had to answer the questions under the following standardised conditions:

- Time available: 1 h 15 min
- Each resident assessed three images per patient in the following sequence: OPG CBCT, 3D model. For each image modality, a questionnaire had to be filled out
- Each resident was shown the region of interest to which the questions related to
- Allowed setup change of OPG: zoom
- Allowed setup change of CBCT: brightness, contrast, zoom, scroll in all three levels (coronal, axial and sagittal
- 3D model: no restrictions

The OPGs of this study were taken either in-house (CRANEX D, Kw73, 10 mA) or extramural. All CBCTs were taken at the Centre of Dental Medicine of the University of Zurich (CBCT: 3D-Accuitomo 170). In order to produce printed 3D models, DICOM data of the region of interest were cropped and STL-files produced using dedicated software (Slicer 4.5.0.) The STL file was printed with a 3D printer (Objet Eden 260 V) in a resolution of 600 dpi with a horizontal layering of 16 μm, using a semi-translucent material (synthetic material, Med610 Stratasys).

For each case and image, the following nine categorical items had to be answered (yes; no; available information not sufficient):

1. Is there a direct contact between teeth/tooth structures and nerve structures?
2. Is the tooth displaced?
3. Is there more than one root?
4. Is there a direct non-physiological contact between the tooth/tooth structure and the adjacent teeth?
5. Is there a pericoronal cyst formation, respectively a cystic formation originating from the tooth/tooth structure?
6. Has more than a third of the root maturation been completed?
7. Is a resorption in the bone or tooth structure visible?
8. Is an ankylosis visible?
9. Is the tooth/tooth structure worth being preserved?

Following questions relating to the treatability were asked after the OPG evaluation:

10. Is this case treatable with this amount of information?
11. Would you request further imaging to improve your diagnostic accuracy?

Even if in the resident's opinion the OPG provided sufficient information to answer all questions, the resident was nevertheless requested to assess the CBCT. The same applied to the 3D model. After every imaging modality assessment, the questionnaires were collected to avoid retrospect changes.

Statistical analysis

Statistical analysis and plots were performed using the statistical software R [12]. To evaluate the differences in the proportions of correct diagnostic answers between OS and ORTH and between different imaging modalities, Fisher's exact tests were used and odds ratios (OR) including confidence intervals (CI) were computed for every question separately. Likewise, Fisher's exact tests were applied to estimate whether there was a difference between the answers given by OS and ORTH on the question if the image provided sufficient information to treat the case (treatability).The same test procedure was also used to investigate if a CBCT after OPG was requested with regard to treatment planning and if specialisation, gender and years of experience as a dentist (dichotomized in 0–4 years of experience versus more) were associated with it. Statistical significance was set to $\alpha = 0.05$ for all analysis.

Results

Diagnostic accuracy (i)

Overall, the majority of the questions were answered correctly, independently to the imaging modality. The percentages of correct answers given by OS were 66.3% for OPG, 83.4% for CBCT and 76.4% for 3D model; and differed slightly to those given by ORTH with 63.7% for OPG, 78.0% for CBCT and 78.7% for 3D model (Figs. 1 and 2). Both OS and ORTH alike answered to around 20% of the questions that the OPG provided insufficient data in order to answer the question.

Assessing a CBCT increased the percentage of correct answers after OPG assessment, both for OS and ORTH. When given a printed 3D model after CBCT, an additional increase in correct answers could be observed for ORTH, but not for OS (Fig. 2 versus Fig. 1).

Evaluating the different questions independently, only three questions were answered significantly different between OS and ORTH (Table 3). The evaluation of a contact between tooth/tooth structure and nerve, the appraisal of root maturation and the diagnosis of a resorption reached in the case of this study higher percentage for the OS group, with odds ratios varying between 1.7 and 3.8. Otherwise, no apparent differences could be detected in the correctness of the answers.

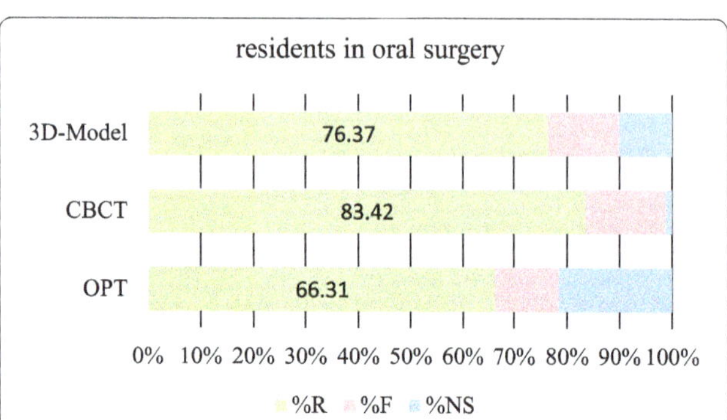

Fig. 1 Accuracy of diagnostic answers from residents in oral surgery (R right, F false, NS not sufficient)

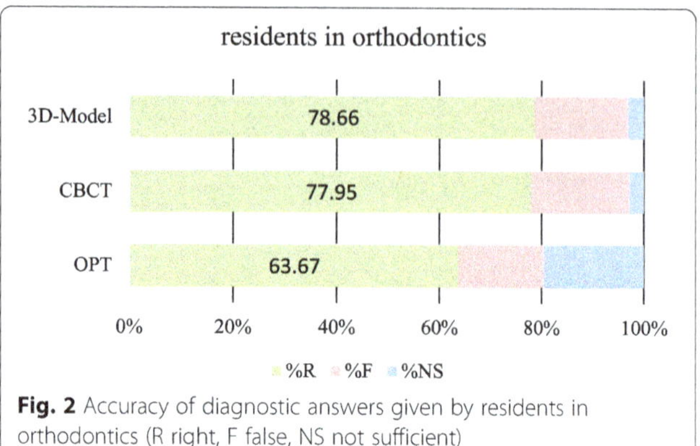

Fig. 2 Accuracy of diagnostic answers given by residents in orthodontics (R right, F false, NS not sufficient)

When comparing the diagnostic accuracy based on OPG and CBCT (following OPG), no differences could be observed for any of the nine questions (Table 4). The same was true when assessing impact of age, gender and years of experience as a dentist on the accuracy of the answers.

Treatability (ii)

At the end of every OPG evaluation, residents were asked whether further imaging was deemed necessary in order to improve diagnostic accuracy. In 81.6% of the cases, further imaging was requested after the OPG. When asked whether the image assessed provided sufficient information to enable a treatment, the ORTH considered the information content of OPGs significantly more often as sufficient compared to the OS group ($p < 0.05$) (Fig. 3). This decision was highly influenced by the residents' background. The odds to request a CBCT were far greater if the OPG assessment was done by a OS (OR 6.3), by a female dentist (OR 3.8) or dentists with only 0 to 4 year of experience (OR 3.0) (Table 5).

Discussion

The aim of this study was twofold: (i) to analyse the diagnostic accuracy of pathologies in three different imaging modalities of the same case and (ii) to analyse the need for further imaging in order to enable treatment. Further, aspects like the impact of specialisation, gender and dental experience were analysed. In contrast to the plethora of scientific literature available dealing with CBCT image accuracy, not much research has been conducted on how CBCT data are being contextually handled. This present investigation was designed to increase our understanding in this specific area.

Diagnostic accuracy (i)

The first objective was not only to analyse if diagnostic accuracy of residents is improved when assessing a CBCT

Table 3 Accuracy of the diagnostic answers given, according to specialisation: residents in oral surgery versus residents in orthodontics

Question pertaining to	OS (%)	ORTH (%)	*p* value	Odds ratio (95% CI)
Contact to nerve	96	87	0.002*	3.8 (1.4–12.0)
Displacement of tooth	92	87	0.089	1.9 (0.9–4.1)
Number of roots	95	95	1.000	–
Contact to adjacent teeth	74	71	0.626	1.1 (0.7–1.9)
Pericoronar cyst	77	72	0.323	1.3 (0.8–2.2)
Maturation of root	89	80	0.029*	2.0 (1.1–3.7)
Resorption (bone or tooth)	76	65	0.040*	1.7 (1.0–2.8)
Ankylosis	83	89	0.176	0.6 (0.3–1.3)
Preservation	79	80	0.793	0.9 (0.5–1.6)

Percentage of correct answers given by residents in oral surgery (OS) and residents in orthodontics (ORTH). To assess the differences between the specialisations, *p* value of Fisher's exact test is given together with odds ratio (OR), including 95% confidence intervals (CI). OR refers to OS with ORTH as reference. $^{*}p < 0.05$

(compared to an OPG), but to dissect the data and evaluate whether the diagnostic accuracy varies when assessing different pathologies, and whether professional background would account for the performance. Although a general increase of more correct answers could be observed for the assessment of CBCT compared to OPG (Figs. 1 and 2), the impact of CBCT was not present in every case when establishing the effect for each clinical question. Somewhat unexpectedly, comparable diagnostic accuracy could be attained already with an OPG for many diagnosed pathologies. Professional background had likewise a very small influence, as specialisation affected only the correctness of three answers moderately, and age, gender and years of experience as a dentist showed no effect at all. In short, only questions relating to resorption of dental or bony tissue, contact to nerve and maturation stage of the root reached significantly higher percentages for the residents in oral surgery group.

Comparable improvement in diagnostic accuracy was shown in previous studies [13] when comparing CBCT to OPG, and there is a broad consensus on the added value of CBCT imaging in diagnostics and treatment planning compared to a two-dimensional imaging [13–23]. Our results are in full agreement with these publications, yet highlight the fact that dental education may influence diagnostic accuracy, depending on the pathology to be assessed.

Moreover, another valuable and novel observation is the divergence seen in the importance of printed 3D models. For residents in oral surgery, printed 3D models caused more uncertainties and led to a decrease of diagnostic accuracy (if assessed in sequential order after OPG and CBCT). In contrast, residents in orthodontics seemed to benefit of an additional assessment of printed 3D models, which resulted in an improvement of their diagnostic ability. This increase in diagnostic accuracy might be partially explained with the larger experience residents in orthodontics share with model assessment.

Treatability (ii)

All residents were asked whether the OPG contained sufficient information to enable a treatment. Interestingly, most residents in orthodontics and nearly all residents in oral surgery stated that the OPG did not provide sufficient information for a treatment plan (Fig. 3), even though the majority of the diagnoses were done correctly. Apparently, this dissonance indicates

Table 4 Accuracy of the diagnostic answers given, according to imaging modality: OPG versus CBCT

Question pertaining to	OPG (%)	CBCT (%)	*p* value	Odds ratio (95% CI)
Contact to nerve	91	93	0.616	0.8 (0.3–2.4)
Displacement of tooth	88	90	0.543	0.7 (0.3–0.5)
Number of roots	95	94	0.775	1.2 (0.3–5.1)
Contact to adjacent teeth	73	70	0.643	1.2 (0.6–2.3)
Pericoronar cyst	73	75	0.764	0.9 (0.5–1.7)
Maturation of root	84	83	1.000	–
Resorption (bone or tooth) toothtooth)	65	72	0.305	0.7 (0.4–1.4)
Ankylosis	86	85	1.000	–
Preservation	83	78	0.510	1.3 (0.6–2.7)

Percentage of correct answers given based on OPG and CBCT (after OPG). To assess the differences between the imaging modality, *p* value of Fisher's exact test is given together with odds ratio (OR), including 95% confidence intervals (CI). OR refers to CBCT with OPG as reference

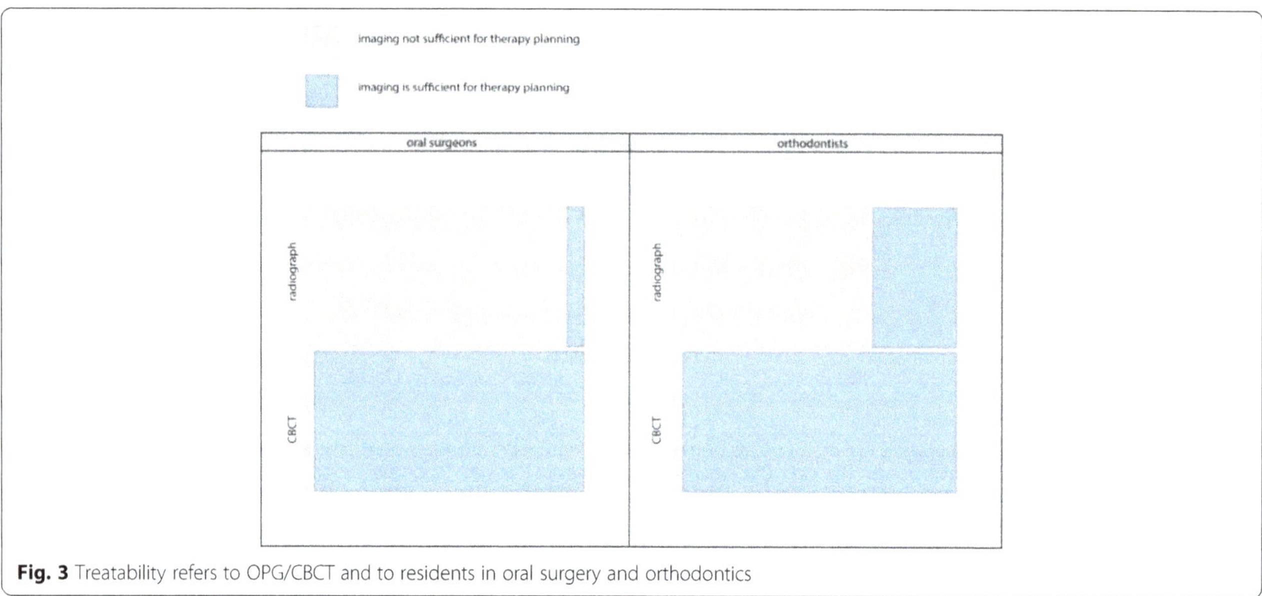

Fig. 3 Treatability refers to OPG/CBCT and to residents in oral surgery and orthodontics

that diagnostic content cannot be equated with the required information needed for treatability. An accurate diagnosis is an essential part of treatment planning, but clinicians obviously look out for more than just a diagnosis when they evaluate and interpret an OPG. The observation that the treatability of the cases is viewed differently after CBCT assessment is in full agreement to previous studies [17, 24, 25].

Perhaps rather surprisingly, residents in orthodontics were significantly more often satisfied with the information given by an OPG for their treatment planning than residents in oral surgery who stated that the case was not treatable with the information provided by an OPG. This trend is probably due to the different goals pursued by each specialisation. The questions that the residents in orthodontics would like to have answered by any imaging modality will probably differ from the queries that the residents in oral surgery aims to have solved. Even when the one and same case is assessed by a resident in oral surgery and orthodontics, every one of them will be focused to answer different questions relating to treatability. Hence, it may be that an OPG will contain enough information for the resident in orthodontist to pen his treatment plan, but may hold only insufficient data for queries related to a surgical approach.

In 81.6% of the cases, further imaging was requested after the OPG. Caution should be applied in the interpretation of this number, as the residents' decision was theoretical and did not imply additional costs or radiation exposure. Nevertheless, it is striking that in the majority of the cases, further imaging was requested. One possible explanation might be the diagnostic difficulty of the chosen cases. This relevant finding indicates a high subjective demand for a CBCT and a lower objective necessity for further imaging after OPG, based on the present cases. However, this conclusion can only be drawn, after performing a CBCT. The onus rests on future scientific endeavours to find means to reduce this discrepancy.

The request for a CBCT was significantly influenced by the residents' professional background (OS vs ORTH) and gender. Residents in oral surgery, female dentists and residents with limited professional experience as dentists indicated up to six times more often the need for further imaging. When analysing the assessment of impacted canines, Lai et al. observed similarly that oral surgeons requested more often CBCT imaging than orthodontists [19]. This might be explained by the fact that oral surgeons are interested in diagnostic information as well as in information for surgical planning. This takes positional relations with regard to surgical approaches into account, being facilitated by 3D imaging. As mentioned above, orthodontics and oral surgery differ in their judgement on treatability. This offers an obvious

Table 5 Request of CBCT after OPG: influence of residents' characteristics

Variable	*p* value	Odds ratio (95% CI)
Specialisation: oral surgery vs orthodontics	< 0.001*	6.3 (1.9–27.2)
Gender: females vs males	0.005*	3.8 (1.4–12.2)
Years of professional experience: 0–4 years vs > 4 year	0.045*	3.0 (1.0–9.9)

p values of Fisher's exact test is given together with odds ratio (OR), including 95% confidence intervals (CI). OR refers to the first listed outcome with the second listed outcome being used as reference. *$p < 0.05$

explanation for the difference regarding the request for further imaging. Residents in oral surgery, who stated more often that the cases were not treatable with the data obtained solely by OPG, were also the same group who requested significantly more CBCT, and vice versa. It is understandable that less experienced clinicians ask for more CBCT scans, but the interpretation why male dentist would request more CBCT scans is not trivial. Hodges et al. [17] demonstrated that clinicians who own CBCT devices requested more CBCT scans than other dentists. This and other reports suggest that dentist-related variables influence the request for CBCT scans at least as much as case-related factors.

Certain limitations affect the generalizability of this study's results. First, only nine cases were assessed with a limited range of pathologies (five retained teeth (canines and molars), two tooth resorptions, one odontoma and one supernumerary tooth). Moreover, the assessment was performed by a small amount of residents of the local university. The fact that all residents shared a similar academic environment might be a source of inadvertent bias. Nevertheless, the odds of some of the portrayed observations are evident and far too important to be ignored on the pretext of the limitations.

Conclusions

This study analysed (i) whether pathologies are accurately diagnosed in three different imaging modalities (OPG, CBCT, 3D model). Diagnostic accuracy was decent with OPG and was improved with CBCT. Next, the study assessed (ii) whether each case was classified as treatable on the basis of the present imaging modality. This result was influenced by the professional background, which influenced whether a CBCT was requested for treatment planning. Further, dentist-related factors like gender and the professional experience as a dentist also took an influence on the request for further imaging.

Abbreviations

3D: Three-dimensional; CBCT: Cone beam computed tomography; DICOM: Digital Imaging and Communications in Medicine; OPG: Orthopantomography; OR: Odds ratio; ORTH: Resident in orthodontics; OS: Resident in oral surgery

Funding

This study was conducted without external funding.

Authors' contributions

JR wrote the ethics application together with BGH and BS. JR performed the data collection. JR performed the data analysis together with DW and prepared the manuscript. RP, BS and BGH designed the study, controlled the study and corrected the manuscript. MR edited the manuscript. DW performed the statistical study setup and analysis. All authors read and approved the final manuscript.

Competing interests

Josipa Radic, Raphael Patcas, Bernd Stadlinger, Daniel Wiedemeier, Martin Rücker and Barbara Giacomelli-Hiestand declare that they have no competing interests.

Author details

[1]Clinic of Cranio-Maxillofacial and Oral Surgery, Centre of Dental Medicine, University of Zurich, Plattenstrasse 11, 8032 Zurich, Switzerland. [2]Clinic for Orthodontics and Paediatric Dentistry, Centre of Dental Medicine, University of Zurich, Plattenstrasse 11, 8032 Zurich, Switzerland. [3]Statistical Services, Centre of Dental Medicine, University of Zurich, Plattenstrasse 11, 8032 Zurich, Switzerland.

References

1. Mason C, Papadakou P, Roberts GJ. The radiographic localization of impacted maxillary canines: a comparison of methods. Eur J Orthod. 2001; 23(1):25–34.
2. Maverna R, Gracco A. Different diagnostic tools for the localization of impacted maxillary canines: clinical considerations. Prog Orthod. 2007;8(1): 28–44.
3. Neves FS, Passos CP, Oliveira-Santos C, Cangussu MC, Campos PS, Nascimento RJ, et al. Correlation between maxillofacial radiographic features and systemic severity as sickle cell disease severity predictor. Clin Oral Investig. 2012;16(3):827–33. https://doi.org/10.1007/s00784-011-0577-0 published Online First: Epub Date]|.
4. Rushton VE, Horner K. The use of panoramic radiology in dental practice. J Dent. 1996;24(3):185–201.
5. Sedaghatfar M, August MA, Dodson TB. Panoramic radiographic findings as predictors of inferior alveolar nerve exposure following third molar extraction. J Oral Maxillofac Surg. 2005;63(1):3–7.
6. Szalma J, Lempel E, Jeges S, Szabo G, Olasz L. The prognostic value of panoramic radiography of inferior alveolar nerve damage after mandibular third molar removal: retrospective study of 400 cases. Oral Surg Oral Med Oral Pathol Oral Radiol Endod. 2010;109(2):294–302. https://doi.org/10.1016/j.tripleo.2009.09.023 published Online First: Epub Date]|.
7. American Academy of O, Maxillofacial R. Clinical recommendations regarding use of cone beam computed tomography in orthodontics. [corrected]. Position statement by the American Academy of Oral and Maxillofacial Radiology. Oral Surg Oral Med Oral Pathol Oral Radiol. 2013; 116(2):238–57. https://doi.org/10.1016/j.oooo.2013.06.002 published Online First: Epub Date]|.
8. Commission E. Radiation Protection No. 172, Cone beam CT for dental and maxillofacial radiology (evidence-based guidelines). Luxembourg: Sedentexct (Hrsg); 2012.
9. Dula K, Bornstein MM, Buser D, Dagassan-Berndt D, Ettlin DA, Filippi A, et al. SADMFR guidelines for the use of cone-beam computed tomography/ digital volume tomography. Swiss Dent J. 2014;124(11):1169–83.
10. Fryback DG. A conceptual model for output measures in cost-effectiveness evaluation of diagnostic imaging. J Neuroradiol. 1983;10(2):94–6.
11. Fryback DG, Thornbury JR. The efficacy of diagnostic imaging. Med Decis Mak. 1991;11(2):88–94. https://doi.org/10.1177/0272989X9101100203 published Online First: Epub Date]|.
12. Team RCR. A language and environment for statistical Computing. Vienna, Austria. URL https://www.R-project.org: R Foundation for Statistical Computing; 2015.
13. Hasani A, Ahmadi Moshtaghin F, Roohi P, Rakhshan V. Diagnostic value of cone beam computed tomography and panoramic radiography in predicting mandibular nerve exposure during third molar surgery. Int J Oral Maxillofac Surg. 2017;46(2):230–5. https://doi.org/10.1016/j.ijom.2016.10.003 published Online First: Epub Date]|.
14. Alqerban A, Jacobs R, Fieuws S, Willems G. Comparison of two cone beam computed tomographic systems versus panoramic imaging for localization of impacted maxillary canines and detection of root resorption. Eur J Orthod. 2011;33(1):93–102. https://doi.org/10.1093/ejo/cjq034 published Online First: Epub Date]|.
15. Botticelli S, Verna C, Cattaneo PM, Heidmann J, Melsen B. Two- versus three-dimensional imaging in subjects with unerupted maxillary canines. Eur J Orthod. 2011;33(4):344–9. https://doi.org/10.1093/ejo/cjq102 published Online First: Epub Date]|.

16. Ghaeminia H, Meijer GJ, Soehardi A, Borstlap WA, Mulder J, Berge SJ. Position of the impacted third molar in relation to the mandibular canal. Diagnostic accuracy of cone beam computed tomography compared with panoramic radiography. Int J Oral Maxillofac Surg. 2009;38(9):964–71. https://doi.org/10.1016/j.ijom.2009.06.007 published Online First: Epub Date]|.
17. Hodges RJ, Atchison KA, White SC. Impact of cone-beam computed tomography on orthodontic diagnosis and treatment planning. Am J Orthod Dentofac Orthop. 2013;143(5):665–74. https://doi.org/10.1016/j.ajodo.2012.12.011 published Online First: Epub Date]|.
18. Katheria BC, Kau CH, Tate R, Chen JW, English J, Bouquot J. Effectiveness of impacted and supernumerary tooth diagnosis from traditional radiography versus cone beam computed tomography. Pediatr Dent. 2010;32(4):304–9.
19. Lai CS, Suter VG, Katsaros C, Bornstein MM. Localization of impacted maxillary canines and root resorption of neighbouring teeth: a study assessing the diagnostic value of panoramic radiographs in two groups of observers. Eur J Orthod. 2014;36(4):450–6. https://doi.org/10.1093/ejo/cjt074 published Online First: Epub Date]|.
20. Pittayapat P, Willems G, Alqerban A, Coucke W, Ribeiro-Rotta RF, Souza PC, et al. Agreement between cone beam computed tomography images and panoramic radiographs for initial orthodontic evaluation. Oral Surg Oral Med Oral Pathol Oral Radiol. 2014;117(1):111–9. https://doi.org/10.1016/j.oooo.2013.10.016 published Online First: Epub Date]|.
21. Ren H, Chen J, Deng F, Zheng L, Liu X, Dong Y. Comparison of cone-beam computed tomography and periapical radiography for detecting simulated apical root resorption. Angle Orthod. 2013;83(2):189–95. https://doi.org/10.2319/050512-372.1 published Online First: Epub Date]|.
22. Tantanapornkul W, Okouchi K, Fujiwara Y, Yamashiro M, Maruoka Y, Ohbayashi N, et al. A comparative study of cone-beam computed tomography and conventional panoramic radiography in assessing the topographic relationship between the mandibular canal and impacted third molars. Oral Surg Oral Med Oral Pathol Oral Radiol Endod. 2007;103(2):253–9. https://doi.org/10.1016/j.tripleo.2006.06.060 published Online First: Epub Date]|.
23. Wriedt S, Jaklin J, Al-Nawas B, Wehrbein H. Impacted upper canines: examination and treatment proposal based on 3D versus 2D diagnosis. J Orofac Orthop. 2012;73(1):28–40. https://doi.org/10.1007/s00056-011-0058-8 published Online First: Epub Date]|.
24. Bjerklin K, Ericson S. How a computerized tomography examination changed the treatment plans of 80 children with retained and ectopically positioned maxillary canines. Angle Orthod. 2006;76(1):43–51. https://doi.org/10.1043/0003-3219(2006)076[0043:HACTEC]2.0.CO;2 published Online First: Epub Date]|.
25. Haney E, Gansky SA, Lee JS, Johnson E, Maki K, Miller AJ, et al. Comparative analysis of traditional radiographs and cone-beam computed tomography volumetric images in the diagnosis and treatment planning of maxillary impacted canines. Am J Orthod Dentofac Orthop. 2010;137(5):590–7. https://doi.org/10.1016/j.ajodo.2008.06.035 published Online First: Epub Date]|.

2

Correlations between clinical parameters in implant maintenance patients: analysis among healthy and history-of-periodontitis groups

Keisuke Seki[1,2*], Shinya Nakabayashi[1], Naoki Tanabe[3], Atsushi Kamimoto[1,2] and Yoshiyuki Hagiwara[1]

Abstract

Background: The pathophysiology and pathology of peri-implantitis remain unclear; however, its similarity to periodontitis has been described. The evaluation of peri-implant tissue and the diagnostic criteria of peri-implant disease are not currently standardized as they are for periodontitis. In this study, we evaluated clinical parameters during the implant maintenance period to determine significant correlations between these parameters.

Methods: We examined 55 implant patients at the time of maintenance visits between April and September 2016 and classified patients into a healthy group (H) and a history-of-periodontitis group (HP). For each implant, we evaluated the modified plaque index, probing pocket depth, and bleeding on probing as clinical parameters. Statistical analyses were performed with Spearman's rank correlation coefficient.

Results: A total of 130 implants were assessed. The mean time since implant placement was 6 years and 6 months. The prevalence of implant-based peri-implantitis was 10.8% of all the implants. All cases of implant-based peri-implantitis came from the HP group, and many were present in patients with a history of severe periodontitis. The probing pocket depth around the implant was significantly greater in the HP group than in the H group. We found weak positive correlations between the probing pocket depth and bleeding on probing ($r_s = 0.401$, $p < 0.05$) in the H group and between the probing pocket depth and bleeding on probing ($r_s = 0.241$, $p < 0.05$) and the modified plaque index ($r_s = 0.228$, $p < 0.05$) in the HP group.

Conclusions: Our findings suggest that probing pocket depth and bleeding on probing as clinical parameters are important indicators for the diagnosis of peri-implant disease during the maintenance period among healthy and history-of-periodontitis groups.

Keywords: Dental implant, Maintenance, Modified plaque index, Probing depth, Bleeding on probing, Correlation

Background

Peri-implant diseases are the main biological complication of implant treatment and greatly influence treatment success [1]. Risk indicators for peri-implantitis include a history of periodontitis, poor oral hygiene, and smoking [2–4]. Peri-implantitis is often encountered clinically, occurring in 12 to 43% of implants and 28 to 47% of implant patients [5–8]. Similarities between the pathology and pathogenic factors of peri-implantitis and those of periodontal disease (such as periodontitis) have been described [9–11]; however, many points remain unclear [12]. For this reason, discussion is ongoing about the clinical criteria and selection of treatment options for peri-implantitis [13, 14].

The diagnostic criteria and treatments for peri-implant diseases such as peri-implantitis are not currently standardized. In contrast, periodontitis is diagnosed by periodontal tissue probing, attachment level, the status of oral hygiene, tooth mobility, occlusion, and furcation and dental X-ray imaging.

* Correspondence: seki.keisuke@nihon-u.ac.jp
[1]Implant Dentistry, Nihon University School of Dentistry Dental Hospital, Tokyo 101-8310, Japan
[2]Department of Comprehensive Dentistry and Clinical Education, Nihon University School of Dentistry, 1-8-13 Kanda-Surugadai, Chiyoda-ku, Tokyo 101-8310, Japan
Full list of author information is available at the end of the article

Ideally, peri-implant mucositis is discovered in its early stages to allow longer maintenance therapy, preventing complications and maintaining a high success rate [15]. No previous study describing clinical examination, such as probing the tissue surrounding implants, has been reported in Japanese patients. In this study, we statistically evaluated various clinical examination parameters during implant maintenance to determine correlations between them.

Methods

Selection of patients

This study enrolled 55 patients (25 men, 30 women; mean age, 63.53 ± 10.51 years) who visited Nihon University School of Dentistry Dental Hospital for implant maintenance from April to September 2016. The inclusion criteria were treatment at the same hospital with two-stage implant placement before 2015, and ongoing maintenance at 3–6-month intervals after superstructure placement. Patients whose superstructure had been in place for less than 3 months were excluded. The dental implants used were Replace Select™/ Steri-Oss® implant system (Novelbiocare, Switzerland), Novel Replace® (Novelbiocare, Switzerland), OsseoSpeed™ (ASTRA TECH Implant System, Switzerland), OSSEOTITE® XP (BIOMET 3i, Indiana, USA), and Brånemark system® Mk III (Novelbiocare, Switzerland); all implants had a rough surface (Table 1). This study was conducted with the approval of the Nihon University School of Dentistry Ethics Committee (Permit Number: 2013-15).

History of periodontitis before implant treatment

Patients with chronic periodontitis were diagnosed based on the latest AAP Classification of Periodontal Diseases and Conditions at the first visit. Clinical attachment level (CAL) was examined for each individual tooth. A CAL of 1–2 mm was defined as mild periodontitis, 3–4 mm was moderate periodontitis, and 5 mm or more was severe periodontitis. The range of the disease was considered to be localized when 30% or less of all teeth were affected, and generalized when more than 30% of teeth were affected [16]. Cases of aggressive periodontitis were not included in this study. Implant therapy was performed after active periodontal treatment with confirmed improvement of the periodontal tissue. We classified patients into two groups based on their medical records: a healthy group without a history-of-periodontitis (H) and a history-of-periodontitis group (HP).

Table 1 Implant systems used

Implant	Number
Replace select ™	44
Novel Replace ®	31
OsseoSpeed ™	25
OSSEOTITE ® XP	18
Brånemark system® Mk III	7
Steri-Oss ® implant system	5
Total	130

Dental history

We recorded the following information from the medical chart: patient sex and age, number of natural teeth at first visit, final number of natural teeth at the beginning of implant treatment, total number of extracted teeth and installed implants, and average maintenance period.

Diagnosis of peri-implantitis

At the time of maintenance, the status of the peri-implant tissue was evaluated. Peri-implantitis is defined as a chronic infection of peri-implant tissue, with resorption of the supporting bone observable radiographically. Peri-implant mucositis is a reversible inflammatory reaction around the implant [17]. We diagnosed peri-implantitis when the probing pocket depth (PPD) around the implant was 6 mm or more, suppuration and bleeding were observed at the time of probing, and bone resorption was present radiographically for 25% or more of the implant length [18].

Maintenance examinations

At the time of optional maintenance, the following parameters were measured for each implant. Data collection and analysis were conducted by two operators who were blind to the research purpose and methods. One operator statistically analyzed the final data set.

Evaluation of plaque adhesion

Plaque adhesion (modified Plaque Index: mPI) on the superstructure of the implant was measured on a 4-point scale (0, no plaque; 1, plaque seen with probing of the tooth surface; 2, moderate accumulation of soft deposits visible with the naked eye; 3, abundance of soft deposits on the tooth). We calculated the average score of four surfaces (buccal, lingual, mesial, and distal aspects).

Probing pocket depth around implants

To standardize the probing force (0.15 N), the operators used a precision scale to calibrate their force with repeated measurements. The same operator inserted a periodontal pocket probe (11 Colorvue® Probe Kit; Hu-Friedy, Chicago, IL, USA) into the pocket around the implant with a force of approximately 0.15 N. PPD was measured in 1-mm increments with the 6-point method (at the mesial and distal angles and at the center of the buccal and lingual aspects of the implant). We calculated the average of the six points for each implant.

Bleeding on probing of peri-implant mucosa

Bleeding on probing (BoP) was evaluated 10 s after the 6-point probing as negative (0, no bleeding) or positive (1, bleeding). We calculated the average of all six points obtained. The minimum BoP score was 0 and the maximum was 1.

Statistical analysis

Data analysis was performed with statistical software (GraphPad Prism 5.0; GraphPad Software Inc., San Diego, CA, USA). Quantitative analysis of differences between the H and HP groups was performed with the Mann–Whitney *U* test. Clinical parameters were analyzed with Spearman's rank correlation coefficient (R_s). A significance level of 95% ($p < 0.05$) was considered statistically significant.

Results

Patients

Of the 55 subjects, 25 were male and 30 were female (H group: 8/10, HP group: 17/20, respectively). A total of 130 implants (H group 39, HP group 91) were included in the analysis (Table 2). The mean maintenance period was 6 years and 6 months. The average number of natural teeth at the first visit and at the beginning of implant treatment were 25.3 ± 2.9 and 22.4 ± 4.5, respectively. Comparison between the H and HP groups revealed a significant difference in patient age at the time of maintenance, number of natural teeth at the beginning of implant treatment, total number of extracted teeth, and time since implant placement.

Prevalence of peri-implantitis, history of periodontitis severity

Among all the subjects, 14 implants (10.8%) had peri-implantitis, all belonging to the HP group (6 patients). Details of periodontitis diagnosis in the HP group were generalized moderate periodontitis (22 patients, 53 implants), generalized moderate periodontitis + localized severe periodontitis (11 patients, 23 implants), and generalized severe periodontitis (4 patients, 15 implants) (Table 3). The proportion of peri-implantitis for each diagnosis were 5.7% (3/53) for generalized moderate periodontitis, 13.0% (3/23) for generalized moderate periodontitis + localized severe periodontitis, and 53.3% (8/15) for generalized severe periodontitis at the implant level. The prevalence of peri-implantitis in the HP group was 15.4% (14/91 at the implant level) and 16.2% (3/37 at the patient level).

Clinical parameters

The data from each subgroup are shown in Table 4.

Modified plaque index

The mPI score for the total study population was 0.21 ± 0.30 (mean ± SD). The mean scores of the H and HP groups were 0.18 (median, 0.25) and 0.23 (median, 0.25), respectively.

Probing pocket depth

The PPD of the total study population was 3.19 ± 0.96 mm (mean ± SD). The mean PPDs of the H and HP groups were 2.87 mm (median, 2.83 mm) and 3.33 mm (median, 3.00 mm), respectively.

Bleeding on probing

The BoP score of the total study population was 0.28 ± 0.29 (mean ± SD). The mean scores of the H and HP groups were 0.30 (median, 0.17) and 0.28 (median, 0.17), respectively.

Correlations between PPD and characteristics of the study population

Because normality and homoscedasticity were not obtained for each clinical parameter between the two groups, a statistical study was conducted using the non-parametric test (Mann–Whitney *U* test) for the difference test between the two groups. PPD was recognized to be significantly greater ($p < 0.01$) in the HP group, but there were no significant differences in mPI and BoP between the two groups. Therefore, we focused on the PPD parameter, in which a significant difference was found between the two groups, and analyzed correlations between PPD and patient characteristics (age, number of teeth, number of extracted teeth, maintenance period). Significant correlation coefficients were observed for the number of extracted teeth in the H group and for all characteristics in the HP group (Table 5).

Table 2 Characteristics of the study population

	H group mean ± SD, or *n* (median)	HP group mean ± SD, or *n* (median)	Significant difference between H and HP group
Age	56.0 ± 11.8 (57.9)	67.2 ± 7.7 (66.9)	**
Number of teeth (at the first visit)	25.3 ± 3.0 (26.5)	25.2 ± 2.9 (26.0)	n.s.
(at the beginning of implant treatment)	23.9 ± 3.6 (25.0)	21.6 ± 4.7 (23.0)	*
Number of extracted teeth	1.6 ± 1.2 (1.0)	4.1 ± 4.0 (2.0)	**
Maintenance period	4 years 3 months (5 years 8 months)	7 years 4 months (8 years 4 months)	**

n.s. not significant, *$p < 0.05$, **$p < 0.01$

Table 3 Prevalence of peri-implantitis and periodontitis diagnosis in the HP group

Diagnosis in HP group (37 patients, 91 implants) Localized: ≤ 30% of site involved, generalized: > 30% of site involved		Numbers of peri-implantitis and prevalence in diagnosis n = 14, 15.4% of HP group
Diagnosis of chronic periodontitis	Implants	Peri-implantitis implants
Generalized moderate (22 patients)	53	3 (5.7 %)
Generalized moderate + Localized severe (11 patients)	23	3 (13.0 %)
Generalized severe (4 patients)	15	8 (53.3%)

Comparison of clinical parameters between the H and HP groups

We analyzed the correlation between PPD and other parameters in each group using Spearman's rank correlation coefficient. We found a weak correlation between PPD and BoP for the H group (r_s = 0.401, p < 0.05). In the HP group, weak correlations were found between PPD and mPI (r_s = 0.228, p < 0.05) and between PPD and BoP (r_s = 0.241, p < 0.05) (Table 6).

Discussion

Patient characteristics

In this study, we reviewed the clinical parameters of 130 implants in 55 patients during ongoing long-term maintenance. We focused on the history of periodontitis and compared the parameters in two groups classified according to a history of periodontitis. A previous study on the prevalence of periodontitis revealed that moderate or severe periodontitis was observed in 64% of people over 65 years of age [19], and that the number of remaining teeth also decreased after the age of 60 [20]. Consistent with these findings, our study suggests that periodontal treatment was started at an older age in the HP group. Previous reports recommended that the follow-up period evaluating the peri-implant tissue should be 5 years or longer. The mean maintenance period of this survey was 6 years and 6 months in total. Therefore, we consider that the observation period of this study was sufficiently long-term and reasonable, resulting in a potentially predictive result [3]. The implant maintenance period of the HP group was longer than that of H group, possibly because the HP group consisted of patients with a history of good compliance who had visited the university hospital for long-term periodontal treatment and understood the importance of periodontal treatment and were likely to continue with maintenance visits after the implant treatment. However, it was expected that patients in the H group are often only partially treated and they had less experienced to receive comprehensive or long-term treatment. We hypothesized that the patients of H group might have felt less necessity of receiving maintenance because they were healthy.

A history of periodontitis has been recognized as an important risk indicator for peri-implantitis [2, 3, 21] and is known to lower the success rate during maintenance. Thus, for long-term implant stability, it is important to perform appropriate periodontal treatment [22–24].

The difference between the number of natural teeth at the first visit and at the beginning of implant treatment indicates that many teeth were extracted in the HP group compared with the H group during the active treatment period. One limitation of this study is that we did not investigate the reasons for tooth extraction. We inferred that in the HP group, many teeth were removed because of periodontitis, whereas a smaller number were extracted in the H group because of root fracture or apical periodontitis. There was no significant difference in the number of implants between the groups. However, the number of natural teeth before implant treatment was smaller in the HP group than in the H group. It is possible that the implants in these patients were used as bridge abutments for wide defects and that the size of the defect was not necessarily reflected in the number of implants.

The severity of periodontitis and peri-implantitis

All the implants with peri-implantitis came from the HP group, not the H group, thus supporting the view that a history of periodontitis is a risk indicator for peri-implantitis. In the diagnosis of periodontitis within the HP group, it is notable that peri-implantitis increased as periodontitis become more severe. This supports the findings of a previous study that reported that the

Table 4 Value of each clinical parameter

Clinical parameters	H group (n = 39) mean ± SD/median	HP group (n = 91) mean ± SD/median	Significance difference between H and HP group
mPI	0.18 ± 0.23/0.25	0.23 ± 0.33/0.25	n.s.
PPD	2.87 ± 0.48/2.83	3.33 ± 1.07/3.00	**
BoP	0.30 ± 0.28/0.17	0.28 ± 0.29/0.17	n.s.

n.s. not significant, *p < 0.05, **p < 0.01

Table 5 Correlations between PPD and characteristics

Characteristics	H group correlation (R_s)	HP group correlation (R_s)
Age	0.040 n.s.	0.209*
Number of teeth (at the beginning of implant treatment)	0.027 n.s.	− 0.355**
Number of extracted teeth	0.369*	0.284**
Maintenance period (month)	0.193 n.s.	0.234*

n.s. not significant, * $p < 0.05$, ** $p < 0.01$

survival rate of implants is inversely proportional to the severity of past periodontitis [25]. In our study of long-term maintenance patients, the findings that the prevalence of peri-implantitis was 10.8% at the implant level and 10.9% at the patient level were similar to previous findings. It was suggested that the criteria for peri-implantitis that we adopted were reasonable. The low prevalence of peri-implantitis in this study (approximately 10%) may be related to the fact that all the subjects received maintenance therapy [26].

Evaluation of clinical parameters

The average mPI was about 0.2 for both groups, indicating little plaque adhesion. One characteristic of patients in this study is that they understood the importance of maintenance and they received oral hygiene instruction. Although poor oral hygiene has been reported to be a risk indicator for peri-implant disease [3], our results suggest that the oral hygiene was maintained in all patients including peri-implantitis patients.

Among all the subjects, 11.5% of the total implant sites had an average PPD of more than 4 mm. Our results were comparable with previous studies, which have reported peri-implant PPDs ranging from 2.52 to 3.8 mm [27–29]. However, we believe that this study was more thorough because of its long-term follow-up. PPD in the HP group was 3.33 ± 1.07 mm, which was significantly greater than that in the H group (2.87 ± 0.48 mm). Interestingly, we found that PPD was greater in patients with a history of periodontitis than in those without this history. It has been reported that worsening periodontal disease of natural teeth affects the pocket depth of adjacent implants [30]. However, although in natural teeth there is a criterion of critical probing depth (4 mm or more) [31], there are no such reference values for implants because the site and placement depth differs and the biological width of the implant is not constant [32].

Table 6 Correlations between PPD and the other parameters

Parameters	H group correlation (R_s)	HP group correlation (R_s)
PPD-mPI	0.182 n.s.	0.228*
PPD-BoP	0.401*	0.241*

n.s. not significant, * $p < 0.05$, ** $p < 0.01$

BoP has been used to evaluate inflammatory conditions of periodontal tissue [33] and can also be an important evaluation item for peri-implant tissues. To avoid diagnosing bleeding resulting from strong probing as a false positive, we set the probing pressure to 0.15 N [34]. BoP values were low, with no significant difference between the groups (H group, 0.30; HP group, 0.28). This result was similar to that of a previous study that reported a low bleeding index in the implant group with a low plaque index [35].

Correlations between probing pocket depth around implants and age, number of teeth, extracted teeth, and maintenance period

There was no significant difference between mPI and BoP when clinical parameters were compared, and there was a significant difference for PPD only in the HP group. For this reason, we analyzed the correlation of the characteristics of patients with significant differences only for PPD. In the H group, a significant correlation with PPD was found only for the number of extracted teeth, suggesting that PPD was correlated with the number of teeth extracted due to reason that it was not periodontitis.

However, in the HP group, age, number of teeth, extracted teeth, and maintenance period all correlated with PPD. This finding suggests that the implant PPD reflects the period required for periodontitis treatment and complexity of treatment before implant placement. Although the number of teeth at the beginning of implant treatment showed only a negative correlation, the small number of teeth present indicates that a large number of teeth were extracted as a result of periodontitis, suggesting that the implant PPD is affected by this. From these results, it can be speculated that the severity of periodontitis before the implant treatment is also reflected in the PPD.

Correlations between clinical parameters

Correlations between PPD and the two other clinical parameters, mPI and BoP, were examined in each group. Because this study targeted all patients who received maintenance, it was predicted that the hygiene around the implants in both groups would be good. However, there was a significant difference between PPD and mPI only in the HP group. It was assumed that the probing depth and oral hygiene around implant appeared to be affected each other in the HP group. In contrast with the target group of our study, there may have been a significant correlation between PPD and mPI in a patient group that had not received maintenance and that had poor oral hygiene.

A correlation between the PPD of the peri-implant tissue and lesion progression has been reported, similar to that seen with periodontitis [27]. Probing around the implant is useful for evaluating soft tissue inflammation and is considered reproducible [36]. Examination of peri-implant bleeding is reported to have higher diagnostic accuracy than probing around natural teeth [37]. However, because measurement results differ depending on the shape of the superstructure and because bleeding can occur even if peri-implant tissue is healthy, implant probing is not completely established as a method to distinguish between healthy and inflamed sites [37, 38]. As in natural teeth, we consider that peri-implant BoP should be assessed after checking for sulcus bleeding. The results of this study, especially the correlation between PPD and BoP, suggest that implant probing is useful for evaluating peri-implant tissue.

In this study, we measured clinical parameters at only one point during the maintenance period. Further investigation is needed with attention not only to the amount of parameter change over time but also to bone resorption on radiological images.

Conclusions

We examined clinical parameters in patients receiving long-term implant maintenance. There were significant differences between the H and HP groups in age at the time of maintenance, number of natural teeth at the beginning of implant treatment, total number of extracted teeth, and maintenance. The prevalence of implant-based peri-implantitis was 10.8% of all the implants. All implants with peri-implantitis came from the HP group, and many belonged to patients with a history of severe periodontitis. The PPD around implants was significantly greater in the HP group than in the H group. We found weak positive correlations between PPD and BoP ($r_s = 0.401$, $p < 0.05$) in the H group and between PPD and BoP ($r_s = 0.241$, $p < 0.05$) and PPD and mPI ($r_s = 0.228$, $p < 0.05$) in the HP group. Our findings suggest that the clinical parameter of probing pocket depth is a critical index for the diagnosis of peri-implant disease during the maintenance period among healthy and history-of-periodontitis groups.

Abbreviations

BoP: Bleeding on probing; mPI: Modified plaque index; PPD: Probing pocket depth

Funding

This study had no funding.

Authors' contributions

KS and SN carried out the clinical examinations and analysis. NT performed statistical analysis. KS wrote the manuscript. AK and YH recommended possible treatments and provided valuable comments on this manuscript. All authors read and approved the final manuscript.

Competing interests

Authors Keisuke Seki, Shinya Nakabayashi, Naoki Tanabe, Atsushi Kamimoto, and Yoshiyuki Hagiwara state that there are no conflicts of interest.

Author details

[1]Implant Dentistry, Nihon University School of Dentistry Dental Hospital, Tokyo 101-8310, Japan. [2]Department of Comprehensive Dentistry and Clinical Education, Nihon University School of Dentistry, 1-8-13 Kanda-Surugadai, Chiyoda-ku, Tokyo 101-8310, Japan. [3]Department of Applied Mathematics and Informatics, Nihon University School of Dentistry, Tokyo 101-8310, Japan.

References

1. Esposito M, Hirsch JM, Lekholm U, Thomsen P. Biological factors contributing to failures of osseointegrated oral implants. (I) Success criteria and epidemiology. Eur J Oral Sci. 1998;106:527–51.
2. Ogata Y, Nakayama Y, Tatsumi J, Kubota T, Sato S, Nishida T, et al. Prevalence and risk factors for peri-implant diseases in Japanese adult dental patients. J Oral Sci. 2017;59:1–11.
3. Heitz-Mayfield LJ. Peri-implant diseases: diagnosis and risk indicators. J Clin Periodontol. 2008;35(Suppl 8):292–304.
4. Roos-Jansåker AM, Renvert H, Lindahi C, Renvert S. Nine- to fourteen-year follow-up of implant treatment. Part III: factors associated with peri-implant lesions. J Clin Periodontol. 2006;33:296–301.
5. Mombelli A, Müller N, Cionca N. The epidemiology of peri-implantitis. Clin Oral Implants Res. 2012;23(Suppl 6):67–76.
6. Zitzmann NU, Berglundh T. Definition and prevalence of peri-implant diseases. J Clin Periodontol. 2008;35(Suppl 8):286–91.
7. Fransson C, Lekholm U, Jemt T, Berglundh T. Prevalence of subjects with progressive bone loss at implants. Clin Oral Implants Res. 2005;16:440–6.
8. Koldsland OC, Scheie AA, Aass AM. Prevalence of peri-implantitis related to severity of the disease with different degrees of bone loss. J Periodontol. 2010;81:231–8.
9. Leonhardt A, Renvert S, Dahlén G. Microbial findings at failing implants. Clin Oral Implants Res. 1999;10:339–45.
10. de Waal YC, van Winkelhoff AJ, Meijer HJ, Raghoebar GM, Winkel EG. Differences in peri-implant conditions between fully and partially edentulous subjects: a systematic review. J Clin Periodontol 2013;40:266-286.
11. Lindhe J, Berglundh T, Ericsson I, Liljenberg B, Marinello C. Experimental breakdown of peri-implant and periodontal tissues. A study in the beagle dog. Clin Oral Implants Res. 1992;3:9–16.
12. Berglundh T, Zitzmann NU, Donati M. Are peri-implantitis lesions different from periodontitis lesions? J Clin Periodontol. 2011;38(Suppl 11):188–202.
13. Ladwein C, Schmelzeisen R, Nelson K, Fluegge TV, Fretwurst TI. The presence of keratinized mucosa associated with periimplant tissue health? A clinical cross-sectional analysis. Int J. Implant Dent. 2015;1:11.
14. Schwarz F, Schmucker A, Becker J. Efficacy of alternative or adjunctive measures to conventional treatment of peri-implant mucositis and peri-implantitis: a systematic review and meta analysis. Int J Implant Dent. 2015;1:22.
15. Monjie A, Aranda L, Diaz KT, Alarcón MA, Bagramian RA, Wang HL, et al. Impact of maintenance therapy for the prevention of peri-implant diseases: a systematic review and meta-analysis. J Dent Res. 2016;95:372–9.
16. Armitage GC. Development of a classification system for periodontal diseases and conditions. Ann Periodontol. 1999;4:1–6.
17. Lang NP, Berglundh T; Working group 4 of Seventh European Workshop on Periodontology. Periimplant diseases: where are we now? Consensus of the Seventh European Workshop on Periodontology. J Clin Periodontol. 2011;38 Suppl 11:178-181.
18. Froum SJ, Rosen PS. A proposed classification for peri-implantitis. Int J Periodontics Restorative Dent. 2012;32:533–40.
19. Eke PI, Dye BA, Wei L, Thornton-Evans GO, Genco RJ; CDC Periodontal Disease Surveillance Workgroup. Prevalence of periodontitis in adults in the United States: 2009 and 2010. J Dent Res 2012;91:914-920.
20. Müller F, Naharro M, Carlsson GE. What are the prevalence and incidence of tooth loss in the adult and elderly population in Europe? Clin Oral Implants Res. 2007;18(Suppl 3):2–14.
21. Renvert S, Giovannoli JL. Risk indicators. In: Renvert S, Giovannoli JL, editors. Peri-Implantitis. Chicago, IL: Quintessence Publishing Co., Inc.; 2012. p. 83–127.

22. Hardt CR, Gröndahl K, Lekholm U, Wennström JL. Outcome of implant therapy in relation to experienced loss of periodontal bone support: a retrospective 5-year study. Clin Oral Implants Res. 2002;13:488–94.
23. Schwartz-Arab D, Herzberg R, Levin L. Evaluation of long-term implant success. J Periodontol. 2005;76:1623–8.
24. Schou S, Holmstrup P, Worthington HV, Esposito M. Outcome of implant therapy in patients with previous tooth loss due to periodontitis. Clin Oral Implants Res. 2006;17(Suppl 2):104–23.
25. Roccuzzo M, Bonino F, Aglietta M, Dalmasso P. Ten-year results of a three-arm prospective cohort study on implants in periodontally compromised patients. Part 2: clinical results. Clin Oral Implants Res. 2012;23:389–95.
26. Derks J, Tomasi C. Peri-implant health and disease. A systematic review of current epidemiology. J Clin Periodontol. 2015;42(Suppl 16):158–71.
27. Lekholm U, Adell R, Lindhe J, Brånemark PI, Eriksson B, Rocker B, et al. Marginal tissue reactions at osseointegrated titanium fixtures. (II) A cross-sectional retrospective study. Int J Oral Maxillofac Surg. 1986;15:53–61.
28. Karousis IK, Salvi GE, Heitz-Mayfield LJ, Brägger U, Hämmerle CH, Lang NP. Long-term implant prognosis in patients with and without a history of chronic periodontitis: a 10-year prospective cohort study of the ITI Dental Implant System. Clin Oral Implants Res. 2003;14:329–39.
29. Mengel R, Flores-de-Jacoby L. Implants in patients treated for generalized aggressive and chronic periodontitis: a 3-year prospective longitudinal study. J Periodontol. 2005;76:534–43.
30. Cho-Yan Lee J, Mattheos N, Nixon KC, Ivanovski S. Residual periodontal pockets are a risk indicator for peri-implantitis patients treated for periodontitis. Clin Oral Implants Res. 2012;23:325–33.
31. Lindhe J, Socransky SS, Nyman S, Haffajee A, Westfelt E. "Critical probing depths" in periodontal therapy. J Clin Periodontol. 1982;9:323–6.
32. Fuchigami K, Munakata M, Kitazume T, Tachikawa N, Kasugai S, Kuroda SA. Diversity of peri-implant mucosal thickness by site. Clin Oral Implants Res. 2017;28:171–6.
33. Greenstein G, Caton J, Polson AM. Histologic characteristics associated with bleeding after probing and visual signs of inflammation. J Periodontol. 1981;52:420–5.
34. Gerber JA, Tan WC, Balmer TE, Salvi GE, Lang NP. Bleeding on probing and pocket probing depth in relation to probing pressure and mucosal health around oral implants. Clin Oral Implants Res. 2009;20:75–8.
35. Buser D, Weber HP, Lang NP. Tissue integration of non-submerged implants. 1-year results of a prospective study with 100 ITI hollow-cylinder and hollow-screw implants. Clin Oral Implants Res. 1990;1:33–40.
36. Schou S, Holmstrup P, Stoltze K, Hjørting-Hansen E, Fiehn NE, Skovgaard LT. Probing around implants and teeth with healthy or inflamed peri-implant mucosa/gingiva. A histologic comparison in cynomolgus monkeys (Macaca fascicularis). Clin Oral Implants Res. 2002;13:113–26.
37. Luterbacher S, Mayfield L, Bragger U, Lang NP. Diagnostic characteristics of clinical and microbiological tests for monitoring periodontal and peri-implant mucosal tissue conditions during supportive periodontal therapy. Clin Oral Implants Res. 2000;11:521–9.
38. Jonathan HD, Klokkevold PR. Supportive implant treatment. In: Newman MG, Takei HH, Klokkevold PR, Carranza FA, editors. Carranza's Clinical Periodontology. 12th ed. St. Louis: Elsevier; 2015. p. 807.

3

Impact of maxillary sinus augmentation on oral health-related quality of life

E. Schiegnitz[1*], P. W. Kämmerer[2], K. Sagheb[1], A. J. Wendt[3], A. Pabst[1], B. Al-Nawas[1] and M. O. Klein[1,4]

Abstract

Background: The aim of this study was to measure the oral health-related quality of life (OHRQoL) after maxillary sinus augmentation to determine the physical and psychological impact of this procedure for the patient.

Methods: Three hundred sixteen patients treated with an external or internal maxillary sinus augmentation and a total of 863 implants in the Department of Oral and Maxillofacial Surgery, Johannes Gutenberg University, Mainz, Germany, between July 2002 and December 2007 were included in this retrospective study. Total implant survival was assessed. Completion of a modified 26-item version of the Oral Health Impact Profile (OHIP-G) for assessing the oral health-related quality of life before and after the treatment was asked for. Subcategories were (1) functional limitations, (2) physical and psychological disabilities, and (3) complaints due to the surgical procedure. In 53 patients available for clinical follow-up examination, assessment of soft tissue parameters was performed.

Results: After an average time in situ of 41.2 ± 27 months (3.4 years), the in situ rate was 95.4%. One-year survival rate and five-year survival rate according to Kaplan Meier were 95.4 and 94.4%. Concerning functional limitations, significant better values for OHRQoL after sinus augmentation procedure than before the treatment ($p < 0.001$) were seen. In the subcategory physical and psychological disabilities, all questions had significant better values after the sinus lift ($p < 0.001$). Concerning complaints due to the surgical procedure, mean total scores were 5.1 ± 5.4 pre-operative, 6.9 ± 6.1 (0–31) post-operative, and 2.4 ± 3.7 recently. This meant a significant difference between "pre-operative" vs. "post-operative" ($p = 0.003$), "pre-operative" vs. "recently" ($p < 0.001$), and "post-operative" vs. "recently" ($p < 0.001$). Concerning the influence of implant indication, edentulous patients showed the most distinct improvement after the procedure. Clinical assessment showed stable soft tissue parameters.

Conclusions: Evaluation of OHRQoL after sinus augmentation showed a significant improvement indicating a remarkable benefit for the patients through this procedure.

Keywords: Dental implant, Maxillary sinus augmentation, Oral health-related quality of life

Background

Rehabilitation of completely and partial edentulous patients with dental implants has proved to be a safe and predictable procedure [1–3]. However, reduced bone height and the proximity of the maxillary sinus are challenging limitations for dental implant placement in the posterior maxilla [3]. Besides the use of short and tilted implants [4], one of the most frequently used surgical techniques for gaining adequate bone height in the posterior maxilla is external or internal maxillary sinus floor elevation. Several systematic reviews of the literature showed high overall implant survival rates well beyond 90% for sinus floor evaluation [1, 5, 6]. In addition, a recent Cochrane Systematic review including 18 randomized controlled trials (RCT) confirmed these high survival results [7]. However, the patients' perspective was mostly not appropriately taken into account in these analyses, although patient satisfaction presents one of the most essential objectives to obtain in oral rehabilitation [8, 9]. Hence, the question remains if the patients benefit from the sinus elevation procedures regarding their oral health-related quality of life (OHRQoL). However, studies evaluating the patient's perception after sinus elevation are very rare.

* Correspondence: eik.schiegnitz@unimedizin-mainz.de
[1]Department of Oral and Maxillofacial Surgery, Plastic Surgery, University Medical Centre of the Johannes Gutenberg-University, Augustusplatz 2, 55131 Mainz, Germany
Full list of author information is available at the end of the article

OHRQoL is a complex patient-centered concept that observes the impact of oral states of health on the well-being of individuals and society and assesses the effects of dental interventions [10, 11]. Different items like age, alcohol or tobacco habits, dental diseases, dentition, tooth loss, and condition of prosthesis affect OHRQoL [10, 12]. In addition, sociodemographic, financial, cultural, educational, psychological, and dietary factors have to be considered [13]. These patient-oriented outcomes can be examined using several different tools, including the Oral Health Impact Profile (OHIP), which is the most widely applied measure [14–16]. The OHIP represents a self-reported questionnaire on OHRQoL consisting of 49 questions under seven subscales [17]. The OHIP was translated to several different languages like German, Spanish, and Chinese, and shortened versions like OHIP-14 were introduced to reduce the response time [18–20]. The validity, sensitivity, and specificity of OHIP as a measuring instrument were validated in a huge variety of settings [21–23].

In conclusion, little information is available about patient's perception of sinus augmentation procedures. The aim of the present study was to assess whether sinus augmentation procedures together with implant placement and prosthetic rehabilitation improve quality of life in dental patients using a modified German OHIP and to examine the survival rates after this procedure.

Methods

Study design and subjects

This retrospective study addresses the oral health-related quality of life after maxillary sinus augmentation. Therefore, all patients that received an implantation after maxillary sinus augmentation in the Department of Oral and Maxillofacial Surgery of the University Medical Centre Mainz, Germany, between July 2002 and December 2007 were included in this study. There were no specific exclusion criteria. In this time period, 863 implants in 316 patients after sinus augmentation were inserted. One hundred forty-two of these patients (44.9%) were men and 174 (55.1%) women. Mean age of men was 57.4 years and mean age of women 55.2 years. Fifty-three patients (33 women and 8 men), with 157 dental implants remaining in situ, attended a clinical follow-up examination (Fig. 1). For these patients, plaque index, gingival index, probing depth, and width of keratinized mucosa were evaluated. The retrospective data analysis was conducted in accordance with the Helsinki Declaration of 1975, as revised in 2008, and all patients signed an informed consent. After consulting the local ethic committee, the decision was that due to the retrospective character of this study with no additional data acquisition, no ethical approval was needed according to the hospital laws of the appropriate state (Landeskrankenhausgesetz Rhineland Palatinate, Germany).

Measurement of OHRQoL

For evaluation of OHRQoL after sinus lift procedures, a modified version of the OHIP-G was applied [24]. This modification was performed to adapt the questionnaire to the specific objective of our study, as we wanted to evaluate the oral health-related quality of life after sinus lift procedures. Therefore, for this treatment, specific questions like "Have you had a maxillary sinusitis" were added to the questionnaire. After providing informed consent, patients completed a questionnaire, consisting of the three subcategories (1) functional limitations, (2) physical and psychological disabilities, and (3) complaints due to the surgical procedure. The implemented questions are shown in Tables 1, 2, and 3. Responses were made on an ordinal 4-point adjectival scale (0=never, 1=occasionally, 2=fairly often, and 3=very often). OHRQoL is described by summary scores of the asked items. Higher scores imply a stronger negative influence on OHRQoL; in contrast, lower scores indicate better OHRQoL. The valuation periods were divided

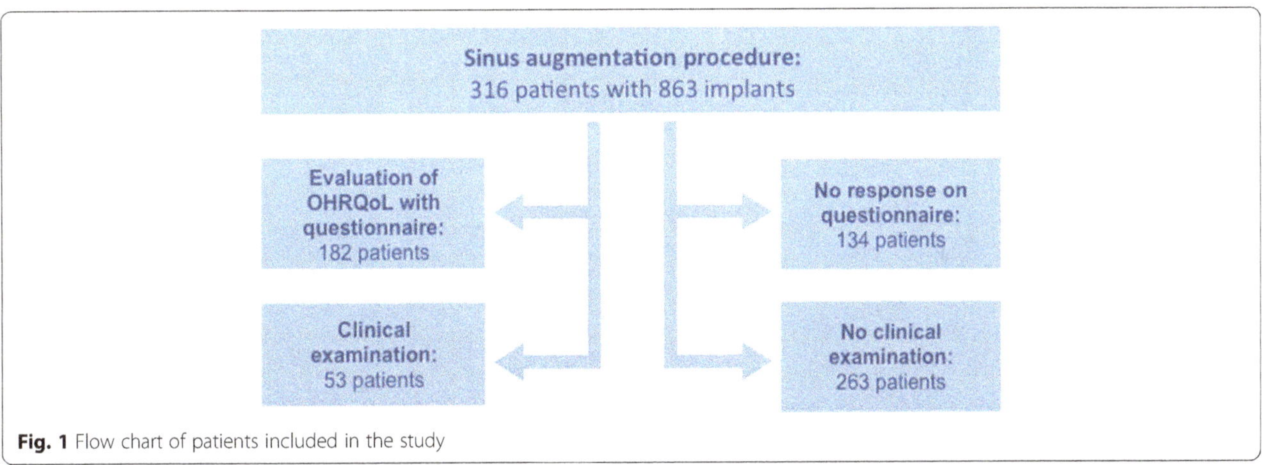

Fig. 1 Flow chart of patients included in the study

Table 1 Mean value and standard deviation for the subcategory functional limitations

Item	Mean ± SD before sinus lift	Mean ± SD after sinus lift	*p* value
Have you had difficulty chewing any foods?	1.6 ± 1.2	0.4 ± 0.7	<0.001
Have you had to avoid eating some foods?	1.1 ± 1.2	0.3 ± 0.7	<0.001
Have you felt that your sense of taste was impaired?	0.4 ± 0.8	0.1 ± 0.5	<0.001
Have you had trouble pronouncing any words?	0.6 ± 0.9	0.2 ± 0.6	<0.001
Have you been unable to brush your teeth properly?	0.6 ± 0.8	0.3 ± 0.6	<0.001
Have you felt that your breath has been stale?	0.7 ± 1.0	0.4 ± 0.6	<0.001

into "pre-operative" and "recently" for subcategories (1) and (2). For subcategory (3), valuation periods were classified into "pre-operative," "post-operative," and "recently."

Statistics

The Kaplan–Meier survival function was applied for the description of survival rates. To examine the statistical difference between survival rates, a log-rank test was used. Implant-related data were calculated. For statistical comparison of the paired questions and the total scores, a Wilcoxon test was applied. The intention of this study was descriptive, exploratory without a primary hypothesis. Consequently, we show descriptive *p* values of tests and no adjustment to multiple testing was done. The analyses were conducted using SPSS version 20.0 (IBM, USA).

Results

Survival analysis

After an average time in situ of 41.2 ± 27 months (3.4 years; range 0–96 months), 40 of the 863 implants were lost. These results indicated an in situ rate of 95.4%. One-year and five-year survival rate according to Kaplan–Meier were 95.4 and 94.4%. In patients receiving an external sinus lift an in situ rate of 95.1% and in patients with an internal sinus lift an in situ rate of 96.4% after the mean follow-up of 3.4 years was achieved. These results indicated a higher survival rate for the internal sinus lift procedure, but this difference was not statistically significant ($p = 0.614$, Fig. 2). The in situ rates were 100% for implants with a length <10 mm, 95.3% for implants with a length 10–13 mm, and 93.9% for implants with a length >13 mm. These differences were not statistically significant ($p = 0.657$). Implant survival for implant diameter <3.6 mm were 100%, for implant diameter 3.6–4.5 mm 96.0%, and for implant diameter >4.5 mm 92.2%, indicating a not statistically significant difference ($p = 0.123$). For patients that were available for clinical follow-up examination, the plaque index showed that 86.6% of implants had a satisfactory degree of oral hygiene (grades 0 and 1). Concerning the gingival index, 76.4% of the implants showed a gingival index grade 0, 19.7% a gingival index grade 1, and 3.8% a gingival index grade 3. A probing depth of less than 3.5 mm at all four measured sites around each implant was determined for 82.8% of the implants. The width of keratinized mucosa was <1 mm in 38.9% of the implants, between 1 and 2 mm in 37.6% of the implants, and >2 mm in 11.4% of the implants. No keratinized mucosa was found in 12.1% of the cases.

Pre- and post-treatment assessment of oral health-related quality of life

In 182 patients, pre- and post-treatment oral health-related quality of life after sinus augmentation procedure using a standardized questionnaire was evaluated. Subcategories

Table 2 Mean value and standard deviation for the subcategory physical and psychological disabilities

Item	Mean ± SD before sinus lift	Mean ± SD after sinus lift	*p* value
Have you felt tense because of problems with your teeth, mouth or dentures?	1.8 ± 1.1	0.8 ± 1.0	<0.001
Have you felt bad because the appearance of your teeth has been affected?	1.2 ± 1.2	0.4 ± 0.7	<0.001
Have you avoided eating with other people?	0.4 ± 0.8	0.1 ± 0.3	<0.001
Have you been a bit irritable with other people?	0.3 ± 0.7	0.1 ± 0.4	<0.001
Have you avoided going out?	0.3 ± 0.7	0.0 ± 0.2	<0.001
Have you had problems managing your daily routine?	0.4 ± 0.8	0.1 ± 0.4	<0.001
Have you been unable to work to your full capacity?	0.4 ± 0.8	0. 1 ± 0.4	<0.001
Have you had difficulties to relax?	0.7 ± 1.1	0.3 ± 0.6	<0.001
Have you felt that your general health has worsened?	0.6 ± 1.0	0.2 ± 0.6	<0.001

Table 3 Mean value and standard deviation for the subcategory complaints due to the surgical procedure

Item	Mean ± SD pre-operative	Mean ± SD post-operative	Mean ± SD in the last time
Have you felt pain in your mouth?	0.9 ± 1.1	1.2 ± 1.0	0.3 ± 0.6
Have you had difficulties with your mouth opening?	0.2 ± 0.6	0.5 ± 0.9	0.1 ± 1.0
Have you had painful gums?	0.9 ± 1.0	1.0 ± 1.1	0.5 ± 0.8
Have you had a sore or infected jaw?	0.7 ± 0.9	0.7 ± 0.9	0.3 ± 0.7
Have you had headaches?	0.5 ± 0.9	0.5 ± 0.8	0.4 ± 0.7
Have you had ostealgia?	0.3 ± 0.7	0.6 ± 1.1	0.2 ± 0.5
Have you had pain in your maxillary sinus?	0.4 ± 1.0	0.5 ± 0.8	0.1 ± 0.5
Have you had a maxillary sinusitis?	0.3 ± 0.7	0.3 ± 0.6	0.2 ± 0.5
Have you had swellings in your mouth?	0.4 ± 0.7	0.9 ± 0.9	0.2 ± 0.5
Have you had numbness in your mouth?	0.2 ± 0.5	0.5 ± 0.9	0.2 ± 0.6
Have you had poor taste in your mouth?	0.6 ± 0.8	0.5 ± 0.8	0.2 ± 0.5

for this evaluation were (1) functional limitations, (2) physical and psychological disabilities, and (3) complaints due to the surgical procedure.

Concerning functional limitations, all posed questions showed significant better values for OHRQoL after sinus augmentation procedure than before the treatment ($p < 0.001$; Table 1). The total score is calculated from the sum of the respective questions with high values indicating worse OHRQoL. The maximum total score achievable in the subcategory functional limitations was 18. Median total scores in the category functional limitations were 4.64 ± 4.3 (range 0–17) before and 1.65 ± 2.4 (0–13) after the treatment, indicating a significant difference ($n = 169$; $p < 0.001$).

In the subcategory physical and psychological disabilities, all questions had significant better values after the sinus lift ($p < 0.001$; Table 2). The total score achievable in this category was 27. Mean total scores were 5.79 ± 6.4 (range 0–27) before and 1.94 ± 3.2 (range 0–21) after the sinus augmentation procedure, indicating a significant difference ($n = 164$; $p < 0.001$).

In the subcategory complaints due to the surgical procedure, the patients were asked to answer the items regarding the periods "pre-operative," "post-operative," and "recently." Six of the 11 items (items 1, 2, 6, 8, 9, and 10) were significant worse "post-operative" compared to "pre-operative" ($n = 126$; $p \leq 0.03$; Table 3; Fig. 3). However, comparing the periods "pre-operative"

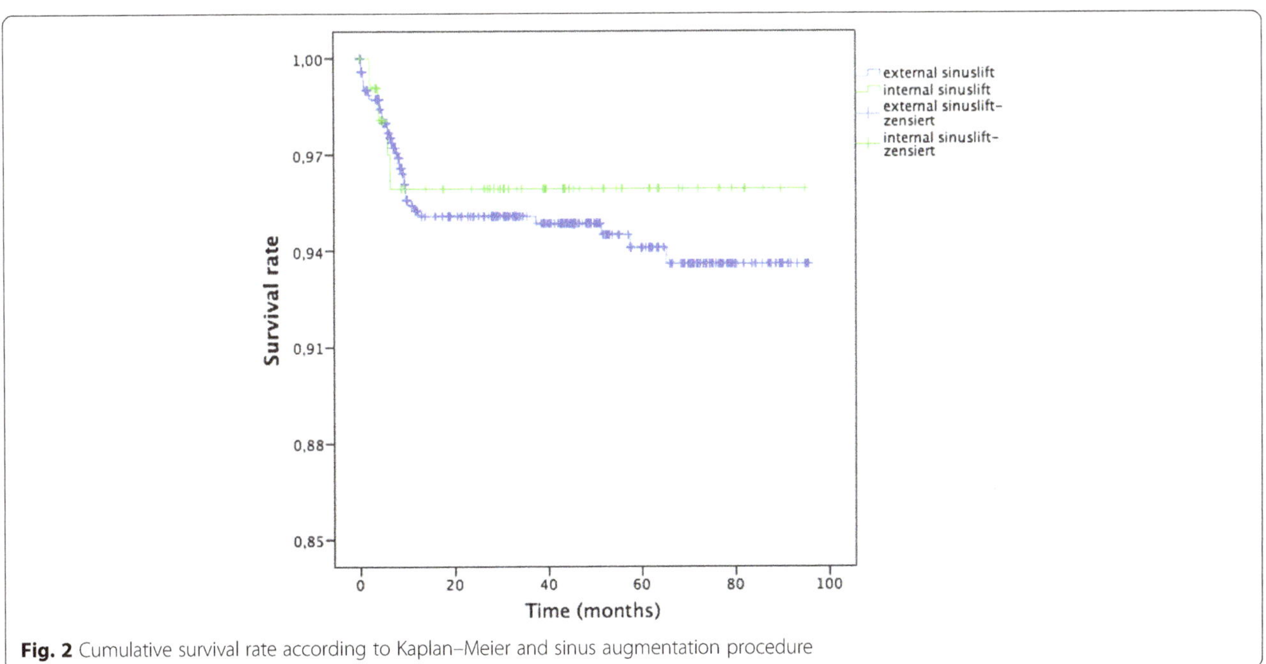

Fig. 2 Cumulative survival rate according to Kaplan–Meier and sinus augmentation procedure

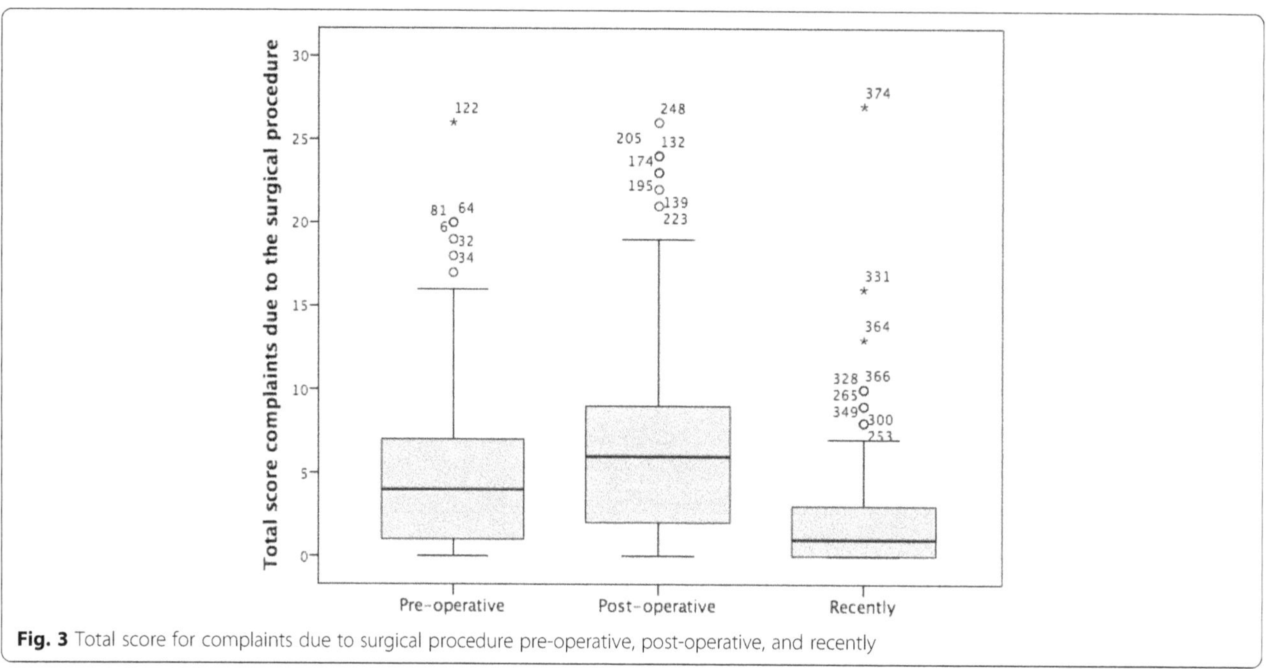

Fig. 3 Total score for complaints due to surgical procedure pre-operative, post-operative, and recently

and "recently," items 1, 3, 4, 6, 7, 8, 9, and 11 showed a significant improvement ($n = 126$; $p \leq 0.002$). Comparison of the periods "post-operative" and "recently," all items were significant better in the period recently ($n = 126$; $p < 0.001$). Mean total scores were 5.1 ± 5.4 (range 0–26) pre-operative, 6.9 ± 6.1 (0–31) post-operative, and 2.4 ± 3.7 (range 0–27) recently. This meant a significant difference between "pre-operative" vs. "post-operative" ($n = 126$; $p = 0.003$), "pre-operative" vs. "recently" ($n = 126$; $p < 0.001$), and "post-operative" vs. "recently" ($n = 126$; $p < 0.001$).

Impact of implant indication on oral health-related quality of life

In edentulous patients, median total scores in the category functional limitations were 8.4 ± 4.1 before and 2.7 ± 2.4 after the treatment, indicating a significant improvement ($p < 0.001$; Fig. 4). In addition, patients with a distal extension situation (4.6 ± 4.0 vs. 1.7 ± 2.7; $p < 0.001$), an extended edentulous gap (3.9 ± 3.8 vs. 1.4 ± 1.9; $p = 0.009$) and a single tooth gap (1.5 ± 2.2 vs. 0.6 ± 1.3; $p = 0.034$) showed significant lower mean total scores after the rehabilitation compared to before

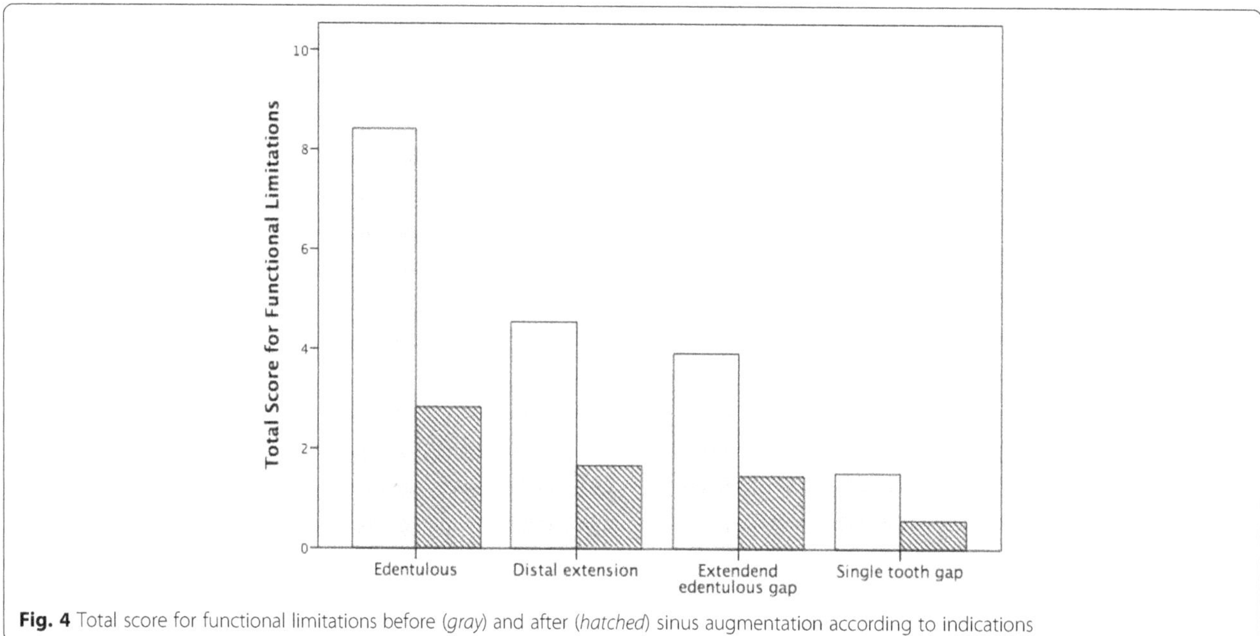

Fig. 4 Total score for functional limitations before (*gray*) and after (*hatched*) sinus augmentation according to indications

the treatment. Concerning the category physical and psychological disabilities, mean total score of edentulous patients showed the most distinct improvement after the procedure (11.1 ± 8.2 vs. 3.7 ± 4.5; $p < 0.001$; Fig. 5). For patients with a distal extension situation (5.5 ± 5.8 vs. 1.8 ± 3.3; $p < 0.001$), with an extended edentulous gap (4.4 ± 4.9 vs. 1.4 ± 1.7; $p = 0.007$) and with a single tooth gap (3.0 ± 3.0 vs. 1.0 ± 1.2; $p = 0.005$), total score were significantly lower after the sinus lift.

Discussion

The clinical and radiological outcomes of sinus augmentation procedures have been published in several studies [1, 3, 6, 7]. However, little data on the physical and psychological impact of this procedure on the patient is available yet. The present study evaluated pre-operative and post-treatment OHRQoL self-assessment scores of patients treated with dental implants after sinus augmentation procedures.

The one-year and five-year survival rates of the investigated implants were 95.4 and 94.4%. These results are in accordance with the recent literature. In a current meta-analysis, mean implant survival rates were 98.6 ± 2.6% for sinus augmentation procedures using bone substitute materials alone, 88.6 ± 4.1% for sinus augmentation procedures using bone substitute materials mixed with autologous bone, and 97.4 ± 2.2% for sinus augmentation procedures using autologous bone alone [1]. The mean follow-up of the investigated studies was 39.7 ± 34.6 months with a range from 4 to 170 months. Corbella et al. showed in a recent systematic review a survival rate from 95.4 to 100% after 3-year follow-up for internal sinus lift and a survival rate from 75.57 to 100% for external sinus lift [5]. Del-Fabbro et al. estimated a mean weighted cumulative implant survival at 1, 2, 3, and 5 years as 98.12, 97.40, 96.75, and 95.81% [6].

In the present study, OHRQoL after sinus augmentation was investigated using a modified version of the G-OHIP. The results showed significant better values for all three subcategories after the treatment, indicating a remarkable benefit for the patients. Concerning the influence of implant indication, edentulous patients showed the most distinct improvement after the procedure. So far, many studies have examined the quality of life in patients treated with dental implants [25–28]. However, to our best knowledge, studies investigating quality of life after sinus augmentation are very rare. Mardinger et al. examined the patient's perception of immediate post-operative recovery after sinus-floor augmentation [29]. In this prospective study, health-related quality of life questionnaire was given to 76 patients evaluating patient perception of recovery in the four areas pain, oral function, general activity, and other symptoms. The results showed that average and maximal pain peaked on post-operative day 1 and improved on post-operative days 4 and 5. Difficulty in mouth opening was greatest on post-operative day 1 and improved on post-operative day 3. Swelling peaked on post-operative day 2 and improved on post-operative day 5. The authors concluded that an average patient undergoing sinus augmentation procedure should expect recovery within 5 days. In a prospective cohort study, Reisine et al. examined quality of life changes among post-menopausal women getting dental implants with bone augmentation procedures using OHIP-14 questionnaire [30]. The results

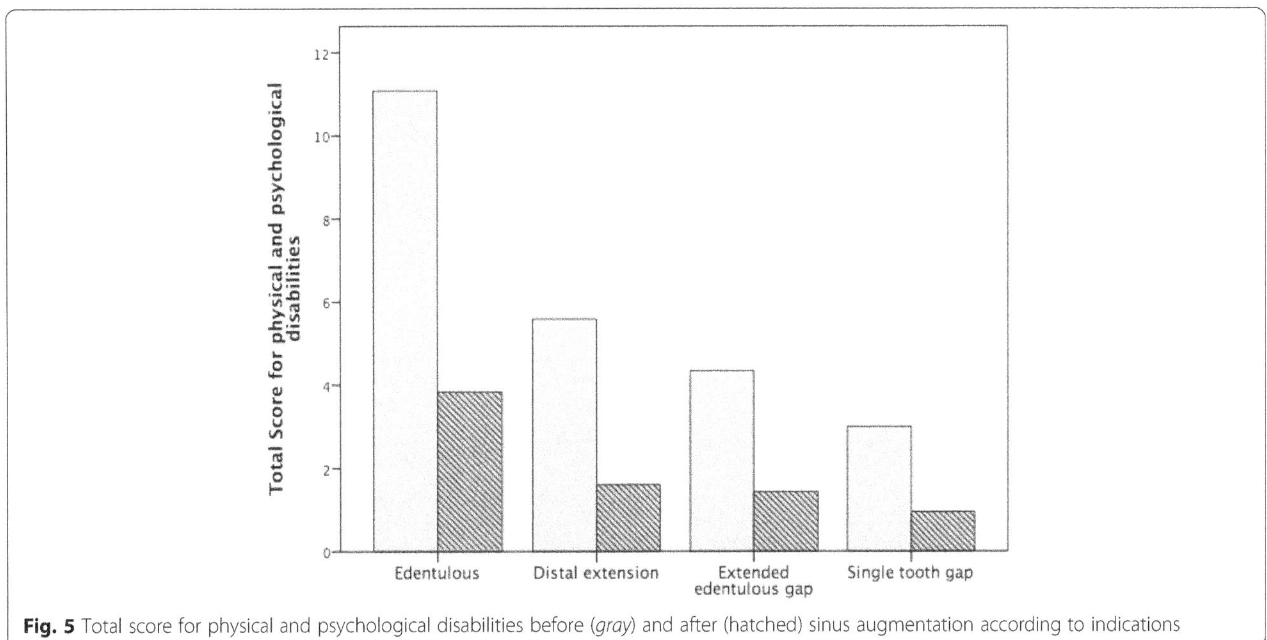

Fig. 5 Total score for physical and psychological disabilities before (*gray*) and after (hatched) sinus augmentation according to indications

showed that patients' quality of life improved continuously from the pre-treatment to the 9-month assessment. Type of augmentation procedure had no significant influence on quality of life. Better et al. included 18 patients in a prospective clinical study to investigate patient's perception of immediate post-operative recovery after sinus augmentation, using a minimally invasive implant device [31]. The minimally invasive implant device consisted of a self-tapping implant which contained an L-shaped internal channel allowing the introduction of liquids through the implant body and into the maxillary sinus. The results showed that patients' perceptions of post-operative symptoms in the tested areas pain, oral function, general activity, and other symptoms were mostly scored "not at all" or "very little" on post-operative day 1, indicating a minimum discomfort through this procedure for the patient. In a prospective non-randomized clinical trial, changes in OHRQoL and health-related quality of life (HRQoL) after bone graft harvesting for dental implants with respect to the donor site were examined [32]. Therefore, autologous bone grafts were harvested in 23 patients either from an intra-oral or an extra-oral donor site, followed by implant placements. OHRQoL was analyzed using the OHIP-49, HRQoL was measured using the short-form 36. In the results, bone harvesting from an extra-oral donor site deteriorated HRQoL substantially more compared with intra-oral donor sites. OHRQoL impaired from baseline to first follow-up in both groups; however, changes were not statistically significant. The authors concluded that in clinical decision-making regarding donor site for bone graft harvesting, patients and clinicians should consider expected decrease in HRQoL if deciding to use extra-oral donor sites. Therefore, the authors recommended to prefer intra-oral donor sites whenever possible. In a recent study of Nickenig et al., OHIP-G 21 was evaluated in 8689 patients with various kinds of indications (free end gap, posterior single-tooth gap, anterior single-tooth gap, dental gap, and edentulous jaw) for dental implants [33]. Comparable to our results, the results showed an improved OHRQoL for all indications after prosthetic reconstruction. The modification of our OHIP score complicates the comparability of the baseline results of the mentioned study with our results. However, also patients with edentulous jaws and patients with an anterior single-tooth gap benefited most significantly from the treatment.

In order to measure OHRQoL in the present study, a specific and shortened questionnaire based on the validated and reliable OHIP score was developed to consider representative impairments of maxillary sinus augmentation like sinusitis and to relieve the clinical application. In a cross sectional study, Allen et McMillan proofed that a shortened OHIP-14 version showed a similar ability to assess OHRQoL compared to the detailed OHIP-49 version [34]. However, there has been some concern that the short-form OHIP-14 may not detect improvements following clinical intervention due to floor effects [35]. The OHIP was used as a measure because it showed high test-retest reliability and was validated in numerous cross-sectional population studies [36].

Conclusions

Within the limitations of this study, the results demonstrated a high long-term survival for sinus augmentation procedures and significant improvement of OHRQoL after this procedure. Therefore, sinus augmentation procedures are highly valuable treatment options in implant dentistry.

Authors' contributions

The data from this study is part of the dissertation work submitted to Johannes Gutenberg University, Mainz as part of doctoral thesis of AJW. ES, PWK, KS, AJW, AP, BAl-N, and MOK contributed to substantial contributions to the conception or design of the work or the acquisition, analysis, or interpretation of data for the work. ES, PWK, KS, AJW, AP, BAl-N, and MOK drafted the work or revising it critically for important intellectual content. ES, PWK, KS, AJW, AP, BAl-N, and MOK approved the final version of the manuscript to be published. ES, PWK, KS, AJW, AP, BAl-N, and MOK agreed to be accountable for all aspects of the work in ensuring that questions related to the accuracy or integrity of any part of the work are appropriately investigated and resolved. All authors read and approved the final manuscript.

Competing interests

The authors Eik Schiegnitz, Peer W. Kämmerer, Keyvan Sagheb, Annika J. Wendt, Andreas Pabst, Bilal Al-Nawas, and Marc O. Klein declare that they have no competing interests.

Author details

[1]Department of Oral and Maxillofacial Surgery, Plastic Surgery, University Medical Centre of the Johannes Gutenberg-University, Augustusplatz 2, 55131 Mainz, Germany. [2]Department of Oral and Maxillofacial Surgery, Plastic Surgery, University of Rostock, Rostock, Germany. [3]Department of Prosthodontics, University of Hamburg-Eppendorf, Hamburg, Germany. [4]Oral and Maxillofacial Surgery, Private Praxis, Düsseldorf, Germany.

References

1. Al-Nawas B, Schiegnitz E. Augmentation procedures using bone substitute materials or autogenous bone—a systematic review and meta-analysis. Eur J Oral Implantol. 2014 Summer;7 Suppl 2:S219-34.
2. Derks J, Hakansson J, Wennstrom JL, Tomasi C, Larsson M, Berglundh T. Effectiveness of implant therapy analyzed in a Swedish population: early and late implant loss. J Dent Res. 2015;94(3 Suppl):44S–51S.
3. Schiegnitz E, Al-Nawas B, Tegner A, Sagheb K, Berres M, Kammerer PW, et al. Clinical and radiological long-term outcome of a tapered implant system with special emphasis on the influence of augmentation procedures. Clin Implant Dent Relat Res. 2016;18(4):810–20.
4. Aparicio C, Perales P, Rangert B. Tilted implants as an alternative to maxillary sinus grafting: a clinical, radiologic, and periotest study. Clin Implant Dent Relat Res. 2001;3(1):39–49.

5. Corbella S, Taschieri S, Del Fabbro M. Long-term outcomes for the treatment of atrophic posterior maxilla: a systematic review of literature. Clin Implant Dent Relat Res. 2015;17(1):120–32.
6. Del Fabbro M, Corbella S, Weinstein T, Ceresoli V, Taschieri S. Implant survival rates after osteotome-mediated maxillary sinus augmentation: a systematic review. Clin Implant Dent Relat Res. 2012;14(Suppl 1):e159–68.
7. Esposito M, Felice P, Worthington HV. Interventions for replacing missing teeth: augmentation procedures of the maxillary sinus. Cochrane Database Syst Rev. 2014;5:CD008397.
8. Brennan M, Houston F, O'Sullivan M, O'Connell B. Patient satisfaction and oral health-related quality of life outcomes of implant overdentures and fixed complete dentures. Int J Oral Maxillofac Implants. 2010;25(4):791–800.
9. Al-Omiri M, Hantash RA, Al-Wahadni A. Satisfaction with dental implants: a literature review. Implant Dent. 2005;14(4):399–406.
10. Bramanti E, Matacena G, Cecchetti F, Arcuri C, Cicciu M. Oral health-related quality of life in partially edentulous patients before and after implant therapy: a 2-year longitudinal study. Oral Implantol. 2013;6(2):37–42. Pubmed Central PMCID: 3808938.
11. Atchison KA, Gift HC. Perceived oral health in a diverse sample. Adv Dent Res. 1997;11(2):272–80.
12. Shimazaki Y, Soh I, Saito T, Yamashita Y, Koga T, Miyazaki H, et al. Influence of dentition status on physical disability, mental impairment, and mortality in institutionalized elderly people. J Dent Res. 2001;80(1):340–5.
13. Locker D. Self-esteem and socioeconomic disparities in self-perceived oral health. J Public Health Dent. 2009 Winter;69(1):1-8.
14. Allen PF, McMillan AS, Walshaw D. A patient-based assessment of implant-stabilized and conventional complete dentures. J Prosthet Dent. 2001;85(2):141–7.
15. Ohrn K, Jonsson B. A comparison of two questionnaires measuring oral health-related quality of life before and after dental hygiene treatment in patients with periodontal disease. Int J Dent Hyg. 2012;10(1):9–14.
16. Brondani MA, MacEntee MI. Thirty years of portraying oral health through models: what have we accomplished in oral health-related quality of life research? Qual Life Res. 2014;23(4):1087–96.
17. Slade GD, Spencer AJ. Development and evaluation of the Oral Health Impact Profile. Community Dent Health. 1994;11(1):3–11.
18. John MT, Miglioretti DL, LeResche L, Koepsell TD, Hujoel P, Micheelis W. German short forms of the Oral Health Impact Profile. Community Dent Oral Epidemiol. 2006;34(4):277–88.
19. Lopez R, Baelum V. Spanish version of the Oral Health Impact Profile (OHIP-Sp). BMC Oral Health. 2006;6:11. Pubmed Central PMCID: 1534011.
20. Wong MC, Lo EC, McMillan AS. Validation of a Chinese version of the Oral Health Impact Profile (OHIP). Community Dent Oral Epidemiol. 2002;30(6):423–30.
21. Locker D, Jokovic A, Clarke M. Assessing the responsiveness of measures of oral health-related quality of life. Community Dent Oral Epidemiol. 2004;32(1):10–8.
22. McGrath C, Comfort MB, Lo EC, Luo Y. Patient-centred outcome measures in oral surgery: validity and sensitivity. Br J Oral Maxillofac Surg. 2003;41(1):43–7.
23. Lam WY, McGrath CP, Botelho MG. Impact of complications of single tooth restorations on oral health-related quality of life. Clin Oral Implants Res. 2014;25(1):67–73.
24. John MT, Patrick DL, Slade GD. The German version of the Oral Health Impact Profile—translation and psychometric properties. Eur J Oral Sci. 2002;110(6):425–33.
25. Allen PF, McMillan AS. A longitudinal study of quality of life outcomes in older adults requesting implant prostheses and complete removable dentures. Clin Oral Implants Res. 2003;14(2):173–9.
26. Sonoyama W, Kuboki T, Okamoto S, Suzuki H, Arakawa H, Kanyama M, et al. Quality of life assessment in patients with implant-supported and resin-bonded fixed prosthesis for bounded edentulous spaces. Clin Oral Implants Res. 2002; 13(4):359–64.
27. Stellingsma K, Bouma J, Stegenga B, Meijer HJ, Raghoebar GM. Satisfaction and psychosocial aspects of patients with an extremely resorbed mandible treated with implant-retained overdentures. A prospective, comparative study. Clin Oral Implants Res. 2003;14(2):166–72.
28. Heydecke G, Locker D, Awad MA, Lund JP, Feine JS. Oral and general health-related quality of life with conventional and implant dentures. Community Dent Oral Epidemiol. 2003;31(3):161–8.
29. Mardinger O, Poliakov H, Beitlitum I, Nissan J, Chaushu G. The patient's perception of recovery after maxillary sinus augmentation: a prospective study. J Periodontol. 2009;80(4):572–6.
30. Reisine S, Freilich M, Ortiz D, Pendrys D, Shafer D, Taxel P. Quality of life improves among post-menopausal women who received bone augmentation during dental implant therapy. Int J Oral Maxillofac Surg. 2012;41(12):1558–62. Pubmed Central PMCID: 3547602.
31. Better H, Slavescu D, Barbu H, Cochran DL, Chaushu G. Patients perceptions of recovery after maxillary sinus augmentation with a minimally invasive implant device. Quintessence Int. 2014;45(9):779–87.
32. Reissmann DR, Dietze B, Vogeler M, Schmelzeisen R, Heydecke G. Impact of donor site for bone graft harvesting for dental implants on health-related and oral health-related quality of life. Clin Oral Implants Res. 2013;24(6):698–705.
33. Nickenig HJ, Wichmann M, Terheyden H, Kreppel M. Oral health-related quality of life and implant therapy: a prospective multicenter study of preoperative, intermediate, and posttreatment assessment. J Craniomaxillofac Surg. 2016;44(6):753–7.
34. Allen PF, McMillan AS. The impact of tooth loss in a denture wearing population: an assessment using the Oral Health Impact Profile. Community Dent Health. 1999;16(3):176–80.
35. Stewart AL, Hays RD, Ware Jr JE. The MOS short-form general health survey. Reliability and validity in a patient population. Med Care. 1988;26(7):724–35.
36. Yuen HK, Nelson SL. Test–retest reliability of Oral Health Impact Profile (OHIP-49) in adults with systemic sclerosis. Spec Care Dentist. 2014;34(1):27–33. Pubmed Central PMCID: 3879960.

4

Effect of different angulations and collar lengths of conical hybrid implant abutment on screw loosening after dynamic cyclic loading

Mai Ahmed Yousry El-Sheikh, Tamer Mohamed Nasr Mostafa* and Mohamed Maamoun El-Sheikh

Abstract

Background: The purpose of this in vitro study was to evaluate the effect of different angulations and collar lengths of the implant abutment on screw loosening by measuring removal torque value (RTV) before and after dynamic cyclic loading using digital torque gauge.

Methods: A total 90 sets of 4.5 mm diameter × 10 mm length bone level implants with conical hybrid connection were used. They were divided equally according to abutment angulation, into three groups: GI 0° abutment, GII 15° abutment, and GIII 25°. Each group was divided into two subgroups, 15 each, according to collar height: subgroup A (2 mm) and subgroup B (4 mm). Each implant and abutment assembly was positioned vertically in the center of the acrylic resin block using stainless steel cylindrical split mold. Initial analysis was made by abutment screw tightened with 30 Ncm torque twice with 10-min intervals using a digital torque gauge. RTV before and after cyclic loading of the abutment screws were measured in newton centimeter using digital torque gauge. One hundred thousand cycles of eccentric dynamic cyclic loading, at 130 N at a rate of 1 Hz, were applied 5 mm away from the central axis of the implant fixture. Percentage of removal torque loss (%RTL) before and after dynamic cyclic loading were calculated and statistically analyzed using the SPSS version 20.

Results: For GI, %initial RTL was 25.0 ± 1.5% and decreased significantly after loading (23.5 ± 2.3%). For GII, %initial RTL was 25.5 ± 1.4% and increased significantly after loading (33.4 ± 3.7%). For GIII, %initial RTL was 25.944 ± 1.2% and increased significantly after loading (40.1 ± 5.1%). There was significant effect on screw loosening for abutment angulations and collar lengths.

Conclusion: Within the limitations of this study, results suggested that screw loosening increases with increasing abutment angulations and collar lengths after dynamic cyclic loading.

Keywords: Removal torque loss, Abutment angulation, Abutment collar height, Dynamic cyclic loading, Digital torque gauge, Screw loosening

* Correspondence: tifournasr@gmail.com
Prosthodontic Department, Faculty of Dentistry, Tanta University, Elgeish St., Tanta, Egypt

Introduction

Successful implant therapy requires a dynamic equilibrium between biological and mechanical factors. The mechanical factors are generally considered multifactorial which are involved in the success of implant rehabilitation. Majority of implant complications nowadays are caused by mechanical factors rather than the implant itself. Mechanical complications of the implant-prosthetic system include loosening and fracture of the maintaining screw, micromovements, fixture fracture, abutment fracture, and fracture of over structure [1].

It was reported that abutment screw loosening is the most common mechanical complication surpassed by loss of osseointegration [2]. Loosening and fracture are potential problems for implant abutments and their fastening screws [3]. Incidence of screw loosening was up to 12.7% in single crowns and 6.7% in fixed partial dentures [4].

Several complications may arise because of loose retaining or abutment screws as granulation tissue between the loose abutment and the implant, leading to fistulae formation and infection of the soft tissue. In addition, loose screws are more liable to fracture under load, leading to long-term prosthesis complications [2].

The whole concept of the dental implant mechanics has been designed in such a way as to have a weak link that will be the first component that will fail in case the system is overloaded. The screw used to fasten the abutment to the implant usually represents this weak link [3].

Considering that the union between prosthesis and implant is promoted by a screw joint, the aim to tight the abutment screw is to keep the components together [5]. A screw is tightened by applying torque as a clamping force to provide a stable joint between the abutment and implant fixture. This clamping force is also known as the preload, which elongates the screw within the material then elastically recovered, increasing the strength with which the abutment and implant are pulled together [6].

When the implant set is submitted to functional loads, occlusal forces to the connection are concentrated at the abutment screw; consequently, the optimum preload is critical for joint stability and to avoid screw loosening [7].

Several factors related to screw design and fabrication can affect the risk of abutment or prosthetic screw loosening in a metal-to-metal screw system; these primarily are related to preload which by itself is affected by multiple factors: torque magnitude, screw head design, thread design, and number and composition of metal [8]. There are some factors that can affect initial torque loss, including tightening torque value, implant system, abutment screw material, errors in casting of metallic alloys, repeated tightening/loosening cycles of the screw, and improper insertion torque. These factors can reduce the frictional fit between the screws and internal threads of the implant, which may lead to screw loosening [9, 10].

Also screw loosening may be caused by inadequate tightening torque, settling of implant components, inappropriate implant position, inadequate occlusal scheme or crown anatomy, poorly fitting frameworks, improper screw design/material, increased abutment angulations, increased collar length, and heavy occlusal forces [11].

Ideally, dental implants should be aligned vertically with the axial forces. When the long axis of the implant fixture and the long axis of the planned prosthetic tooth are not aligned, due to improper jaw relationship or compromised osseous anatomy, angled abutment is often the abutment of choice for prosthodontic restorations [4]; it helps to avoid vital anatomical structures [12]. Angled abutments are used in all-on-four and all-on-six approaches in completely edentulous patients [13]. They can be used for esthetics reasons [8]. Angled abutments reduce treatment time, fees, and the need to perform guided bone regeneration procedure [14].

Kallus et al. [15] demonstrated prototype angled abutments of the Branemark. Nowadays, angled abutments vary from 15 to 45° angulation. Researches showed that angled abutment developed transverse force under loads in the direction of angled abutment resulting in off-axis forces. When functional or parafunctional load is applied to angled abutment, it generates micromovement which might play a role in screw loosening [4].

Collar length is the distance between the implant platform and the gingival margin. Sometimes, significant vertical space that has not been corrected with vertical ridge augmentation may necessitate selection of longer abutments, which would lead to an increased vertical cantilever. Furthermore, selection of the length of abutment collar would be affected if different distances between the implant platform and the gingival margin exist. Despite consistent occlusogingivial dimension, the thickness of soft tissue around the abutment affects abutment collar length selection. Therefore, in posterior regions where reduction of surrounding soft tissues thickness does not interfere with esthetic results, this reduction may be beneficial from a biomechanical point of view [9]. Selection of the suitable abutment collar length from a prosthetic/esthetic point of view is influenced by the length of the implant collar used. Abutment collar length is determined based on the height of the emergence profile and prosthetic restoration type (cemented, screw-retained, or overdenture) [16].

Abutment selection according to collar length index is a critical mechanical factor; selection of longer abutments leads to an increased vertical cantilever which acts as a force magnifier [8]. Vertical cantilever designs increase forces on screws due to the lever effect and, therefore, should be avoided [17, 18]. Although increased restorative vertical space with longer collar length could play a role in screw loosening, there is no certain evidence that increase in abutment collar length can affect screw loosening. However, considering the abutment height from implant platform to the top of abutment (including abutment collar), an increase in the collar length might result in an increase in the vertical cantilever. To reduce the possibility of screw loosening, reducing the cantilever length has been recommended [9].

The application of dynamic cyclic loading is used to simulate masticatory function mimic oral cavity that might lead to a failure of implant–abutment connection. Also, it is a reliable method to test the effect of mechanical fatigue on the implant–abutment stability [4].

To date, there are limited publications regarding the investigation of screw loosening according to abutment angulations and collar lengths before and after dynamic cyclic loading. Sethi and colleagues [19] noted no implant fractures or screw loosening during a 96-month monitoring period for 2261 implants ($N = 467$ patients) with angulations ranging from 0 to 45°. While Asvanund and colleagues [4] addressed screw loosening with increasing abutment angulations, Siadat and coworkers [9] concluded that increase in height of the abutment collar could adversely affect the torque loss of the abutment screw.

So, the aim of this in vitro study was to evaluate the effect of different angulations and collar lengths of the implant abutment on screw loosening by measuring removal torque value before and after dynamic cyclic loading using digital torque gauge.

Materials and methods

Total 90 stock titanium abutments (Anyridges; MEGAGEN, Seoul, Korea) with different angulations and collar lengths were used in this study and divided into three groups, 30 each according to the degree of abutment angulations GI 0° abutment, GII 15° abutment, and GIII 25°. Each group was divided into two subgroups, 15 each according to implant abutment collar lengths: subgroup A (2 mm) and subgroup B (4 mm). For each sample conical hybrid connection implant, 4.5 mm diameter × 10 mm length bone level implants with platform-switching were used. Titanium abutment screw was used (Fig. 1).

Ninety auto-polymerized acrylic resin blocks were prepared for this study using a stainless steel split cylindrical mold with 20 mm length, 20 mm width, and 2.5 in. thickness. A stainless steel base was made wider than the split cylinder, so it can be seated inside this base. At the center of the base, small opening with the same diameter of implant abutment was made so it can help implant abutment assembly to be centralized vertically in the acrylic resin block. Split cylindrical mold was cleaned and dried; then, vaseline was applied into the whole internal surface to ensure separation of acrylic block from the mold. Implant fixture and abutment were screwed through the hole in the stainless steel base.

The auto-polymerized acrylic resin powder and liquid were mixed according to the manufacturer's recommendation, poured inside the split cylindrical mold, and left for polymerization. After polymerization, implant fixture was unscrewed from abutment to separate the split cylinder from the stainless steel base; then, the cylinder was removed showing the acrylic resin block with implant fixture centralized vertically and perpendicular to the base and the platform was flushed with acrylic resin block level. Finishing and polishing were made, using micromotor, by red and white stone (Fig. 2).

Ninety stock titanium abutments were selected with post length of 7 mm; each abutment had titanium screw with same length, diameter, thread, and head

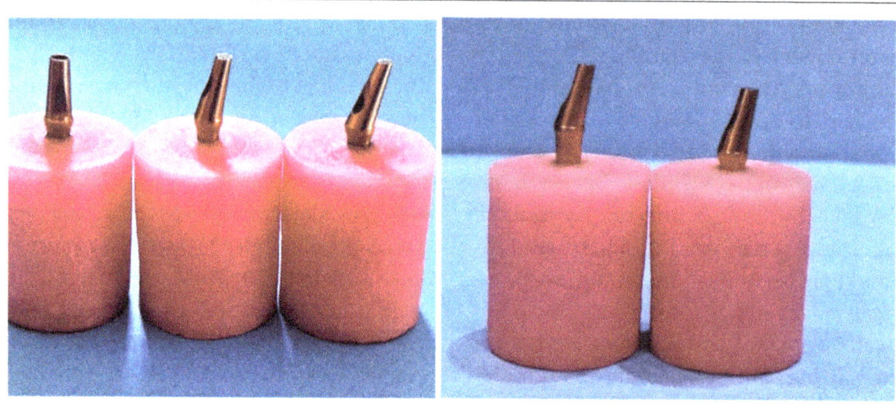

Fig. 1 Different abutment angulations and collar lengths

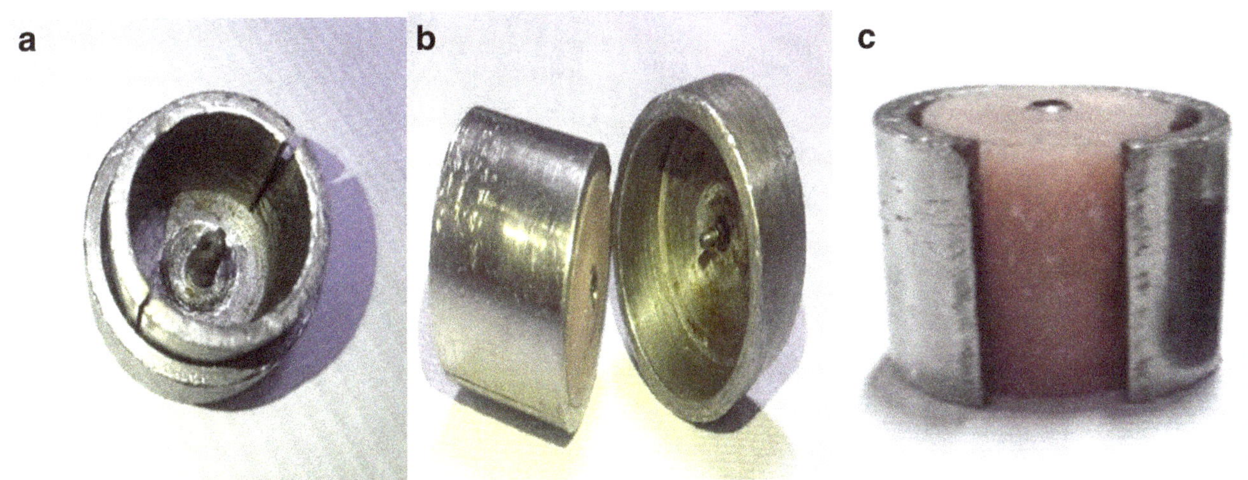

Fig. 2 **a** Stainless steel split cylindrical mold with implant fixture screwed to abutment. **b** Implant fixture unscrewed from abutment after polymerization. **c** Implant fixture centralized vertically and perpendicular to the base with platform flushed with resin block level

design for each group. For each selected abutment, metal tube was fabricated to fit accurately on the abutment. The titanium abutment was mounted on the fixture which was prepared to be scanned with a 3D scanner (Smart optics, England). The desired design and dimensions of metal tube was designed by CADCAM software (Dentcreate, Exocad) in wax (CopraDur, White peaks dental solution, Germany), with flat occlusal surface (10 mm in diameter) which was parallel to the horizontal plane and perpendicular to the implant fixture long axis to permit contact with the testing machine piston in a flat horizontal plane. In the center of the flat occlusal surface, a small rounded hole was designed exactly opposite to the abutment screw hole that facilitates screw driver accessibility for easy tightening and removal. Then, this accurately designed wax pattern was casted to a nickel chromium alloy tube (Fig. 3).

Self-adhesive resin cement (G- CEM, USA) was used for fixing of metal tube to the abutment. A customized rigid metal mounting jig was designed, as a holding device, to ensure solid fixation of the sample while recording the measures.

Recording RTV before loading

Abutment screws were tightened in all the groups to 30 Ncm using a digital torque gauge (HTG2 - 200Nc, IMADA, Toyohashi, Japan) according to the manufacturer's recommendations to ensure an accurate application of reproducible force to each abutment screw every time for standardization. Ten minutes after first torque application, all screws were retightened to the same tightening torque (30 Ncm). Ten minutes later, RTV before loading was measured and recorded.

Recording RTV after loading

At each group, after measuring the initial removal torque value, the abutment screw was tightened again to the recommended torque value (30 Ncm).

The acrylic resin block was firmly mounted in a holder of the lower fixed compartment of a computer-controlled universal testing machine (Model 3345; Instron Industrial Products, Norwood, MA, USA) for 100,000 cycles of eccentric dynamic cyclic loading.

Dynamic cyclic loading was performed with a metallic rod with a round tip which was attached to the upper movable compartment of the machine, under a load of

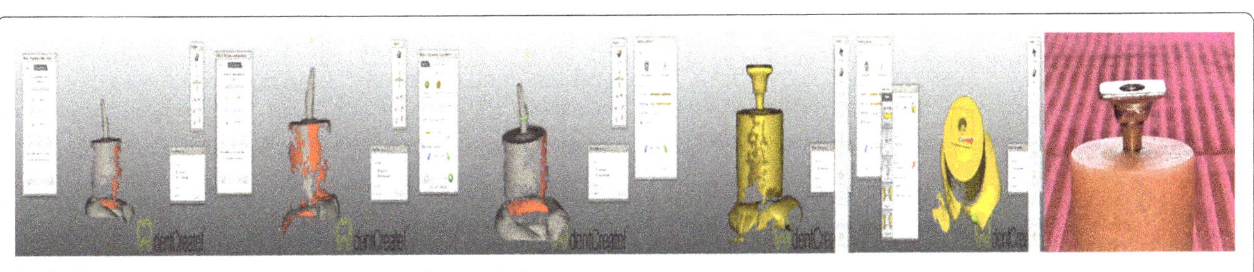

Fig. 3 3D scanning for abutment and designing for metal tube

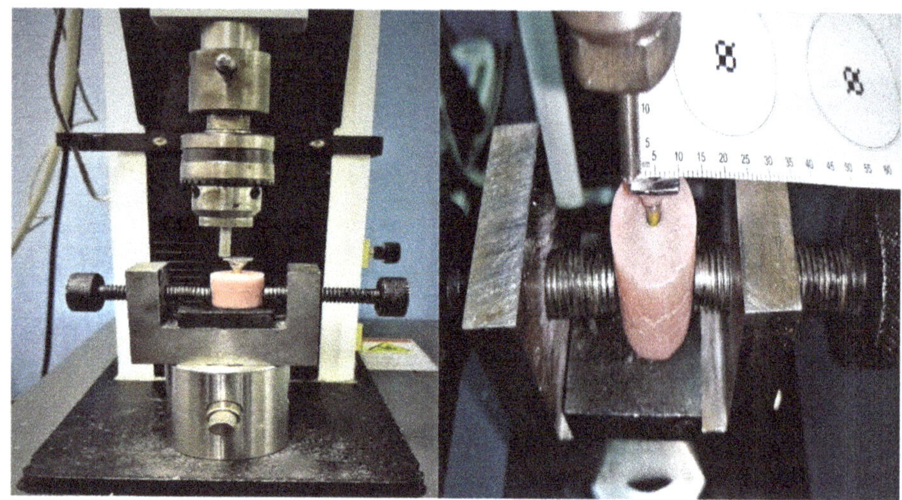

Fig. 4 Application of cyclic loading with universal testing machine

130 N with contact time between the rod and the metal tube 0.2 s at a rate of 1 Hz which simulates the tooth contact duration of each masticatory cycle. The load was perpendicular to the metal tube and 5 mm away from the center axis of the implant (Fig. 4). After that, the acrylic resin block with fixture and abutment was transferred again to the metal jig to measure RTV after loading.

Calculation of RTL ratio of abutment screw before and after dynamic cyclic loading

Screw loosening of each assembly (implant–abutment) was analyzed by measuring RTV before and after dynamic cyclic load by using the digital torque gauge. RTL can be an indicator of how much loosening takes place.

Each RTL ratio was calculated using the following formula:

Removal torque loss ratio before loading (%initial RTL)

$$= \frac{\text{Tightening torque} - \text{removal torque before loading}}{\text{Tightening torque}} \times 100$$

Removal torque loss ratio after loading (%postload RTL)

$$= \frac{\text{Tightening torque} - \text{removal torque after loading}}{\text{Tightening torque}} \times 100$$

Removal torque loss ratio between before and after loading (%difference between initial and postload RTL)

$$= \frac{\text{Removal torque before loading} - \text{removal torque after loading}}{\text{Removal torque before loading}} \times 100$$

Student *T* test and ANOVA were used to compare mean of %initial and %postload RTL between different groups and subgroups followed by pair-wise Tukey's post hoc tests at 0.05 level of significance. Differences between mean greater than Tukey post hoc value were considered significant ($P < 0.05$). Statistical analysis was performed by using SPSS program version 20 (SPSS 20; Inc. Chicago, USA).

Results

One-way ANOVA and pair-wise Tukey's post hoc tests showed that %initial RTL among the groups was not significantly different ($P > .05$), while %postload RTL was significantly different among the three groups ($P < .05$). GIIIB had the highest %postload RTL (42.8% ± 5.6) while GIA had the lowest (22.8% ± 2.9). For GIA and B, %postload RTL was lower than %initial RTL. %postload RTL is significantly different between different abutment groups (< 0.001*) except between Group IA and Group IB which was not significantly different ($P > .05$). %difference RTL between the three groups is significantly different (< 0.001*) (Tables 1, 2, 3, and 4 and Figs. 4, 5, and 6).

Discussion

Conical hybrid connection was used in this study as it was proven that the conical hybrid demonstrated the best stress distribution [20]. This connection has a conical union between the implant fixture and the abutment. In the conical abutment, lateral force is resisted by the taper design of the Morse taper connection. Thus,

Table 1 One-way ANOVA and post hoc Tukey test results for mean ± SD of the %initial RTL, %postload RTL, and %difference between initial and postload RTL between all groups

	%initial RTL	%postload RTL		%difference between initial and postload RTL	
	Mean ± SD				
Subgroups					
GIA	24.9% ± 1.7	22.8% ± 2.9		− 2.7% ± 2.0	
GIB	25.1% ± 1.5	24.1% ± 1.3		− 1.3% ± 1.0	
GIIA	25.1% ± 1.3	30.6% ± 1.6		7.3% ± 0.7	
GIIB	25.9% ± 1.5	36.2% ± 3.1		13.9% ± 2.5	
GIIIA	25.9% ± 1.0	37.4% ± 2.9		15.6% ± 2.8	
GIIIB	25.9% ± 1.5	42.8% ± 5.6		22.9% ± 6.2	
ANOVA					
F	1.5	88.0		153.9	
P value	0.1	< 0.001*		< 0.001*	
After value	Tukey's test				
	GIA	GIB	GIIA	GIIB	GIIIA
GIB	0.8				
GIIA	< 0.001*	< 0.001*			
GIIB	< 0.001*	< 0.001*	< 0.001*		
GIIIA	< 0.001*	< 0.001*	< 0.001*	0.9	
GIIIB	< 0.001*	< 0.001*	< 0.001*	< 0.001*	< 0.001*

− negative means decreased post loading RTL ratio (removal torque gain)
*statistical significant differences (*P* <.05)

Table 2 One-way ANOVA and post hoc Tukey test results for mean ± SD of the initial RTV, postload RTV, and difference between initial and postload RTV between all groups

	Initial RTV	Postload RTV		Difference between initial and postload RTV	
	Mean ± SD				
Subgroups					
GIA	22.5 ± 0.5	23.1 ± 0.8		− 0.6 ± 0.4	
GIB	22.4 ± 0.4	22.7 ± 0.4		− 0.2 ± 0.2	
GIIA	22.4 ± 0.4	20.8 ± 0.5		1.6 ± 0.1	
GIIB	22.2 ± 0.4	19.1 ± 0.9		3.0 ± 0.5	
GIIIA	22.2 ± 0.3	18.7 ± 0.8		3.4 ± 0.5	
GIIIB	22.2 ± 0.4	17.1 ± 1.6		5.0 ± 1.2	
ANOVA					
F	1.5	88.0		153.9	
P value	0.1	< 0.001*		< 0.001*	
After value	Tukey's test				
	GIA	GIB	GIIA	GIIB	GIIIA
GIB	0.8				
GIIA	< 0.001*	< 0.001*			
GIIB	< 0.001*	< 0.001*	< 0.001*		
GIIIA	< 0.001*	< 0.001*	< 0.001*	0.9	
GIIIB	< 0.001*	< 0.001*	< 0.001*	< 0.001*	< 0.001*

− negative means decreased post loading RTL ratio (removal torque gain)
*statistical significant differences (*P* <.05)

Table 3 Comparison between short and high collar length (A and B)

Collar length		Subgroups		T test	
		A (2 mm collar length)	B (4 mm collar length)	t	P value
Initial RTV	Mean ± SD	22.3 ± 0.4	22.3 ± 0.5	0.9	0.3
Postload RTV	Mean ± SD	20.9 ± 1.9	19.6 ± 2.5	2.5	0.014*
Difference between initial and postload RTV	Mean ± SD	1.4 ± 1.7	2.6 ± 2.3		
Paired test	P value	< 0.001*	< 0.001*		

*statistical significant differences ($P < .05$)

the stress concentration is resisted by the side-wall contact surface of its taper design. This stress concentration increases at the apical end of the side-wall contact surface where the implant fixture is thicker. This thickness might provide more resistance to the force, especially the off-axis loading force (as in case of angled abutment). Thus, in abutments with conical hybrid connection design, the screw is not the only source of resistance to loading force, as it is in abutments with an internal hexagonal design [21, 22].

In this study, abutment screws were tightened to 30 Ncm according to the manufacturer's instructions with digital torque gauge. Application of the optimum torque to the implant–abutment complex is critical for long-term successful prosthetic implant restoration. Applied torque develops a force within the screw called preload [23].

Ten-minute interval was left after the first torque application, and all screws were retightened to the same tightening torque (30 Ncm) with the same digital torque gauge to compensate for the preload loss due to settling effect of the screw thus ensure achieving optimal preload as only 10% of the initial torque is transformed into preload, where the remaining 90% is used to overcome the friction between the surface irregularities [23].

The results of this study indicated that there is some torque loss after applying two insertion torques with a 10-min interval before any loading as RTVs were less than 30 Ncm. This finding matches previous studies that reported initial torque loss after 2–10 min [4, 9, 10]. Although there was an increase in %RTL before loading in every group, loosening of screws could not be detected clinically. This may indicate that the remaining tightening torque would serve clinically for a longer period.

In the current study, the results showed that there is a significant difference in %RTL before and after application of dynamic cyclic loading for all angulations and collar lengths. These results are in an agreement with previous researches that found a significant difference between %initial and %postload RTL after mechanical cyclic loading [24, 25]. This result was explained by Bickford et al. [26] as the process of screw loosening occurs in two stages. Initially, external forces cause sliding between the threads, partially relieving the stretching of the screw and reducing preload. At this stage, the higher the preload (within a certain limit), the greater will be the resistance to loosening. The second stage is attained by a gradual reduction of preload below a critical level, in which external forces cause the turning of the screw in an anti-clockwise direction, and it loses its function.

The results of this study showed that, the removal torque loss ratios, with 15° and 25° angulations, were significantly increased. The removal torque loss ratio was increased significantly with increasing angulation as with the 25° angulation the removal torque loss ratio was significantly higher than 15° angulation.

On the other hand, these results disagree with studies that yielded no significant difference between straight and angled abutments for deflection, rotation, and torque required to loosen abutment screws for any parameter at any time [12, 27]. Hsu et al. [28] showed that the clinical performance of angled abutments is comparable to that of straight abutments with respect to both soft tissue responses and general survival rates. However, in vitro studies of stress/strain analyses of angled abutments can only agree that stress/strain levels increase as abutment angulation increases.

These results are in agreement with previous studies which stated that the difference in abutment screw RTV after load showed better results when less angulation abutment was used and studies have failed to show any contraindication to their use [4, 19, 29]. Ha et al. [30], in an evaluation of the influence of abutment angulation on screw loosening of implants in the anterior maxilla, found that the angled abutments showed higher RTV ($P < .05$) than the straight and gold premachined UCLA-type abutments and the difference between them was not significant. This can be attributed to the off-axis force as loading on angled abutments is mostly off-axis, which raises the concern of how angled abutments generally perform with such an unfavorable loading regimen [28].

The increase in RTL with increasing abutment angulation can be attributed to the off-axis force as loading on angled abutments is mostly off-axis, which raises the concern of how angled abutments generally perform with such an unfavorable loading regimen [28]. Forces

Table 4 The raw data in all six experimental groups

N	Groups	Subgroups	Initial RTV	Postload RTV	Initial RTL	Postload RTL	% of change RTV	% of change RTL
1	GI	A	23	24.1	23.33	19.67	− 4.78	15.69
2	GI	A	22.4	23.04	25.33	23.2	− 2.86	8.41
3	GI	A	22.3	22.9	25.67	23.67	− 2.69	7.79
4	GI	A	21.8	21.5	27.33	28.33	1.38	− 3.66
5	GI	A	23	24.2	23.33	19.33	− 5.22	17.15
6	GI	A	22.1	22.8	26.33	24	− 3.17	8.85
7	GI	A	22.8	23.15	24	22.83	− 1.54	4.88
8	GI	A	22.9	24	23.67	20	− 4.8	15.5
9	GI	A	22.2	22.9	26	23.67	− 3.15	8.96
#	GI	A	22	21.6	26.67	28	1.82	− 4.99
#	GI	A	21.9	22.4	27	25.33	− 2.28	6.19
#	GI	A	22	22.8	26.67	24	− 3.64	10.01
#	GI	A	22.8	23.2	24	22.67	− 1.75	5.54
#	GI	A	22.9	23.9	23.67	20.33	− 4.37	14.11
#	GI	A	23.5	24.5	21.67	18.33	− 4.26	15.41
#	GI	B	23	23.1	23.33	23	− 0.43	1.41
#	GI	B	22.9	23	23.67	23.33	− 0.44	1.44
#	GI	B	22.5	22.7	25	24.33	− 0.89	2.68
#	GI	B	22.4	22.5	25.33	25	− 0.45	1.3
#	GI	B	21.8	22.4	27.33	25.33	− 2.75	7.32
#	GI	B	23	23.1	23.33	23	− 0.43	1.41
#	GI	B	22.8	23	24	23.33	− 0.88	2.79
#	GI	B	22.5	22.7	25	24.33	− 0.89	2.68
#	GI	B	22.7	22.9	24.33	23.67	− 0.88	2.71
#	GI	B	22.8	23.2	24	22.67	− 1.75	5.54
#	GI	B	21.4	21.5	28.67	28.33	− 0.47	1.19
#	GI	B	22.1	22.8	26.33	24	− 3.17	8.85
#	GI	B	22.2	22.97	26	23.43	− 3.47	9.88
#	GI	B	22.5	22.6	25	24.67	− 0.44	1.32
#	GI	B	22.3	22.8	25.67	24	− 2.24	6.51
#	GII	A	22.9	21.4	23.67	28.67	6.55	− 21.12
#	GII	A	22.5	20.9	25	30.33	7.11	− 21.32
#	GII	A	22.4	20.8	25.33	30.67	7.14	− 21.08
#	GII	A	22.1	20.6	26.33	31.33	6.79	− 18.99
#	GII	A	21.9	19.9	27	33.67	9.13	− 24.7
#	GII	A	23	21.5	23.33	28.33	6.52	− 21.43
#	GII	A	22.6	21	24.67	30	7.08	− 21.61
#	GII	A	22.4	20.8	25.33	30.67	7.14	− 21.08
#	GII	A	22	20.5	26.67	31.67	6.82	− 18.75
#	GII	A	22.3	20.7	25.67	31	7.17	− 20.76
#	GII	A	21.8	19.8	27.33	34	9.17	− 24.41
#	GII	A	22.8	21.1	24	29.67	7.46	− 23.63
#	GII	A	22.7	21	24.33	30	7.49	− 23.3

Table 4 The raw data in all six experimental groups *(Continued)*

N	Groups	Subgroups	Initial RTV	Postload RTV	Initial RTL	Postload RTL	% of change RTV	% of change RTL
#	GII	A	22.2	20.6	26	31.33	7.21	− 20.5
#	GII	A	23.1	21.5	23	28.33	6.93	− 23.17
#	GII	B	22.8	20.4	24	32	10.53	− 33.33
#	GII	B	22.1	19.2	26.33	36	13.12	− 36.73
#	GII	B	22	18.7	26.67	37.67	15	− 41.24
#	GII	B	21.8	17.8	27.33	40.67	18.35	− 48.81
#	GII	B	22.7	20.1	24.33	33	11.45	− 35.64
#	GII	B	22.1	18.9	26.33	37	14.48	− 40.52
#	GII	B	22.9	20.4	23.67	32	10.92	− 35.19
#	GII	B	22.2	19.4	26	35.33	12.61	− 35.88
#	GII	B	21.5	17.7	28.33	41	17.67	− 44.72
#	GII	B	21.6	17.8	28	40.67	17.59	− 45.25
#	GII	B	22.7	19.5	24.33	35	14.1	− 43.86
#	GII	B	21.9	18.5	27	38.33	15.53	− 41.96
#	GII	B	22.8	20.3	24	32.33	10.96	− 34.71
#	GII	B	22.3	19.5	25.67	35	12.56	− 36.35
#	GII	B	22	18.8	26.67	37.33	14.55	− 39.97
#	GIII	A	22.6	20.1	24.67	33	11.06	− 33.77
#	GIII	A	22.4	19.2	25.33	36	14.29	− 42.12
#	GIII	A	22.3	19.1	25.67	36.33	14.35	− 41.53
#	GIII	A	21.9	17.7	27	41	19.18	− 51.85
#	GIII	A	21.9	17.9	27	40.33	18.26	− 49.37
#	GIII	A	22.5	19.3	25	35.67	14.22	− 42.68
#	GIII	A	22.3	19	25.67	36.67	14.8	− 42.85
#	GIII	A	22.7	20.2	24.33	32.67	11.01	− 34.28
#	GIII	A	21.8	17.8	27.33	40.67	18.35	− 48.81
#	GIII	A	21.8	17.8	27.33	40.67	18.35	− 48.81
#	GIII	A	22	18.1	26.67	39.67	17.73	− 48.74
#	GIII	A	22.2	18.6	26	38	16.22	− 46.15
#	GIII	A	22.6	20.1	24.67	33	11.06	− 33.77
#	GIII	A	22.2	18.3	26	39	17.57	− 50
#	GIII	A	22.1	18.2	26.33	39.33	17.65	− 49.37
#	GIII	B	22.7	18.8	24.33	37.33	17.18	− 53.43
#	GIII	B	22	17	26.67	43.33	22.73	− 62.47
#	GIII	B	22	16.9	26.67	43.67	23.18	− 63.74
#	GIII	B	21.9	15.7	27	47.67	28.31	− 76.56
#	GIII	B	21.8	15.8	27.33	47.33	27.52	− 73.18
#	GIII	B	22.6	18.7	24.67	37.67	17.26	− 52.7
#	GIII	B	22.1	18.2	26.33	39.33	17.65	− 49.37
#	GIII	B	21.7	14.05	27.67	53.17	35.25	− 92.16
#	GIII	B	22	15.9	26.67	47	27.73	− 76.23
#	GIII	B	22.8	18.9	24	37	17.11	− 54.17
#	GIII	B	22.9	19	23.67	36.67	17.03	− 54.92

Table 4 The raw data in all six experimental groups *(Continued)*

N	Groups	Subgroups	Initial RTV	Postload RTV	Initial RTL	Postload RTL	% of change RTV	% of change RTL
#	GIII	B	21.6	14.5	28	51.67	32.87	– 84.54
#	GIII	B	23	19.24	23.33	35.87	16.35	– 53.75
#	GIII	B	22	16.8	26.67	44	23.64	– 64.98
#	GIII	B	22.1	17.7	26.33	41	19.91	– 55.72

applied off-axis may be expected to overload the bone surrounding single-tooth implants, as shown by means of finite element analysis, which affects abutment screw leading to its loosening [31].

The greater the angulation, the greater the off-axis force that generates more stress and strain in implant components specially the screw [30] When off-axis loading is applied to an implant, the magnitude of the stress will be increased three times or more [28]. There was a statistically significant increase in stress and strain when abutment angulation increased. This supports the concept of eliminating unnecessary occlusal and off-axial forces on implant-supported restorations [4]. With clinical loading of implants restored using angled abutments, lateral occlusal forces may increase creating torsional force which increases screw loosening [12, 29]. Any direction of load that is not in the long axis of the implant will magnify the crestal stresses to the implant–bone interface and to the abutment screws in the restoration [8].

On the other hand, concerning the area of contact between screw thread and abutment, the increase of abutment angulation leads to decrease area of friction that leads to retention and thus screw loosening occurs. Comparing micromotion level between a straight abutment, a 15° to 25° abutment angulation, an increase in the micromotion level by 30% was observed. This micromotion may explain the screw failure. However, no screw failure occurred in a study with 2261 angled abutment evaluated for 96 months [29, 32].

According to the results of this study, it was showed that with straight abutments, %postload RTL was lower than %initial RTL. This result could be explained by Squier et al. [33] who stated that abutments of the conical hybrid connection showed detorque values higher than the initial torque due to the cold solder on the implant–abutment interface, which agrees with the results of this study. This condition arises from the friction between the two surfaces, which differ slightly; the pressure created by the insertion force determines the maintenance of the connection even after stopping the applied force for insertion.

Several studies have been conducted on this type of implant–abutment connection [23, 34]. Sutter et al. [35] demonstrated reverse torque values of this hybrid implant–abutment connection that were 124% of the initial tightening torque. These authors suggested that cold welding occurred in the conical hybrid implant–abutment connection.

Schmitt et al. [36] compared conical and nonconical implant–abutment connection systems in terms of their in vitro and in vivo performances. In vitro studies indicate that conical and nonconical abutments exhibited sufficient resistance to the maximal bending forces and fatigue loading. However, conical abutments were

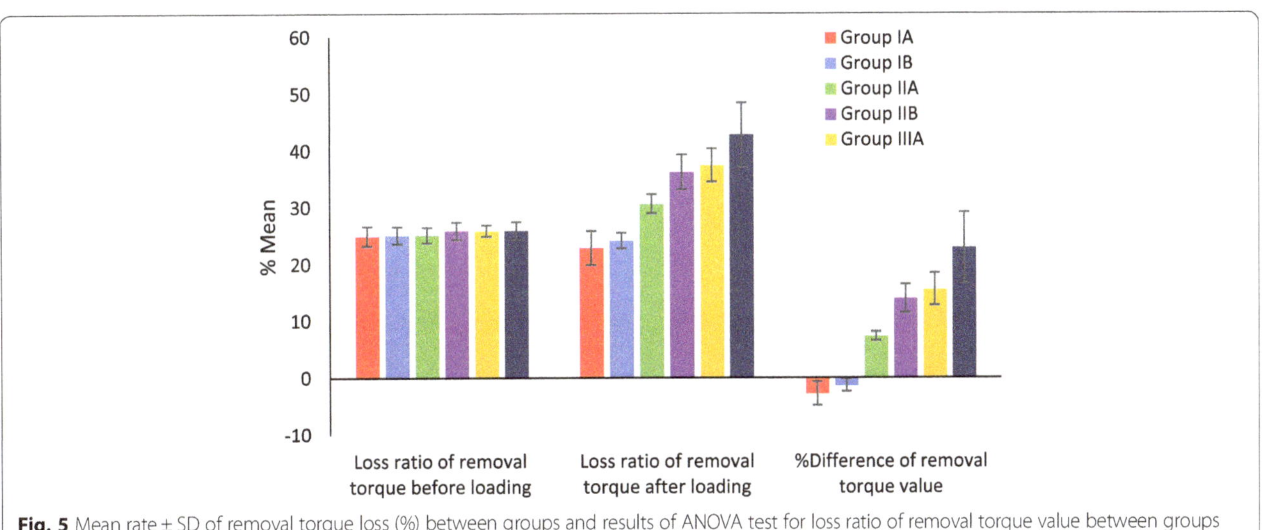

Fig. 5 Mean rate ± SD of removal torque loss (%) between groups and results of ANOVA test for loss ratio of removal torque value between groups

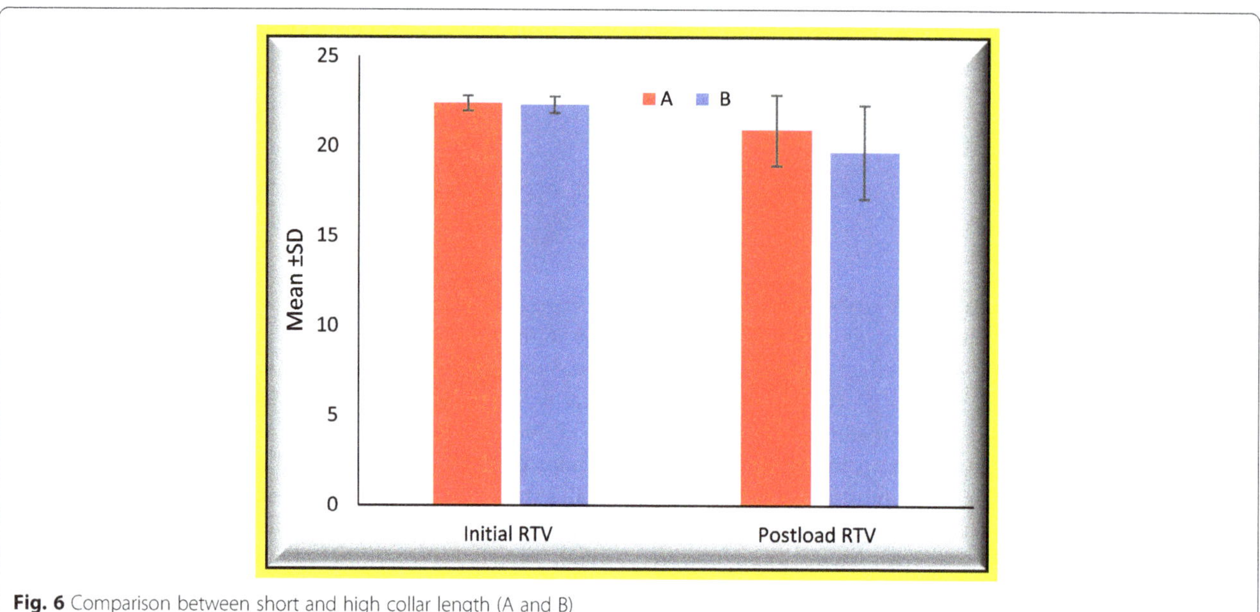

Fig. 6 Comparison between short and high collar length (A and B)

superior in terms of sealing, microgap formation, torque maintenance, and abutment stability.

According to the results of this study, %RTL increased significantly with increasing collar length and the percentage of removal torque gaining after load with 0° abutments with collar height 4 mm was less than that of 2 mm. This finding matches what was found by Siadat et al. [9] who evaluated the effect of collar length on screw loosening and concluded that an increase in the abutment collar length significantly increase the torque loss of abutment–implant screw after cyclic loading. The abutment collar length acts as vertical cantilever, so increasing abutment collar would lead to an increased vertical cantilever which acts as a force magnifier [8]. Cantilever designs increase bending forces on screws due to the lever effect [17, 18].

Conclusions

Within the limitations of this in vitro study, it can be concluded that:

- Screw loosening increases with increasing abutment angulation and collar length after 100,000 cycles of dynamic cyclic loading.
- Results of this study showed that conical hybrid connection design provides more biomechanically stable screw joint with straight abutments than angled abutments.

Acknowledgements
Not applicable

Funding
Not applicable.

Authors' contributions
ME carried out the sample preparation, measurements, data collection, and drafting of the manuscript. TM participated in the design of experiment and performed the statistical analysis and interpretation of data, and ME participated in the conception, design, and critical revision of the manuscript for important intellectual content. All authors read and approved the final manuscript.

Competing interests
Mai El-sheikh, Tamer Mostafa, and Mohamed El-Sheikh declare that they have no competing interests.

References

1. Prado CJ, Neves FD, Soares CJ, Dantas KA, Dantas TS, Naves LZ. Influence of abutment screw design and surface coating on the bending flexural strength of the implant set. J Oral Implantol. 2014;40:123–8.
2. Goodacre CJ, Bernal G, Rungcharassaeng K, Kan JY. Clinical complications with implants and implant prostheses. J Prosthet Dent. 2003;90:121–32.
3. Michalakis KX, Calvani PL, Muftu S, Pissiotis A, Hirayama H. The effect of different implant-abutment connections on screw joint stability. J Oral Implantol. 2014;40:146–52.
4. Asvanund P, Cheepsathit L. Effect of different angulation angled abutment on screw loosening of implants under cyclic loading. M Dent J. 2016;36: 337–24.
5. Ferreira MB, Delben JA, Barao VA, Faverani LP, Dos Santos PH, Assuncao WG. Evaluation of torque maintenance of abutment and cylinder screws with Morse taper implants. J Craniofac Surg. 2012;23:631–4.
6. Geckili E, Geckili O, Bilhan H, Kutay O, Bilgin T. Clinical comparison of screw-retained and screwless Morse taper implant-abutment connections: one-year postloading results. Int J Oral Maxillofac Implants. 2017;32:1123–31.
7. Schwarz MS. Mechanical complications of dental implants. Clin Oral Implants Res. 2000;11:156–8.
8. Misch CE. Principles for abutment and prosthetic screws and screw-retained components and prostheses. In: Elsevier Mosby. 2nd ed; 2015. p. 724–52.
9. Siadat H, Pirmoazen S, Beyabanaki E, Alikhasi M. Does abutment collar length affect abutment screw loosening after cyclic loading? J Oral Implantol. 2015;41:346–51.
10. Delben JA, Gomes EA, Barao VA, Assuncao WG. Evaluation of the effect of retightening and mechanical cycling on preload maintenance of retention screws. Int J Oral Maxillofac Implants. 2011;26:251–6.

11. Cho WR, Huh YH, Park CJ, Cho LR. Effect of cyclic loading and retightening on reverse torque value in external and internal implants. J Adv Prosthodont. 2015;7:288–93.
12. Eger DE, Gunsolley JC, Feldman S. Comparison of angled and standard abutments and their effect on clinical outcomes: a preliminary report. Int J Oral Maxillofac Implants. 2000;15:819–23.
13. Antoun H, Belmon P, Cherfane P, Sitbon JM. Immediate loading of four or six implants in completely edentulous patients. Int J Periodontics Restorative Dent. 2012;32:1–9.
14. Cavallaro JG, Greenstein G. Angled implant abutments. A Practical Application of Available Knowledge J Am Dent Assoc. 2011;142:150–8.
15. Kallus T, Henry P, Jemt T, Jorneus L. Clinical evaluation of angulated abutments for the Branemark system: a pilot study. Int J Oral Maxillofac Implants. 1990;5:39–45.
16. Herrero-Climent M, Romero-Ruiz MM, Diaz-Castro CM, Bullon P, Rios-Santos JV. Influence of two different machined-collar heights on crestal bone loss. Int J Oral Maxillofac Implants. 2014;29:1374–9.
17. Stuker RA, Teixeira ER, Beck JP, Costa NP. Preload and torque removal evaluation of three different abutment screws for single standing implant restorations. J Appl Oral Sci. 2008;15:55–8.
18. Kim NG, Kim YS, Kim CW, Jang KS, Lim YJ. The effect of abutment height on screw loosening in single implant-supported prothesis after dynamic cyclic loading. J Korean Acad Prosthodont. 2004;42:664–70.
19. Sethi A, Kaus T, Sochor P. The use of angulated abutments in implant dentistry: five-year clinical results of an ongoing prospective study. Int J Oral Maxillofac Implants. 2000;15:801–10.
20. Tonella BP, Pellizzer EP, Ferraco R, Falcon-Antenucci RM, Carvalho PS, Goiato MC. Photoelastic analysis of cemented or screwed implant-supported prostheses with different prosthetic connections. J Oral Implantol. 2011;37:401–10.
21. Akca K, Cehreli MC, Iplikcioglu H. Evaluation of the mechanical characteristics of the implant abutment complex of a reduced-diameter Morsetaper implant. A nonlinear finite element stress analysis. Clin Oral Implants Res. 2003;14:444–54.
22. Bozkaya D, Muftu S. Mechanics of the tapered interference fit in dental implants. J Biomech. 2003;36:1649–58.
23. Pardal-Pelaez B, Montero J. Preload loss of abutment screws after dynamic fatigue in single implant-supported restorations. A systematic review. J Clin Exp Dent. 2017;9:1355–61.
24. Mohammed HH, Lee JH, Bae JM, Cho HW. Effect of abutment screw length and cyclic loading on removal torque in external and internal hex implants. J Adv Prosthodont. 2016;8:62–9.
25. Shin HM, Huh JB, Yun MJ, Jeon YC, Chang BM, Jeong CM. Influence of the implant-abutment connection design and diameter on the screw joint stability. J Adv Prosthodont. 2014;6:126–32.
26. Bickford JH, Nassar S. Handbook of bolts and bolted joints. New York: Marcel Dekker, Inc; 1998.
27. Dixon DL, Breeding LC, Sadler JP, McKay ML. Comparison of screw loosening, rotation, and deflection among three implant designs. J Prosthet Dent. 1995;74:270–8.
28. Hsu ML, Chung TF, Kao HC. Clinical applications of angled abutments - a literature review. Chin Dent J. 2005;24:15–21.
29. Morsch CS, Rafael CF, Dumes HF, Juanito GM, Bianchini MA. Failure of prosthetic screws on 971 implants. Braz J Oral Sci. 2015;14:195–8.
30. Ha CY, Lim YJ, Kim MJ, Choi JH. The influence of abutment angulation on screw loosening of implants in the anterior maxilla. Int J Oral Maxillofac Implants. 2011;26:45–55.
31. Papavasiliou G, Kamposiora P, Bayne SC, Felton DA. Three-dimensional finite element analysis of stress-distribution around single tooth implants as a function of bony support, prosthesis type, and loading during function. J Prosthet Dent. 1996;76:633–40.
32. Szmukler-Moncler S, Salama H, Reingewirtz Y, Dubruille JH. Timing of loading and effect of micromotion on bone-dental implant interface: review of experimental literature. J BiomedMater Res. 1998;43:192–203.
33. Squier RS, Psoter WJ, Taylor TD. Removal torques of conical, tapered implant abutments: the effects of anodization and reduction of surface area. Int J Oral Maxillofac Implants. 2002;17:24–7.
34. Norton MR. In vitro evaluation of the strength of the conical implant to abutment joint in two commercially available implant systems. J Preosthet Dent. 2000;83:567–71.
35. Sutter F, Weber HP, Sorensen J, Belser U. The new restorative concept of the ITI dental implant system: design and engineering. Int J Periodontics Restorative Dent. 1993;13:408–31.
36. Schmitt CM, Nogueira-Filho G, Tenenbaum HC, Lai JY, Brito C, Doring H. Performance of conical abutment (Morse taper) connection implants: a systematic review. J Biomed Mater Res A. 2014;102:552–74.

5

Calprotectin and cross-linked N-telopeptides of type I collagen levels in crevicular fluid from implant sites with peri-implant diseases

Eijiro Sakamoto[1], Rie Kido[1], Yoritoki Tomotake[2], Yoshihito Naitou[2], Yuichi Ishida[3] and Jun-ichi Kido[1*]

Abstract

Background: Peri-implant crevicular fluid (PICF) contains calprotectin and NTx, which are markers for inflammation and bone resorption, respectively. The aims of this pilot study were to compare calprotectin and NTx levels in PICF from implant sites with or without peri-implant diseases and to evaluate the usefulness of calprotectin and NTx as diagnostic markers for peri-implant diseases.

Methods: Thirty-five patients with dental implants participated in this pilot study. PICF samples were collected from peri-implant disease sites ($n = 40$) and non-diseased (healthy) sites ($n = 34$) after clinical indicators including probing depth (PD), bleeding on probing (BOP), gingival index (GI), and bone loss (BL) rate were investigated. Calprotectin and NTx amounts in PICF were measured using their respective ELISA kits and then compared between diseased and healthy samples. The relationship between PICF calprotectin or NTx levels and clinical indicator levels was investigated. A receiver operating characteristic (ROC) curve analysis of calprotectin and NTx was performed to predict peri-implant diseases.

Results: Calprotectin and NTx levels in PICF were significantly higher from peri-implant disease sites than from healthy sites. PICF calprotectin amounts correlated with PD, and its levels were significantly higher in the GI-1 and GI-2 groups than in the GI-0 group. PICF NTx amounts correlated with PD and the BL rate. ROC curves indicated that PICF calprotectin and NTx are useful biomarkers for peri-implant diseases.

Conclusions: Calprotectin and NTx in PICF have potential as biomarkers for the diagnosis of peri-implant diseases.

Keywords: Calprotectin, NTx, Peri-implant crevicular fluid, Peri-implant diseases

Background

Dental treatments with implants are now being widely performed due to advances in the development of surgical procedures for dental implants and prosthodontics. However, the incidence of peri-implant diseases has been increasing with implant placement [1], and thus, the early detection of these diseases is important for maintaining dental implants. Peri-implant diseases with inflammation and the destruction of peri-implant tissues have mainly been classified into peri-implantitis with the resorption of alveolar bone around osseointegrated dental implants and peri-implant mucositis without pathological bone resorption [2]. Peri-implant diseases are diagnosed by clinical indicators including probing depth (PD), bleeding on probing (BOP), suppuration, the mobility of an implant, and radiographic bone loss (BL) [3, 4]. Clinical indicators for a diagnosis of peri-implant diseases are similar to the diagnostic indicators for periodontal diseases of natural teeth. However, the measurement of PD using a dental probe is more difficult around dental implants than around natural teeth because peri-implant tissues have less attached gingiva compared with periodontal tissue, and implant structures and prosthetic superstructures sometimes

* Correspondence: kido.jun-ichi@tokushima-u.ac.jp
[1]Department of Periodontology and Endodontology, Institute of Biomedical Sciences, Tokushima University Graduate School, 3-18-15 Kuramoto, Tokushima 770-8504, Japan
Full list of author information is available at the end of the article

prevent a probing [3, 5]. BL of 2–3 mm on radiographs has been used as a diagnostic standard in cumulative interceptive supportive therapy (CIST) [6]; however, difficulties are associated with obtaining accurate information on slight BL on radiographs in conventional X-ray examinations. The prevalence of peri-implant mucositis and peri-implantitis was previously reported to be between 19 and 65% and between 1 and 47%, respectively [1, 7], and showed a wide range because case definition of peri-implant diseases was different among those studies in which peri-implant diseases were diagnosed using clinical indicators. These reports suggest that the case definition with the diagnosis of peri-implant diseases using clinical indicators is not sufficiently accurate or clear to evaluate pathological conditions.

The diagnosis of peri-implant diseases using biomarkers in peri-implant crevicular fluid (PICF) has recently been examined and may be more accurate than that of clinical indicators to evaluate inflammation and the degradation of tissue surrounding dental implants [4, 7, 8]. PICF contains similar components to gingival crevicular fluid (GCF), namely pro-inflammatory cytokines such as interleukin-1β (IL-1β) and tumor necrosis factor-α (TNF-α), enzymes including aspartate aminotransferase (AST) and collagenase-2 (matrix metalloproteinase-8 (MMP-8)), and bone-related proteins such as cross-linked C-telopeptide of type I collagen (ICTP) and receptor activator of nuclear factor-κB (NF-κB) ligand (RANKL) [9–13]. These factors and proteins in PICF and GCF are regarded as diagnostic biomarkers for peri-implant diseases as well as periodontal diseases.

Calprotectin (S100A8/S100A9) is an inflammation-related protein that is produced in leukocytes, macrophages/monocytes, and epithelial cells, and its level increases in several inflammatory diseases including ulcerative colitis, rheumatoid arthritis, and cystic fibrosis [14, 15]. Calprotectin was previously detected in GCF, and its level was significantly higher in GCF from periodontal disease sites than in that from healthy non-diseased sites [16, 17]. Furthermore, GCF calprotectin levels correlated with clinical indicator levels, such as PD, GI, and BOP [17, 18], and was shown to predict periodontal disease activity [19]. These findings indicate that calprotectin is a useful inflammatory biomarker for periodontal diseases. Calprotectin was also detected in PICF, but its levels in PICF samples from healthy and peri-implant disease sites were not compared [20].

Cross-linked N-telopeptide of type I collagen (NTx) is a product of bone type I collagen degradation by cathepsin K in osteoclasts, is released into blood and urine, and is a specific biomarker of bone resorption [21–23]. NTx levels have been shown to increase in the blood and urine of patients with osteoporosis, hyperparathyroidism, and bone metastasis of cancer and are used as a diagnostic marker for these bone metabolism diseases [23, 24]. GCF contains NTx, and significant differences were not detected in its levels in GCF between healthy and periodontitis sites [25–27]. In contrast, Aruna [28] examined NTx in GCF samples from periodontitis sites and did not detect NTx in GCF from healthy sites. Although Friedmann et al. [20] measured NTx amounts in PICF and GCF, its levels in PICF did not correlated with changes of alveolar bone levels.

This pilot study aims to investigate whether calprotectin and NTx levels in PICF reflect inflammation and alveolar BL in peri-implant tissues, respectively, and also if these proteins are useful biomarkers for the diagnosis of peri-implant diseases.

Methods

Patients and clinical examinations

The present clinical study was approved by the Ethics Committees of Tokushima University Hospital (nos. 2368 and 2719) in accordance with the Helsinki Declaration of 2013 and performed from November 2016 to August 2017. Patients who received dental implants from 3 to 9 years ago, had healthy or diseased implants with peri-implant diseases, and visited at Tokushima University Hospital for the maintenance of dental implants and treatment were recruited for the present clinical study. Thirty-five patients (10 males and 25 females; aged 68.7 ± 6.5 years) gave written informed consent after receiving an explanation of this study (Table 1). Participants with healthy and diseased dental implants did not have any systemic inflammatory diseases or a history of antibiotic therapy within 3 months. PD, BOP, and gingival index (GI) were examined as clinical indicators after the collection of PICF. GI scores were evaluated according to modifications of the standard of Löe and Silness [29]. The BL rate of alveolar bone was assessed on radiographic films according to modifications of Schei et al.'s method [30]. Diseased sites with peri-implant diseases were defined as periodontal sites with PD ≥ 3 mm, BOP negative or positive, and GI score

Table 1 Characteristics of participants and examining sites

Participants		
Number of participants	35	
Gender (male/female)	10:25	
Age (years)	68.7 ± 6.5	
Examining sites	Healthy	Diseased
Number of PICF samples	34	40
PD (mm)	2.32 ± 0.58	4.70 ± 1.36†
Gingival index	0.0 ± 0.0	1.5 ± 0.5†
BOP-positive rate (%)	0.0 ± 0.0	40.0 ± 15.2*
Bone loss rate (%)	19.7 ± 9.8	42.7 ± 18.0†

*$P < 0.01$ and †$P < 0.001$ vs healthy group

≥ 1. Healthy implant sites were defined as sites with PD < 3 mm, BOP negative, and GI score = 0.

PICF sampling and sample preparation

PICF samples were collected from peri-implant sites using sterile paper strips according to a modified procedure of our previous method [31]. Briefly, PICF sampling sites were isolated with cotton rolls, supra-gingival plaque was removed, and sites were then very gently air-dried. Periopaper® (Oraflow Inc., NY, USA) was gently inserted into a peri-implant crevice and held for 30 s. The volume of PICF was measured using a Periotron® 8000 (Harco Electronics, Winnipeg, MB, Canada). Paper strips containing blood and pus were not used in the present study. PICF in the paper strip was extracted in 100 μl of phosphate-buffered saline (pH = 7.4) containing 0.2 μM phenylmethylsulfonyl fluoride by centrifugation and used in ELISA for calprotectin and NTx.

Protein determination by ELISA

Calprotectin in PICF samples was determined using Calprotectin Human ELISA kit® (Hycult Biotech, PB Uden, the Netherlands) according to the instruction manual. Briefly, the extracted PICF solution was diluted to 100–200-fold using dilution buffer provided in the kit. The diluted PICF solution was added to wells coated with an antibody of human calprotectin and incubated at room temperature for 1 h. After washing the wells, a biotinylated anti-calprotectin antibody was added and incubated at room temperature for 1 h. An immune complex in the wells was reacted with a streptavidin-peroxidase conjugate for 1 h and further incubated with 3,3′,5,5′-tetramethylbenzidine (TMB) for 15 min in the dark. After stopping the reaction using a stop solution, the absorbance of the reacting solution in wells was determined using a microplate reader at 450 nm.

NTx in PICF samples was measured using Human NTx-I ELISA kit® (LifeSpan Biosciences Inc., Seattle, WA, USA) according to the instruction manual. Briefly, extracted PICF samples were added to wells and incubated at 37 °C for 90 min. A biotinylated anti-NTx antibody was added to the wells containing PICF sample solution and incubated at 37 °C for 1 h with gentle agitation. After washing the wells, HRP conjugate was added, incubated at 37 °C for 30 min, and then reacted with TMB substrate solution at 37 °C for 15 min. After stopping the reaction, the absorbance of the reacting solution was determined using at 450 nm. The concentrations of calprotectin and NTx were expressed as nanograms per microliter of PICF.

Statistical analysis

Differences in PD, GI, the BL rate, calprotectin levels, and NTx levels between healthy and diseased groups were statistically analyzed by the Mann-Whitney *U* test. Differences in the BOP-positive rate between healthy and diseased groups were statistically evaluated using Fisher's exact test. Difference in calprotectin amounts among the GI score 0, 1, and 2 groups were analyzed by the Mann-Whitney *U* test. The relationships between PD and calprotectin or NTx amounts and between the BL rate and NTx amount were analyzed by Spearman's rank correlation test. Receiver operating characteristic (ROC) curves was constructed for calprotectin and NTx amounts in the healthy and diseased groups. Data were analyzed using statistical analysis software (SPSS version 20, IBM, Chicago, IL, USA). *P* values less than 0.05 were considered to indicate significance.

Results

Characteristics of PICF samples and sites of PICF collection

Thirty-four of PICF samples were collected from healthy peri-implant sites and forty samples from diseased sites (Table 1). The mean PD in diseased sites was 4.70 mm, which was significantly deeper than that of healthy sites (2.32 mm). The mean GI score of diseased sites was 1.5, which was significantly higher than that of healthy sites. A significant difference was observed in the BOP-positive rate between diseased and healthy sites (diseased = 40.0 vs healthy = 0.0; $P < 0.01$). Furthermore, the mean BL rate of peri-implant disease sites was 42.7%, which was approximately 2.2-fold that of healthy sites (19.7%).

Comparison of calprotectin and NTx levels between diseased and healthy sites

Mean calprotectin amounts in PICF samples from diseased and healthy sites were 171.9 and 40.1 ng per site, respectively (Fig. 1a), and their mean concentrations were 231.7 and 113.2 ng/μl PICF, respectively (Fig. 1b). Calprotectin amounts and concentrations in the diseased group were significantly higher than those in the healthy group by approximately 4.3-fold and 2.1-fold, respectively (healthy vs diseased; $P < 0.01$).

NTx amounts in PICF samples from healthy sites ranged between 0.03 and 14.34 ng per site, while those in samples from diseased sites were between 0.85 and 16.38 ng per site (Fig. 2a). Mean NTx amounts were 6.16 and 2.94 ng per site in PICF samples from the diseased and healthy groups, respectively, while the mean concentrations of NTx in the diseased and healthy groups were 9.27 and 6.62 ng/μl PICF, respectively (Fig. 2b). NTx levels in PICF samples were significantly higher from diseased sites than from healthy sites (healthy vs diseased: NTx amount $P < 0.01$, NTx concentration $P < 0.05$).

Relationship between calprotectin amounts in PICF and clinical indicators

The PD range in all PICF sampling sites was 1–8 mm and calprotectin amounts ranged between 0.1 and 534.1 ng per

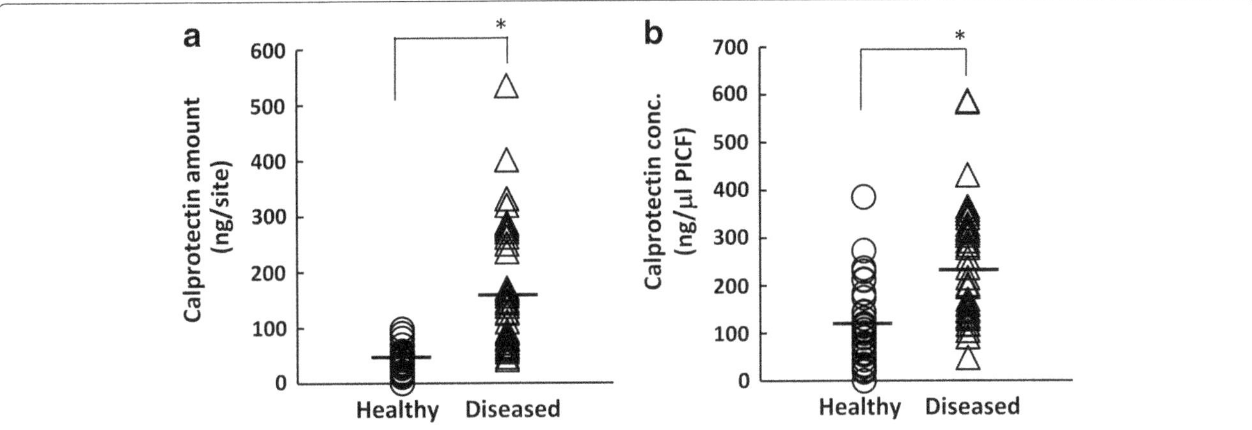

Fig. 1 Comparison of calprotectin levels in PICF. PICF samples were collected from peri-implant disease sites ($n = 40$, diseased) and non-diseased sites ($n = 34$, healthy). Calprotectin amounts (**a**) were measured by ELISA, and its concentration (**b**) was normalized by the volume of PICF. Horizontal bars show the mean values of each group. $^*P < 0.01$

site (Fig. 3a). A positive correlation was observed between calprotectin amounts in PICF samples and PD ($\rho = 0.709$, $P < 0.001$). The relationship between calprotectin amounts in PICF samples and GI scores was investigated (Fig. 3b). The median of calprotectin amounts in PICF samples were 36.8, 110.3, and 159.3 ng at GI-0, GI-1, and GI-2 sites, respectively. Calprotectin amounts in PICF samples from sites with GI-1 and GI-2 were significantly higher than those from sites with GI-0 (GI-0 vs GI-1 or GI-2, $P < 0.001$); however, no significant difference was noted in calprotectin amounts between GI-1 and GI-2.

Relationship between NTx amounts in PICF and PD or BL rate

NTx amounts in PICF samples correlated with PD at PICF sampling sites ($\rho = 0.434$, $P < 0.001$, Fig. 4a). The BL rate in healthy sites ranged between 6.9 and 41.8%, while that in diseased sites was between 7.7 and 80.0% (Fig. 4b). A positive correlation was observed between NTx amounts and the BL rate ($\rho = 0.570$, $P < 0.001$).

ROC analysis for cutoff values of calprotectin and NTx amounts in PICF

ROC curves for calprotectin and NTx levels in PICF were plotted in order to predict peri-implant diseases. The area under the ROC curve (AUC) for calprotectin amounts was 0.964 (95% CI = 0.913–0.996, $P < 0.001$) and the cutoff value was 60.4 ng per site, with a sensitivity of 92.5% and specificity of 90.9% (Fig. 5a). The AUC for NTx amounts was 0.784 (95% CI = 0.672–0.891, $P < 0.001$) and the cutoff value was 1.88 ng per site, with a sensitivity of 82.5% and specificity of 63.6% (Fig. 5b).

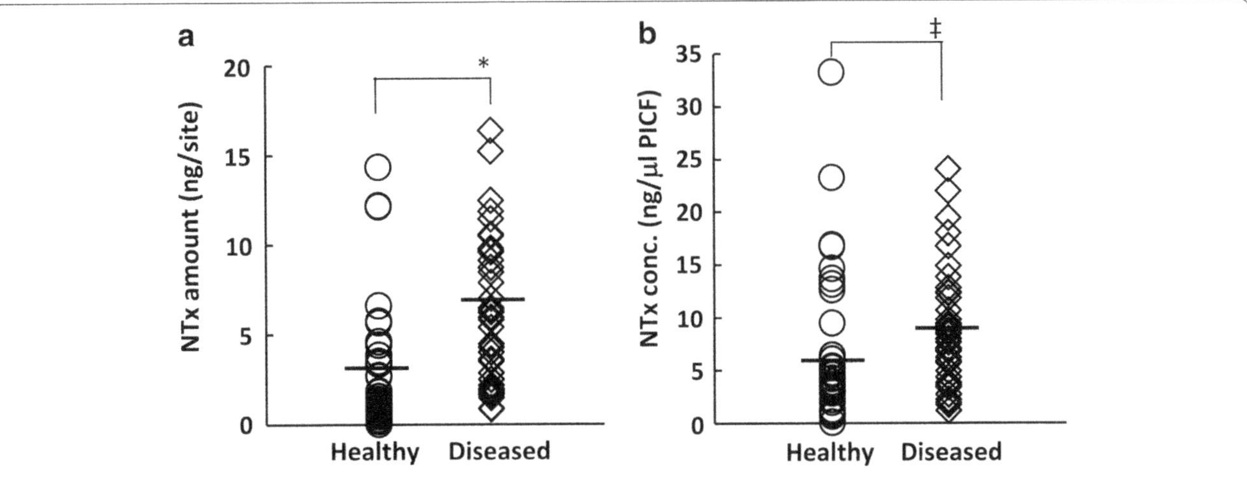

Fig. 2 Comparison of NTx levels in PICF. NTx amounts (**a**) in PICF samples from peri-implant disease sites ($n = 40$, diseased) and non-diseased sites ($n = 34$, healthy) were measured by ELISA, and its concentration (**b**) was normalized by the volume of PICF. Horizontal bars show the mean values of each group. $^‡P < 0.05$, $^*P < 0.01$

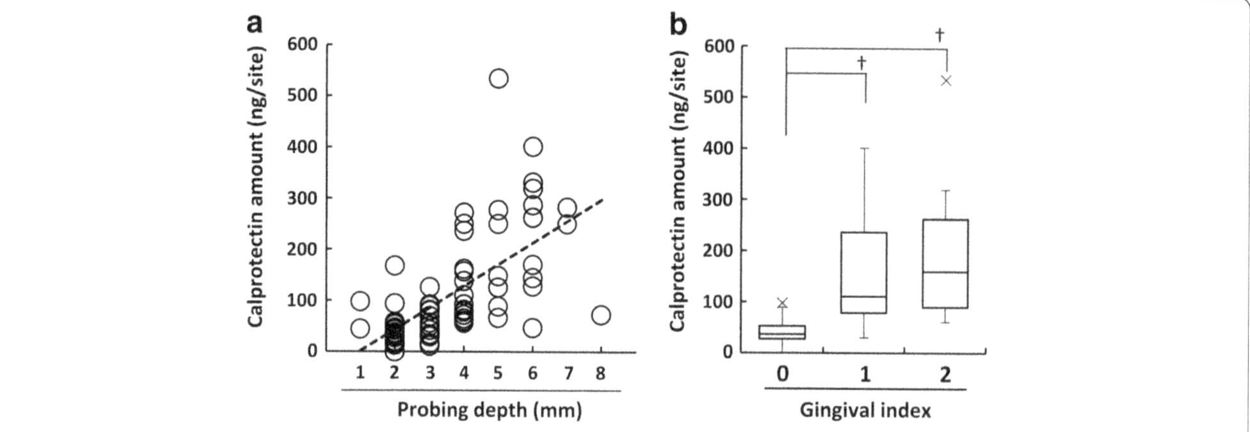

Fig. 3 Relationship between PICF calprotectin amounts and PD or GI scores. **a** The relationship between PICF calprotectin amounts and PD was evaluated in PICF samples from peri-implant disease and healthy groups ($n = 74$, $\rho = 0.709$, $P < 0.001$). **b** Relationship between PICF calprotectin amounts and GI scores. Calprotectin amounts in PICF samples from sites with GI-0 ($n = 34$), GI-1 ($n = 20$), and GI-2 ($n = 20$) were statistically analyzed. Horizontal bars show the median of each group. $^{\dagger}P < 0.001$

Discussion

Diagnostic studies on peri-implant diseases using biomarkers in PICF have been performing because clinical indicators do not necessarily lead to an accurate evaluation of peri-implant diseases [5, 7, 8, 32]. Calprotectin levels were significantly higher in periodontitis GCF than in healthy GCF, and thus, calprotectin is regarded as a useful inflammatory marker for periodontal diseases [16, 17, 19]. Calprotectin amounts in PICF were measured, and its levels did not significantly change between 2 and 3 years after the functional loading of dental implants [20]. However, calprotectin levels in PICF samples from sites with and without peri-implant diseases have not yet been investigated. The present study demonstrated that calprotectin amounts and concentrations in PICF samples were significantly higher from diseased sites than from healthy sites, and a positive association was observed between calprotectin levels and clinical indicators such as PD and GI scores. This result for peri-implant diseases was similar to previous findings obtained in diagnostic studies on periodontal diseases [16, 33]. A significant difference was noted in calprotectin amounts between GI-0 group and GI-1 or GI-2 group, suggesting that PICF calprotectin indicates initial, weak inflammation in peri-implant diseases because calprotectin is mainly existed in leukocytes that more express at early stage of inflammation and acute inflammation [14, 15]. In contrast, there was a little difference of the median of calprotectin level between the GI-1 and GI-2 groups, but not significant difference, supposing that calprotectin amounts may reach to almost the maximum level at inflammation sites with GI-1 and GI-2. The ability of some biomarkers including pro-inflammatory cytokines, inflammation-related factors, and proteolytic enzymes to diagnose peri-implant diseases has been examined [5, 7, 8, 32]. IL-1β, IL-6, and PGE_2 levels

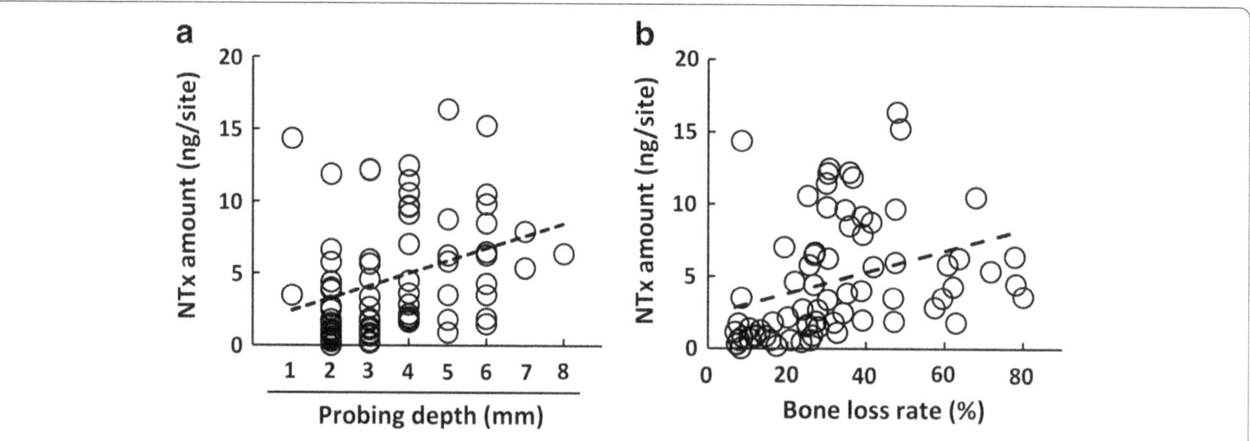

Fig. 4 Correlation between NTx amounts and PD or BL rates. **a** The correlation between PICF NTx amounts and PD was evaluated in PICF samples from peri-implant disease and healthy groups ($n = 74$, $\rho = 0.434$, $P < 0.001$). **b** The correlation between PICF NTx amounts and BL rates (%) was evaluated in PICF samples from peri-implant disease and healthy groups ($n = 74$, $\rho = 0.570$, $P < 0.001$)

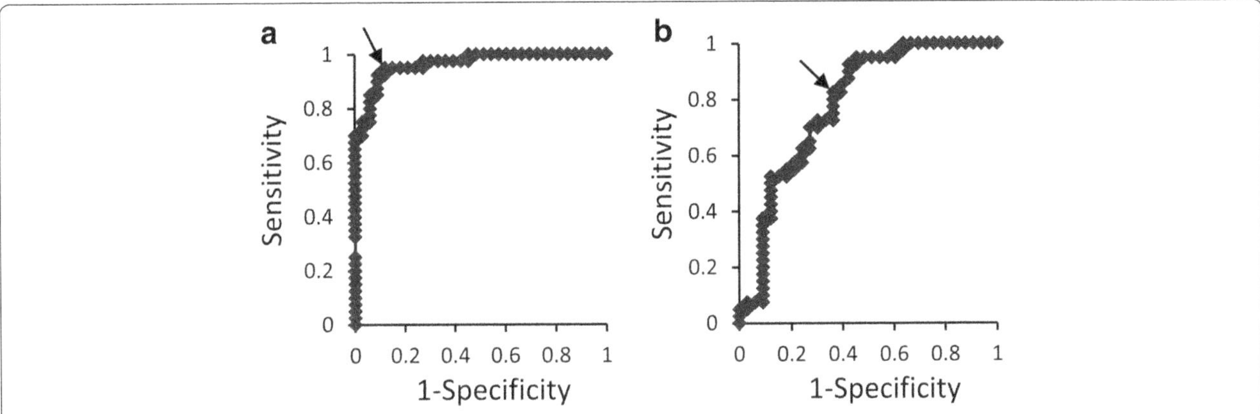

Fig. 5 ROC analyses of PICF calprotectin and NTx to predict peri-implant diseases. PICF samples were collected from sites with and without peri-implant diseases ($n = 74$). Calprotectin (**a**) and NTx (**b**) amounts in PICF samples were subjected to ROC curve analysis. AUC values for calprotectin and NTx amounts were 0.964 (95% CI = 0.913–0.996, $P < 0.001$) and 0.784 (95% CI = 0.672–0.891, $P < 0.001$), respectively, when cutoff values were 60.4 ng/site (arrow in **a**) and 1.88 ng/site (arrow in **b**)

in PICF were significantly higher from peri-implantitis sites than from healthy implant sites [10, 34, 35]. However, Aboyoussef et al. [36] and Melo et al. [37] showed no significant differences in IL-1β, IL-6, and PGE_2 levels between peri-implantitis and healthy groups. These reports indicate an opposite result, which IL-1β, IL-6, and PGE_2 are reliable markers to detect peri-implant diseases or not. In contrast, PICF calprotectin levels showed very high sensitivity (92.5%) and specificity (90.9%) for a diagnosis of peri-implant diseases when the cutoff value was 60.4 ng per site. The sensitivity and specificity of PICF calprotectin were higher than those of AST activity, which was higher in PICF from peri-implant diseases sites than from healthy sites, with a sensitivity = 81% and specificity = 74% [12]. MMP-8 levels were previously reported to be increased in PICF from sites with peri-implantitis [11], and MMP-8 levels in PICF from peri-implant disease sites correlated with GI scores ($\rho = 0.772$, $P < 0.001$) [38]. The correlation observed between PICF calprotectin levels and GI scores in the present study ($\rho = 0.744$, $P < 0.001$, data not shown) was similar to the relationship between MMP-8 levels and GI scores.

We did not classify peri-implant diseases into peri-implant mucositis and peri-implantitis in this pilot study. Peri-implant mucositis does not show BL, whereas peri-implantitis shows BL of more than 2.5 or 3 mm on intra-oral radiographs [39, 40]. Figuero et al. [2] introduced plural diagnostic criteria for peri-implant mucositis and peri-implantitis. Rakic et al. [5] defined peri-implantitis as a PD of more than 5 mm, BOP positive, and BL of at least two threads of implant. Furthermore, Sanz et al. [41] proposed their opinion for the radiographic assessment of alveolar bone in peri-implant treatment. However, difficulties are associated with accurately measuring 2–3 mm of alveolar BL on a radiograph taken by a regular method and assessing BL levels by implant threads when implant species differ. We evaluated BL around dental implants using Schei et al.'s method [30], which has been used to evaluate BL rate in periodontal diseases. The mean BL rate was significantly higher at peri-implant disease site than at healthy sites without inflammation and deep PD. Therefore, we did not distinguish peri-implant mucositis and peri-implantitis that were diagnosed by measuring bone level on radiograph in the present pilot study. Biomarkers for BL may be more accurate than clinical BL indicators because PICF NTx amounts were found to correlate with BL rates determined by Schei et al.'s method ($\rho = 0.570$, $P < 0.001$). Biomarkers for bone metabolism in PICF and clinical, radiological assessment of bone level may accurately diagnose peri-implant mucositis and peri-implantitis.

Bone-related proteins including ICTP, osteocalcin (OCN), and RANKL have been studied as BL biomarkers in peri-implantitis. ICTP, a cross-linked C-telopeptide of type I collagen, is a marker for bone degradation, and its levels in PICF were significantly higher from peri-implantitis sites than from healthy sites [9, 42]. However, Tümer et al. [13] did not detect a significant difference in PICF ICTP levels between peri-implantitis and healthy sites. RANKL is a main mediator of osteoclast formation and associated with bone resorption [43]. Soluble RANKL (sRANKL) concentrations in PICF were significantly higher from peri-implantitis sites than from healthy implant sites ($P < 0.01$), and its levels correlated with clinical indicators such as PD ($\rho = 0.309$, $P = 0.034$) and BOP ($\rho = 0.327$, $P = 0.024$) [44]. In the present study, NTx amounts and concentrations showed similar significant differences to sRANKL between the peri-implant disease and healthy groups (amount: $P < 0.01$, concentration: $P < 0.05$), and a stronger correlation was observed between NTx amounts and PD ($\rho = 0.434$, $P < 0.001$). In contrast, Arikan et al. [9] showed that sRANKL concentrations in PICF were significantly higher in healthy groups, while Sarlati et al. [45] reported no significant difference in PICF sRANKL concentrations among healthy, peri-implant mucositis, and peri-implantitis groups. OCN is a major non-collagenous protein in bone and is associated with bone metabolism [46]. The mean OCN concentration in PICF from peri-implantitis sites was approximately 1.5-fold that of healthy groups [13], and this finding was similar to the result for NTx in PICF. Although OCN levels in PICF samples were significantly higher from peri-implant mucositis sites without BL than from healthy sites, OCN levels in PICF from peri-implantitis with BL was not significantly different from those in PICF from healthy and peri-implant mucositis sites [47]. These conflicting findings do not necessarily suggest that ICTP, sRANKL, and OCN are reliable biomarkers for alveolar BL. Few studies showed a relationship between the PICF levels of bone-related markers and those of clinical indicators for alveolar BL. NTx levels in GCF samples were significantly higher from periodontitis sites than from healthy sites [28]; however, the relationship between NTx levels in PICF or GCF and BL levels has not yet been investigated. NTx in PICF may be a reliable biomarker for evaluating BL in peri-implantitis because PICF NTx levels correlated with the BL rate as well as PD and had high sensitivity and specificity for predicting peri-implant diseases.

Treatments for peri-implant diseases are selected by CIST [6], in which clinical indicators including PD, BOP, implant mobility, and BL on radiographs are used to diagnose peri-implant diseases. However, these clinical indicators are not considered to be sufficiently accurate or objective for the diagnosis of peri-implant diseases. Biomarkers in PICF contribute to the diagnosis of peri-implant diseases by clinical indicators and may provide a reliable diagnosis of onset, progression, and prognosis of disease as well as the selection of treatments. This pilot study suggests that calprotectin and NTx in PICF may be useful biomarkers for the diagnosis of peri-implant diseases, and future study using a large number of PICF samples will support the results obtained herein.

Conclusions

Calprotectin and NTx in PICF are markers of inflammation and bone resorption in peri-implant tissues and may be useful diagnostic markers for peri-implant diseases.

Abbreviations

AST: Aspartate aminotransferase; BL: Bone loss; BOP: Bleeding on probing; CIST: Cumulative interceptive supportive therapy; GCF: Gingival crevicular fluid; GI: Gingival index; ICTP: Cross-linked C-telopeptide of type I collagen; IL-1β: Interleukin-1β; MMP-8: Matrix metalloproteinase-8; NF-κB: Nuclear factor-κB; NTx: Cross-linked N-telopeptide of type I collagen; OCN: Osteocalcin; PD: Probing depth; PICF: Peri-implant crevicular fluid; RANKL: Receptor activator of NF-κB ligand; sRNAK: Soluble RANKL; TMB: 3,3′,5,5′-Tetramethylbenzidine; TNF-α: Tumor necrosis factor-α

Acknowledgements

We thank Dr. Toyoko Tajima (Oral Implant Center, Tokushima University Hospital) and Dr. Toshihiko Nagata, Dr. Koji Naruishi, Dr. Hiromichi Yumoto, Dr. Masami Ninomiya, Dr. Mika Bando, Dr. Yuji Inagaki, Dr. Chie Mihara, Dr. Takahisa Ikuta, Mr. Ryosuke Takagi, and Mr. Kohei Nonaka (Department of Periodontology and Endodontology, Institute of Biomedical Sciences, Tokushima University Graduate School) for the collection of PICF and support of the statistical analysis.

Funding

This study was supported by Grant-in-Aid for Scientific Research (no. 15K15767) from the Japan Society for the Promotion of Science (Tokyo, Japan) and in part by Shofu Inc. (Kyoto, Japan).

Authors' contributions

ES and RK collected the PICF, evaluated the clinical indicators, and determined the calprotectin and NTx in PICF samples. YT, YN, and YI diagnosed peri-implant diseases and supported to plan the clinical study. JK planted the present study, performed the statistical analysis of data, and wrote the manuscript. All authors read and approved the final manuscript.

Competing interests

Authors Eijiro Sakamoto, Rie Kido, Yoritoki Tomotake, Yoshihito Naitou, Yuichi Ishida and Jun-ichi Kido declare that they have no competing interests.

Author details

[1]Department of Periodontology and Endodontology, Institute of Biomedical Sciences, Tokushima University Graduate School, 3-18-15 Kuramoto, Tokushima 770-8504, Japan. [2]Oral Implant Center, Tokushima University Hospital, Tokushima, Japan. [3]Department of Oral and Maxillofacial Prosthodontics, Institute of Biomedical Sciences, Tokushima University Graduate School, Tokushima, Japan.

References

1. Mombelli A, Müller N, Cionca N. The epidemiology of peri-implantitis. Clin Oral Implants Res. 2012;23(Suppl 6):67–76.
2. Figuero E, Graziani F, Sanz I, Herrera D, Sanz M. Management of peri-implant mucositis and peri-implantitis. Periodontol. 2000;2014(66):255–73.
3. Hämmerle CHF, Glauser R. Clinical evaluation of dental implant treatment. Periodontol. 2000;2004(34):230–9.
4. Heitz-Mayfield LJA. Peri-implant diseases: diagnosis and risk indicators. J Clin Periodontol. 2008;35(Suppl 8):292–304.
5. Rakic M, Struillou X, Petkovic-Curcin A, Matic S, Canullo L, Sanz M, et al. Estimation of bone loss biomarkers as a diagnostic tool for peri-implantitis. J Periodontol. 2014;85:1566–74.
6. Mombelli A, Lang NP. The diagnosis and treatment of peri-implantitis. Periodontol. 2000;1998(17):63–76.
7. Dursun E, Tözüm TF. Peri-implant crevicular fluid analysis, enzymes and biomarkers: a systematic review. J Oral Maxillofac Res. 2016;7:e9.
8. Faot F, Nascimento GG, Bielemann AM, Campão TD, Leite FRM, Quirynen M. Can peri-implant crevicular fluid assist in the diagnosis of peri-implantitis? A systematic review and meta-analysis. J Periodontol. 2015;86:631–45.
9. Arikan F, Buduneli N, Lappin DF. C-telopeptide pyridinoline crosslinks of type I collagen, soluble RANKL, and osteoprotegerin levels in crevicular fluid of dental implants with peri-implantitis: a case-control study. Int J Oral Maxillofac Implants. 2011;26:282–9.
10. Ata-Ali J, Flichy-Fernández AJ, Alegre-Domingo T, Ata-Ali F, Palacio J, Peñarrocha-Diago M. Clinical, microbiological, and immunological aspects of healthy versus peri-implantitis tissue in full arch reconstruction patients: a prospective cross-sectional study. BMC Oral Health. 2015;15:43.
11. Nomura T, Ishii A, Shimizu H, Taguchi N, Yoshie H, Kusakari H, et al. Tissue inhibitor of metalloproteinases-1, matrix metalloproteinases-1 and -8, and collagenase activity levels in peri-implant crevicular fluid after implantation. Clin Oral Implants Res. 2000;11:430–40.

12. Paolantonio M, Di Placido G, Tumini V, Di Stilio M, Contento A, Spoto G. Aspartate aminotransferase activity in crevicular fluid from dental implants. J Periodontol. 2000;71:1151–7.
13. Tümer C, Aksoy Y, Güncü GN, Nohutcu RM, Kilinc K, Tözüm TF. Possible impact of inflammatory status on C-telopeptide pyridinoline cross-links of type I collagen and osteocalcin levels around oral implants with peri-implantitis: a controlled clinical trial. J Oral Rehabil. 2008;35:934–9.
14. Fagerhol MK, Andersson KB, Naess-Andersen CF, Brandtzaeg P, Dale I. Calprotectin (the L1 leukocyte protein). In: Smith UL, Dedman JR, editors. Stimulus response coupling: the role of intracellular calcium-binding proteins. Boca Raton, FL: CRC Press; 1990. p. 187–210.
15. Stříž I, Trebichavský I. Calprotectin—a pleiotropic molecule in acute and chronic inflammation. Physiol Res. 2004;53:245–53.
16. Kido J, Nakamura T, Kido R, Ohishi K, Yamuchi N, Kataoka M, et al. Calprotectin, a leukocyte protein related to inflammation, in gingival crevicular fluid. J Periodontal Res. 1998;33:434–7.
17. Kido J, Nakamura T, Kido R, Ohishi K, Yamuchi N, Kataoka M, et al. Calprotectin in gingival crevicular fluid correlates with clinical and biochemical markers of periodontal disease. J Clin Periodontol. 1999;26:653–7.
18. Nakamura T, Kido J, Kido R, Ohishi K, Yamuchi N, Kataoka M, et al. The association of calprotectin level in gingival crevicular fluid with gingival index and the activities of collagenase and aspartate aminotransferase in adult periodontitis patients. J Periodontol. 2000;71:361–7.
19. Kaner D, Bernimoulin JP, Dietrich T, Kleber B-M, Friedmann A. Calprotectin levels in gingival crevicular fluid predict disease activity in patients treated for generalized aggressive periodontitis. J Periodontal Res. 2011;46:417–26.
20. Friedmann A, Friedrichs M, Kaner D, Kleber B-M, Bernimoulin J-P. Calprotectin and cross-linked N-terminal telopeptides in peri-implant and gingival crevicular fluid. Clin Oral Implants Res. 2006;17:527–32.
21. Clemens JD, Herrick MV, Singer FR, Eyre DR. Evidence that serum NTx (collagen-type I N-telopeptides) can act as an immunochemical marker of bone resorption. Clin Chem. 1997;43:2058–63.
22. Hanson DA, Weis MA, Bollen AM, Maslan SL, Singer FR, Eyre DR. A specific immunoassay for monitoring human bone resorption: quantitation of type I collagen cross-linked N-telopeptides in urine. J Bone Miner Res. 1992;7:1251–8.
23. Herrmann M, Seibel M. The amino- and carboxyterminal cross-linked telopeptides of collagen type I, NTX-I and CTX-I: a comparative review. Clin Chim Acta. 2008;393:57–75.
24. Joerger M, Huober J. Diagnostic and prognostic use of bone turnover markers. Recent Results Cancer Res. 2012;192:197–223.
25. Becerik S, Afacan B, Öztürk VÖ, Atmaca H, Emingil G. Gingival crevicular fluid calprotectin, osteocalcin and cross-linked N-terminal telopeptide levels in health and different periodontal diseases. Dis Markers. 2011;31:343–52.
26. Becerik S, Gürkan A, Afacan B, Özgen ÖV, Atmac H, Töz H, et al. Gingival crevicular fluid osteocalcin, N-terminal telopeptides, and calprotectin levels in cyclosporine A-induced gingival overgrowth. J Periodontol. 2011;82:1490–7.
27. Wilson AN, Schmid MJ, Marx DB, Reinhardt RA. Bone turnover markers in serum and periodontal microenvironments. J Periodontal Res. 2003;38:355–61.
28. Aruna G. Estimation of N-terminal telopeptides of type I collagen in periodontal health, disease and after nonsurgical periodontal therapy in gingival crevicular fluid: a clinic- biochemical study. Indian J Dent Res. 2015;26:152–7.
29. Löe H, Silness J. Periodontal disease in pregnancy. I Prevalence and severity. Acta Odontol Scand. 1963;21:533–51.
30. Schei O, Waerhaug J, Lovdal A, Arno A. Alveolar bone loss as related to oral hygiene and age. J Periodontol. 1959;30:7–16.
31. Kido J, Bando Y, Bando M, Kajiura Y, Hiroshima Y, Inagaki Y, et al. YKL-40 level in gingival crevicular fluid from patients with periodontitis and type 2 diabetes. Oral Dis. 2015;21:667–73.
32. Duarte PM, Serrão CR, Miranda TS, Zanatta LC, Bastos MF, Faveri M, et al. Could cytokine levels in the peri-implant crevicular fluid be used to distinguish between healthy implants and implants with peri-implantitis? A systematic review. J Periodontal Res. 2016;51:689–98.
33. Kajiura Y, Lew J-H, Ikuta T, Nishikawa Y, Kido J, Nagata T, et al. Clinical significance of GCF sIL-6R and calprotectin to evaluate the periodontal inflammation. Ann Clin Biochem. 2017;54:664–70.
34. Yaghobee S, Khorsand A, Rasouli Ghohroudi AA, Sanjari K, Kadkhodazadeh M. Assessment of interleukin-1beta and interleukin-6 in the crevicular fluid around healthy implants, implants with peri-implantitis, and healthy teeth: a cross-sectional study. J Korean Assoc Oral Maxillofac Surg. 2014;40:220–4.
35. Yalçn S, Baseğmez C, Mijiritsky E, Yalçn F, Isik G, Onan U. Detection of implant crevicular fluid prostaglandin E2 levels for the assessment of peri-implant health: a pilot study. Implant Dent. 2005;14:194–200.
36. Aboyoussef H, Carter C, Jandinski JJ, Panagakos FS. Detection of prostaglandin E2 and matrix metalloproteinases in implant crevicular fluid. Int J Oral Maxillofac Implants. 1998;13:689–96.
37. Melo RF, Lopes BM, Shibli JA, Marcantonio E Jr, Marcantonio RA, Galli GM. Interleukin-1β and interleukin-6 expression and gene polymorphisms in subjects with peri-implant disease. Clin Implant Dent Relat Res. 2012;14:905–14.
38. Kivelä-Rajamäki MJ, Teronen OP, Maisi P, Husa V, Tervahartiala TI, Pirilä EM, et al. Laminin-5γ2-chain and collagenase-2 (MMP-8) in human peri-implant sulcular fluid. Clin Oral Implants Res. 2003;14:158–65.
39. Renvert S, Lindahl C, Roos Jansåker AM, Persson GR. Treatment of peri-implantitis using an Er:YAG laser or an air-abrasive device: a randomized clinical trial. J Clin Periodontol. 2011;38:65–73.
40. Schwarz F, Sahm N, Iglhaut G, Becker J. Impact of the method of surface debridement and decontamination on the clinical outcome following combined surgical therapy of peri-implantitis: a randomized controlled clinical study. J Clin Periodontol. 2011;38:276–84.
41. Sanz M, Chapple IL, on behalf of Working Group 4 of the VIII European Workshop on Periodontology. Clinical research on peri-implant diseases: consensus report of working group 4. J Clin Periodontol. 2012;39(Suppl. 12):202–6.
42. Giannobile WV. C-telopeptide pyridinoline cross-links. Sensitive indicators of periodontal tissue destruction. Ann N Y Acad Sci. 1999;878:404–12.
43. Boyce BF, Xing L. Functions of RANKL/RANK/OPG in bone modeling and remodeling. Arch Biochem Biophys. 2008;473:139–46.
44. Rakic M, Lekovic V, Nikolic-Jakoba N, Vojvodic D, Petkovic-Curcin A, Sanz M. Bone loss biomarkers associated with peri-implantitis. A cross-sectional study. Clin Oral Implants Res. 2013;24:1110–6.
45. Sarlati F, Sattari M, Gazar AG, Rafsenjani AN. Receptor activator of nuclear factor kappa B ligand (RANKL) levels in peri-implant crevicular fluid. Iran J Immunol. 2010;7:226–33.
46. Lian JB, Gundberg CM. Osteocalcin. Biochemical considerations and clinical applications. Clin Orthop Relat Res. 1988;226:267–91.
47. Murata M, Tatsumi J, Kato Y, Suda S, Nunokawa Y, Kobayashi Y, et al. Osteocalcin, deoxypyridinoline and interleukin-1β in peri-implant crevicular fluid of patients with peri-implantitis. Clin Oral Implants Res. 2002;13:637–43.

6

CAD/CAM implant surgical guides: maximum errors in implant positioning attributable to the properties of the metal sleeve/osteotomy drill combination

Dimitrios Apostolakis* and Georgios Kourakis

Abstract

Background: The purpose of this study is to provide the relevant equations and the reference tables needed for calculating the maximum errors in implant positioning attributed to the properties of the mechanical parts of any CAD/CAM implant surgical guide, especially the in-office manufactured ones.

Methods: An algorithm was developed and implemented in C programming language in order to accurately calculate the maximum error at the apex, error at the neck, vertical error at the apex and deviation of implant axis, between the planned and the actual implant position. The calculations were based on the parameters of total length (= implant length + offset), offset (distance from neck of implant to the lip of the metal sleeve), clearance (space between the bur and the sleeve), sleeve length. The variability of the parameters was constrained: (1) implant length, 8–18 mm; (2) sleeve length, 4–7 mm; (3) clearance, 50–410 μm; and (4) offset values, 6–17 mm. Multiple regression analysis was conducted to quantify the relationship between the error at the apex and the error at the neck and various predictors.

Results: The equations used for the bespoke estimation of the errors in implant positioning along with three reference tables of the various errors tabulated are presented. The maximum error at the apex of the implant was computed 2.8 mm, the maximum deviation of the implant axis 5.9° and the maximum error at the neck (entrance) of the implant was estimated 1.5 mm. The vertical error between the planned and actual implant position can be considered negligible (< 0.1 mm).

Conclusions: The results of this study compute part of the expected differences in final clinical implant position when any CAD/CAM surgical guide is used. Given that the implantologist, with the capability of an in-office digital designed and 3d printed surgical guide, can readily decide upon the dimensions of the metal sleeve, the clearance between the osteotomy bur and the sleeve, and the design of the guide in relation to the distance of the lip of the sleeve to the implant neck (offset), in order to minimise the inevitable errors.

Keywords: CAD, CAM, Implant guide, 3d printing, Osteotomy, Stereolithography

Background

Computer-aided designed and computer-aided manufactured (CAD/CAM) implant surgical guides are long recommended to reliably transfer a virtual treatment plan to the surgical field [1, 2]. The 3d-printed guide stands a basic part of a process commonly referred to as guided implant surgery (GIS) [3]. The outcome of this process has been shown to be relatively accurate [4, 5], even when the guide is in the hands of inexperienced surgeons [6].

The error in guided implant surgery, when defined as the difference between the planned and the actual position of the implant, is the cumulative result of flaws along the different stages of the procedure. Inaccuracies in the CBCT or CT acquisition process [7], the DICOM to STL conversion [8], the registration process of the different modes [3], the procedure followed for designing and manufacturing the surgical guide [9], the method

* Correspondence: dentalradiology@hotmail.com
Private Practice, Dental Radiology in Crete, Plateia 1866, No 39, 73100 Chania, Crete, Greece

used to stabilise the guide in the mouth (i.e. teeth, mucosa, bone) [10], the way the guide is manipulated by the surgeon and finally the quality and quantity and morphology of the local bone [4].

All of the current research concerning the mechanical parts of a CAD/CAM surgical guide has so far investigated the accuracy of implant guides designed and manufactured professionally by companies specialising in the field of medicine and dentistry [11–16]. These companies usually provide, in addition to the guide and software, their own correspondent surgical kit, especially designed to perform solely with their guide.

In-office 3d printing with low-cost fused deposition modelling (FDM) or desktop stereolithography apparatus (SLA) printers and freeware provides a cheaper alternative for manufacturing surgical guides with materials and components supplied from the free market. In-office 3d printing gives the opportunity to the implantologist to readily produce a CAD/CAM guide and place implants using the surgical kit at his current disposal. The production of such a 3d guide may pertain the same errors as a commercially constructed guide does, with the exception that now the implantologist is oblivious to the magnitude and, as a result, the clinical significances of these errors.

It is the aim of this paper to compute the maximum errors in the positioning of the implants with relation to the basic mechanical components of a 3d surgical guide/surgical kit combination taking into account the positional and dimensional properties of the guide's metal part (sleeve) and the dimensional properties of any osteotomy bur used. The analytical equations for the bespoke computation of the errors for any conceivable combination of the relevant parameters will be provided. Reference tables will be reported facilitating the in-office production of any 3d surgical implant guide.

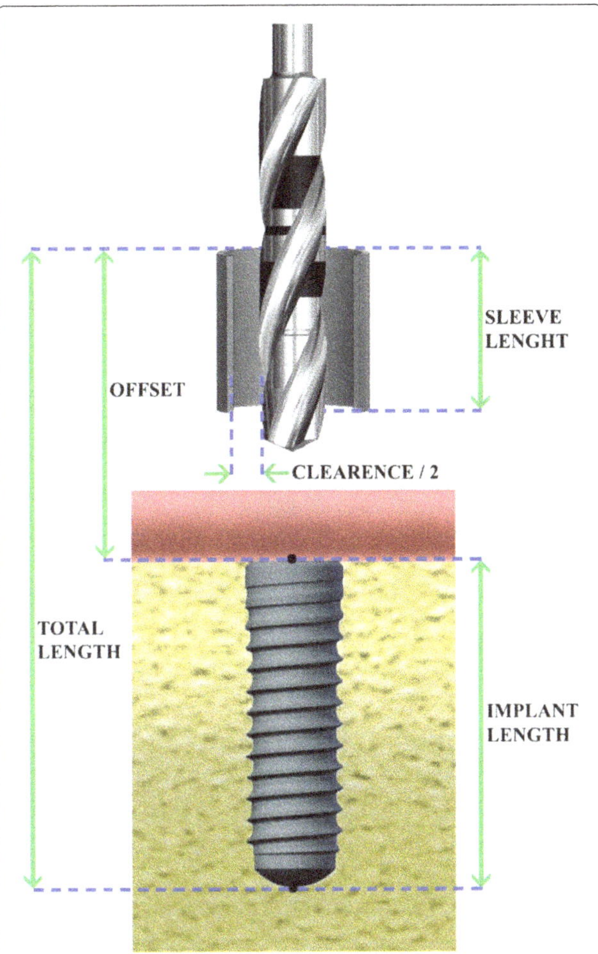

Fig. 1 The parameters used for the calculation of the various errors and the deviation of implant axis

Methods

For the estimation of the errors in implant positioning due to the properties of the metal sleeve/osteotomy drill combination, four [4] parameters are necessary: (1) sleeve length, (2) clearance (space between the bur and the sleeve), (3) implant length, and (4) offset (distance of the lip of the metal sleeve to the neck of the implant) (Figs. 1 and 2).

Definitions

1. Basic size: the nominal size of the metal sleeve and the osteotomy drill given by the manufacturer.
2. Sleeve length: the total length of the metal sleeve inserted into the surgical guide, including any lip protruding on the occlusal surface of the guide.
3. Offset: the distance between the neck of the implant and the occlusal surface of the lip of the metal sleeve.
4. Clearance: the difference between the inner diameter of the metal sleeve and the diameter of the osteotomy bur.
5. Implant length: the nominal length of the implant from the neck to the apex.
6. Total length: the sum of implant length and offset.
7. Error at the apex: the Euclidian distance between the apex of the implant at the planned position and the apex at the more extreme position permissible by the sleeve/drill combination (measured from the central implant axis).
8. Error at the neck: the Euclidian distance between the neck of the implant at the planned position and the neck of the implant at the more extreme position permissible by the sleeve/drill combination (measured from the central implant axis).
9. Deviation: the angle in degrees between the central axis of the implant on the planned position and the same axis on the most extreme permissible position.
10. Vertical error at the apex: the distance of the final position of the apex of the implant to the horizontal

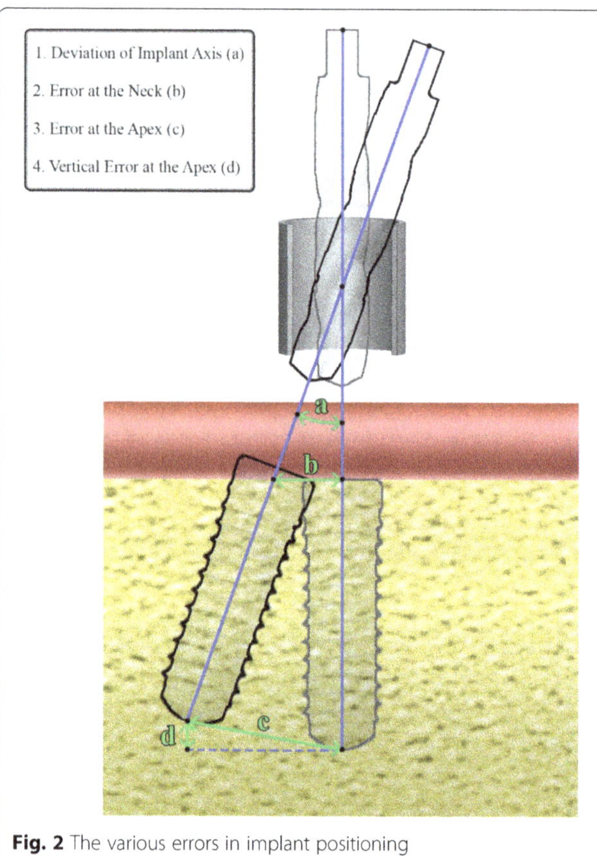

Fig. 2 The various errors in implant positioning

plane where the point of the planned position of the implant is included.

Based on the geometric analysis of the problem in hand, an algorithm was developed and implemented in C programming language. The purpose of this program was to readily and accurately compute the following maximum positioning errors, permissible by the different sleeve/drill/guide properties (Fig. 2):

1. Deviation of the implant axis in degrees,
2. Error at the neck in mm,
2. Error at the apex in mm,
4. Vertical error at the apex in mm.

These computations were based on the four parameters: (1) implant length, (2) sleeve length, (3) clearance and (4) offset (Fig. 1), and the results were tabulated in reference tables. The implant length and the offset were added together to form a new variable termed total length used exclusively on the calculations related to the error at the apex.

The variability of the parameters was constrained to reflect probable clinical conditions: (1) implant length between 8 and 18 mm, in 1 mm steps; (2) sleeve length between 4 and 7 mm, in 1 mm steps; (3) clearance between 50 and 410 μm, in 30 μm steps; and (4) offset values between 6 and 17 mm, in 1 mm steps. The minimum distance between the bottom of the metal sleeve (towards the bone) and the neck of the implant was set at the considered clinically appropriate distance of 2 mm.

Multiple regression was employed twice, with three independent variables each time to separate the effects of clearance, total length, sleeve length and offset on the values of the error at the apex and the error at the neck.

Microsoft® Excel 2016 32 bit was used for the statistical analysis. Significance level was set to $p < 0.05$.

All the values in the reference tables were rounded to one significant digit after the decimal point.

Results

The range of the various maximum permissible errors due to the metal sleeve/osteotomy drill combination is presented in Table 1.

Concerning the error at the apex, two reference tables were reported (Tables 2 and 3). In these tables, the deviation of the implant axis was also tabulated. A separate table (Table 4) tabulated the error at the neck.

Multiple regression analysis was conducted to examine the relationship between the error at the apex, the error at the neck and the various predictors. Table 5 summarises the analysis results. The multiple regression model for the error at the apex with all three predictors (total length, sleeve length, clearance) produced $R^2 = 0.98$, $F\ (3, 751) = 12{,}754$, $p < 0.0005$. The multiple regression model for the error at the neck with all three predictors (offset, clearance, sleeve length) produced $R^2 = 0.97$, $F\ (3, 543) = 5677$, $p < 0.0005$.

The models:

$$\begin{aligned}\text{Error at the apex (mm)} = {} & 0.046 * (\text{total length}) \\ & + 0.0038 \\ & * (\text{clearance}) - 0.19 \\ & * (\text{sleeve length})\end{aligned}$$

$$\begin{aligned}\text{Error at the neck (mm)} = {} & 0.046 * (\text{offset}) + 0.0018 \\ & * (\text{clearance}) - 0.10 \\ & * (\text{sleeve length})\end{aligned}$$

The values of total length and offset are in mm whilst the values of clearance are in μm.

As it is shown in Table 5, the total length, clearance and offset have positive and significant regression weights indicating that guided surgery with higher scores on these scales is expected to have higher errors in the implant positioning after controlling for the other variables in the model. The sleeve length has a significant negative weight indicating that after accounting for the rest of the variables, surgical guides with increased sleeve length are expected to have lower errors in implant positioning.

Table 1 Range of various maximum permissible errors as calculated in the present study

	Axis deviation (°)	Error at the neck (mm)	Error at the apex (mm)	Vertical error at the apex (mm)
Min	0.4	0.1	0.1	0.0
Max	5.9	1.5	2.8	0.1

Discussion

The purpose of a computer designed and computer manufactured (CAD/CAM) surgical guide is to provide the means for an accurate and reliable transfer of the computer-realised virtual treatment plan to the actual surgical field. The availability of the CBCT imaging modality should have led to an explosion of the usage of these guides, since they have been shown to be more accurate than freehand placement [17] and offer, in addition to the possibility of flapless surgery, the opportunity for a truly prosthetically driven implant placement [18]. However, increased costs, related to software acquisition and guide manufacturing, along with the special instrumentation required in most of the commercially available systems, in combination with an increased lead time between the completion of the virtual treatment plan and the delivery of the actual guide, make a lot of implantologists reluctant to the use of this technique.

Low-cost technologies for the in-office production of 3d guides already exist (SLA and FDM). A low-cost SLA 3d printer is advertised as the ideal for a dental practice with the same printer being tested for training in medical procedures [19]. Freeware for the design and the low-cost export of an STL file of the guide is available. The metal sleeves that are usually incorporated into the guide in order to accommodate the drill are offered in large numbers of internal and external dimensions. The dentist, almost by definition, possesses a high level of engineering and material skills [20]. He/she is currently able to accommodate their surgical need with a low-cost, fast-produced and fully CAD/CAM surgical guide. In the present study,

Table 2 Error at the apex (mm) and deviation of implant axis (°) for sleeve lengths 4 and 5 mm

Sleeve length (mm)	Clearance (μm)	Deviation (degrees)	Total length (mm)															
			14	15	16	17	18	19	20	21	22	23	24	25	26	27	28	29
4.00	50.00	0.72	0.2	0.2	0.2	0.2	0.2	0.2	0.2	0.2	0.3	0.3	0.3	0.3	0.3	0.3	0.3	0.3
	80.00	1.15	0.2	0.3	0.3	0.3	0.3	0.3	0.4	0.4	0.4	0.4	0.4	0.5	0.5	0.5	0.5	0.5
	110.00	1.58	0.3	0.4	0.4	0.4	0.4	0.5	0.5	0.5	0.6	0.6	0.6	0.6	0.7	0.7	0.7	0.7
	140.00	2.00	0.4	0.5	0.5	0.5	0.6	0.6	0.6	0.7	0.7	0.7	0.8	0.8	0.8	0.9	0.9	0.9
	170.00	2.43	0.5	0.6	0.6	0.6	0.7	0.7	0.8	0.8	0.9	0.9	0.9	1.0	1.0	1.1	1.1	1.1
	200.00	2.86	0.6	0.7	0.7	0.8	0.8	0.9	0.9	1.0	1.0	1.1	1.1	1.2	1.2	1.3	1.3	1.4
	230.00	3.29	0.7	0.7	0.8	0.9	0.9	1.0	1.0	1.1	1.2	1.2	1.3	1.3	1.4	1.4	1.5	1.6
	260.00	3.72	0.8	0.8	0.9	1.0	1.0	1.1	1.2	1.2	1.3	1.4	1.4	1.5	1.6	1.6	1.7	1.8
	290.00	4.15	0.9	0.9	1.0	1.1	1.2	1.2	1.3	1.4	1.5	1.5	1.6	1.7	1.7	1.8	1.9	2.0
	320.00	4.57	1.0	1.0	1.1	1.2	1.3	1.4	1.4	1.5	1.6	1.7	1.8	1.8	1.9	2.0	2.1	2.2
	350.00	5.00	1.1	1.1	1.2	1.3	1.4	1.5	1.6	1.7	1.8	1.8	1.9	2.0	2.1	2.2	2.3	2.4
	380.00	5.43	1.1	1.2	1.3	1.4	1.5	1.6	1.7	1.8	1.9	2.0	2.1	2.2	2.3	2.4	2.5	2.6
	410.00	5.85	1.2	1.3	1.4	1.5	1.6	1.7	1.8	1.9	2.1	2.2	2.3	2.4	2.5	2.6	2.7	2.8
5.00	50.00	0.57		0.1	0.1	0.1	0.2	0.2	0.2	0.2	0.2	0.2	0.2	0.2	0.2	0.2	0.3	0.3
	80.00	0.92		0.2	0.2	0.2	0.2	0.3	0.3	0.3	0.3	0.3	0.3	0.4	0.4	0.4	0.4	0.4
	110.00	1.26		0.3	0.3	0.3	0.3	0.4	0.4	0.4	0.4	0.5	0.5	0.5	0.5	0.5	0.6	0.6
	140.00	1.60		0.4	0.4	0.4	0.4	0.5	0.5	0.5	0.5	0.6	0.6	0.6	0.7	0.7	0.7	0.7
	170.00	1.95		0.4	0.5	0.5	0.5	0.6	0.6	0.6	0.7	0.7	0.7	0.8	0.8	0.8	0.9	0.9
	200.00	2.29		0.5	0.5	0.6	0.6	0.7	0.7	0.7	0.8	0.8	0.9	0.9	0.9	1.0	1.0	1.1
	230.00	2.63		0.6	0.6	0.7	0.7	0.8	0.8	0.9	0.9	0.9	1.0	1.0	1.1	1.1	1.2	1.2
	260.00	2.98		0.7	0.7	0.8	0.8	0.9	0.9	1.0	1.0	1.1	1.1	1.2	1.2	1.3	1.3	1.4
	290.00	3.32		0.7	0.8	0.8	0.9	1.0	1.0	1.1	1.1	1.2	1.2	1.3	1.4	1.4	1.5	1.5
	320.00	3.66		0.8	0.9	0.9	1.0	1.1	1.1	1.2	1.2	1.3	1.4	1.4	1.5	1.6	1.6	1.7
	350.00	4.00		0.9	0.9	1.0	1.1	1.2	1.2	1.3	1.4	1.4	1.5	1.6	1.6	1.7	1.8	1.9
	380.00	4.35		1.0	1.0	1.1	1.2	1.3	1.3	1.4	1.5	1.6	1.6	1.7	1.8	1.9	1.9	2.0
	410.00	4.69		1.0	1.1	1.2	1.3	1.4	1.4	1.5	1.6	1.7	1.8	1.8	1.9	2.0	2.1	2.2

Table 3 Error at the apex (mm) and deviation of implant axis (degrees) for sleeve lengths 6 and 7 mm

Sleeve length (mm)	Clearance (μm)	Deviation (°)	Total length (mm)													
			16	17	18	19	20	21	22	23	24	25	26	27	28	29
6	50	0.5	0.1	0.1	0.1	0.1	0.1	0.2	0.2	0.2	0.2	0.2	0.2	0.2	0.2	0.2
	80	0.8	0.2	0.2	0.2	0.2	0.2	0.2	0.3	0.3	0.3	0.3	0.3	0.3	0.3	0.3
	110	1.1	0.2	0.3	0.3	0.3	0.3	0.3	0.3	0.4	0.4	0.4	0.4	0.4	0.5	0.5
	140	1.3	0.3	0.3	0.4	0.4	0.4	0.4	0.4	0.5	0.5	0.5	0.5	0.6	0.6	0.6
	170	1.6	0.4	0.4	0.4	0.5	0.5	0.5	0.5	0.6	0.6	0.6	0.7	0.7	0.7	0.7
	200	1.9	0.4	0.5	0.5	0.5	0.6	0.6	0.6	0.7	0.7	0.7	0.8	0.8	0.8	0.9
	230	2.2	0.5	0.5	0.6	0.6	0.7	0.7	0.7	0.8	0.8	0.8	0.9	0.9	1.0	1.0
	260	2.5	0.6	0.6	0.7	0.7	0.7	0.8	0.8	0.9	0.9	1.0	1.0	1.0	1.1	1.1
	290	2.8	0.6	0.7	0.7	0.8	0.8	0.9	0.9	1.0	1.0	1.1	1.1	1.2	1.2	1.3
	320	3.1	0.7	0.7	0.8	0.9	0.9	1.0	1.0	1.1	1.1	1.2	1.2	1.3	1.3	1.4
	350	3.3	0.8	0.8	0.9	0.9	1.0	1.1	1.1	1.2	1.2	1.3	1.3	1.4	1.5	1.5
	380	3.6	0.8	0.9	1.0	1.0	1.1	1.1	1.2	1.3	1.3	1.4	1.5	1.5	1.6	1.6
	410	3.9	0.9	1.0	1.0	1.1	1.2	1.2	1.3	1.4	1.4	1.5	1.6	1.6	1.7	1.8
7	50	0.4		0.1	0.1	0.1	0.1	0.1	0.1	0.1	0.1	0.2	0.2	0.2	0.2	0.2
	80	0.7		0.2	0.2	0.2	0.2	0.2	0.2	0.2	0.2	0.2	0.3	0.3	0.3	0.3
	110	0.9		0.2	0.2	0.2	0.3	0.3	0.3	0.3	0.3	0.3	0.4	0.4	0.4	0.4
	140	1.1		0.3	0.3	0.3	0.3	0.4	0.4	0.4	0.4	0.4	0.5	0.5	0.5	0.5
	170	1.4		0.3	0.4	0.4	0.4	0.4	0.4	0.5	0.5	0.5	0.5	0.6	0.6	0.6
	200	1.6		0.4	0.4	0.4	0.5	0.5	0.5	0.6	0.6	0.6	0.6	0.7	0.7	0.7
	230	1.9		0.4	0.5	0.5	0.5	0.6	0.6	0.6	0.7	0.7	0.7	0.8	0.8	0.8
	260	2.1		0.5	0.5	0.6	0.6	0.7	0.7	0.7	0.8	0.8	0.8	0.9	0.9	0.9
	290	2.4		0.6	0.6	0.6	0.7	0.7	0.8	0.8	0.8	0.9	0.9	1.0	1.0	1.1
	320	2.6		0.6	0.7	0.7	0.8	0.8	0.8	0.9	0.9	1.0	1.0	1.1	1.1	1.2
	350	2.9		0.7	0.7	0.8	0.8	0.9	0.9	1.0	1.0	1.1	1.1	1.2	1.2	1.3
	380	3.1		0.7	0.8	0.8	0.9	1.0	1.0	1.1	1.1	1.2	1.2	1.3	1.3	1.4
	410	3.4		0.8	0.8	0.9	1.0	1.0	1.1	1.1	1.2	1.3	1.3	1.4	1.4	1.5

we focus on the errors made during the manufacturing of such a guide and especially those depending on the way the metal components of the guide interrelate with the osteotomy bur and with the planned position of the implant. However, it should be stressed that the results of this study remain relevant for every implant surgical guide irrespective of the way it is manufactured, 3d-printed or other.

Computer-aided implant surgery is not flawless, even when the guides are manufactured by experts in 3d printing. Three recent systematic reviews have demonstrated errors between the planned and the final implant position. In the study of Schneider et al. [5], the review revealed a mean deviation of 1.07 mm (95% CI 0.76–1.22 mm) at the entry point, 1.6 mm (95% CI 1.26–2 mm) at the apex and a mean angular deviation of the implant axis of 5.3° (95% CI 3.94–6.581). In the study of Van Assche et al. [21], the mean error at the entry point was 0.99 mm (range 0–6.5 mm), at the apex 1.2 mm (range 0–6.9 mm) and the mean axis deviation was 3.81° (range 0–24.9 degrees). In the study of Tahmaseb et al. [17], the mean error at the entry point was 1.12 mm (maximum 4.5 mm) and 1.39 mm at the apex (maximum 7.1 mm). These reported errors are the summation of flaws in every stage of the procedure in the guided implant surgery: scanning, processing, manufacturing, surgery and not exclusively because of the properties of the mechanical parts of the guide.

A relatively small number of studies are concerned with the errors in the implant positioning due to the mechanical components of the guides. All of them refer to commercially available systems and try to evaluate or even improve these existing systems, elaborating in the mechanical errors of the particular system used [11–16].

Our study is free from the constraints of commercially available systems, but our equations and tables can be used to estimate errors generated by these systems when certain parameters are known. Our study calculates the maximum errors expected by the mechanical components of the computerised implant surgery process, with

Table 4 Error at the neck (mm)

Sleeve length (mm)	Clearance (µm)	Offset (mm)											
		6	7	8	9	10	11	12	13	14	15	16	17
4	50	0.1	0.1	0.1	0.1	0.1	0.1	0.1	0.1	0.2	0.2	0.2	0.2
	80	0.1	0.1	0.1	0.1	0.2	0.2	0.2	0.2	0.2	0.3	0.3	0.3
	110	0.1	0.1	0.2	0.2	0.2	0.2	0.3	0.3	0.3	0.4	0.4	0.4
	140	0.1	0.2	0.2	0.2	0.3	0.3	0.4	0.4	0.4	0.5	0.5	0.5
	170	0.2	0.2	0.3	0.3	0.3	0.4	0.4	0.5	0.5	0.6	0.6	0.6
	200	0.2	0.3	0.3	0.4	0.4	0.5	0.5	0.6	0.6	0.7	0.7	0.8
	230	0.2	0.3	0.3	0.4	0.5	0.5	0.6	0.6	0.7	0.7	0.8	0.9
	260	0.3	0.3	0.4	0.5	0.5	0.6	0.7	0.7	0.8	0.8	0.9	1.0
	290	0.3	0.4	0.4	0.5	0.6	0.7	0.7	0.8	0.9	0.9	1.0	1.1
	320	0.3	0.4	0.5	0.6	0.6	0.7	0.8	0.9	1.0	1.0	1.1	1.2
	350	0.4	0.4	0.5	0.6	0.7	0.8	0.9	1.0	1.1	1.1	1.2	1.3
	380	0.4	0.5	0.6	0.7	0.8	0.9	1.0	1.0	1.1	1.2	1.3	1.4
	410	0.4	0.5	0.6	0.7	0.8	0.9	1.0	1.1	1.2	1.3	1.4	1.5
5	50		0.0	0.1	0.1	0.1	0.1	0.1	0.1	0.1	0.1	0.1	0.1
	80		0.0	0.1	0.1	0.1	0.1	0.2	0.2	0.2	0.2	0.2	0.2
	110		0.1	0.1	0.1	0.2	0.2	0.2	0.2	0.3	0.3	0.3	0.3
	140		0.1	0.2	0.2	0.2	0.2	0.3	0.3	0.3	0.4	0.4	0.4
	170		0.2	0.2	0.2	0.3	0.3	0.3	0.4	0.4	0.4	0.5	0.5
	200		0.2	0.2	0.3	0.3	0.3	0.4	0.4	0.5	0.5	0.5	0.6
	230		0.2	0.3	0.3	0.3	0.4	0.4	0.5	0.5	0.6	0.6	0.7
	260		0.2	0.3	0.3	0.4	0.4	0.5	0.5	0.6	0.7	0.7	0.8
	290		0.3	0.3	0.4	0.4	0.5	0.6	0.6	0.7	0.7	0.8	0.8
	320		0.3	0.4	0.4	0.5	0.5	0.6	0.7	0.7	0.8	0.9	0.9
	350		0.3	0.4	0.5	0.5	0.6	0.7	0.7	0.8	0.9	0.9	1.0
	380		0.3	0.4	0.5	0.6	0.6	0.7	0.8	0.9	1.0	1.0	1.1
	410		0.4	0.5	0.5	0.6	0.7	0.8	0.9	0.9	1.0	1.1	1.2
6	50			0.0	0.1	0.1	0.1	0.1	0.1	0.1	0.1	0.1	0.1
	80			0.0	0.1	0.1	0.1	0.1	0.1	0.1	0.2	0.2	0.2
	110			0.1	0.1	0.1	0.1	0.2	0.2	0.2	0.2	0.2	0.3
	140			0.1	0.1	0.2	0.2	0.2	0.2	0.3	0.3	0.3	0.3
	170			0.1	0.2	0.2	0.2	0.3	0.3	0.3	0.3	0.4	0.4
	200			0.2	0.2	0.2	0.3	0.3	0.3	0.4	0.4	0.4	0.5
	230			0.2	0.2	0.3	0.3	0.3	0.4	0.4	0.5	0.5	0.5
	260			0.2	0.3	0.3	0.3	0.4	0.4	0.5	0.5	0.6	0.6
	290			0.2	0.3	0.3	0.4	0.4	0.5	0.5	0.6	0.6	0.7
	320			0.3	0.3	0.4	0.4	0.5	0.5	0.6	0.6	0.7	0.7
	350			0.3	0.4	0.4	0.5	0.5	0.6	0.6	0.7	0.8	0.8
	380			0.3	0.4	0.4	0.5	0.6	0.6	0.7	0.8	0.8	0.9
	410			0.3	0.4	0.5	0.5	0.6	0.7	0.8	0.8	0.9	1.0
7	50				0.0	0.0	0.1	0.1	0.1	0.1	0.1	0.1	0.1
	80				0.0	0.1	0.1	0.1	0.1	0.1	0.1	0.1	0.2
	110				0.1	0.1	0.1	0.1	0.1	0.2	0.2	0.2	0.2
	140				0.1	0.1	0.2	0.2	0.2	0.2	0.2	0.3	0.3

Table 4 Error at the neck (mm) *(Continued)*

Sleeve length (mm)	Clearance (μm)	Offset (mm)											
		6	7	8	9	10	11	12	13	14	15	16	17
	170				0.1	0.2	0.2	0.2	0.2	0.3	0.3	0.3	0.3
	200				0.2	0.2	0.2	0.2	0.3	0.3	0.3	0.4	0.4
	230				0.2	0.2	0.2	0.3	0.3	0.3	0.4	0.4	0.4
	260				0.2	0.2	0.3	0.3	0.4	0.4	0.4	0.5	0.5
	290				0.2	0.3	0.3	0.4	0.4	0.4	0.5	0.5	0.6
	320				0.3	0.3	0.3	0.4	0.4	0.5	0.5	0.6	0.6
	350				0.3	0.3	0.4	0.4	0.5	0.5	0.6	0.6	0.7
	380				0.3	0.4	0.4	0.5	0.5	0.6	0.6	0.7	0.7
	410				0.3	0.4	0.4	0.5	0.6	0.6	0.7	0.7	0.8

the understanding that the implantologist involved in the in-office printing has to have a knowledge of the dimensions, the design and the tolerances of the components he will use for the manufacturing of the guide. Cassetta et al. [13] estimated that 62.7% of the total implant positioning error was due to the properties of the sleeve/ drill combination, when the Materialise Safe® guide system was used. Even though it is recommended that the osteotomy should be performed without exerting force to the guide [12] and with the bur led parallel to the long axis of the sleeve, this is not possible in a number of cases, especially where the mouth opening is a limiting factor or when an oblique bone ridge is encountered. It is, therefore, probable that during surgery, the drill is tilted inside the sleeve, changing the final position of the implant. Then the metallic components with their dimensions and tolerances define the maximum permissible errors. Obviously, if the drill rotates exactly at the centre of the sleeve, no error is expected. It should be noted that when a sleeve/key/drill combination is used, the expected errors of the mechanical parts should be estimated taking into account the bigger clearance value created by the key usage. To our knowledge, this is the first study to comprehensibly calculate the errors by taking into consideration the parameters that contribute to the 62.7% of the total error in guided implant surgery, as Cassetta et al. [13] stated.

We provide the analytical equations that give the opportunity to the implantologist to calculate the errors of interest for every conceivable situation, even for cases not tabulated by us. Using our simple models, the surgeon is provided with unique information about a large part of the probable errors expected in guided surgery and he/she can include these values in a risk assessment model for the results of the implant surgery.

Table 5 Multiple regression coefficients ($p < 0.0005$)

	Sleeve length	Clearance	Total length	Offset
Error at the apex	– 0.1854	0.0037	0.0453	
Error at the neck	– 0.1041	0.0018		0.0461

Elaborating further on the equations, it can be seen that for every 1 mm of increase in total length (implant length and/or offset), the errors increase by 46 μm. For every 50 μm increase in clearance, our models predict an increase in the error at the apex of 190 μm and in the error at the neck of 90 μm. Finally, for every 1 mm increase in the sleeve length, we anticipate a decrease in the error of implant positioning in the apex of 190 μm and in the error at the position of the implant neck of 100 μm. The Deviation of the implant axis is exclusively dependent on the sleeve length and the clearance and can easily be calculated. We found, in tantum with other studies, and as expected by the mathematical properties of the computation, that a longer implant with a short metal sleeve away from the neck of the implant (large offset) and a sleeve/bur combination with a large clearance will result in a large error at the neck of the implant, a larger error at the apex and a large deviation angle of the implant axis.

As an example on the implementation of our equations, we could simulate the (pilot) osteotomy for the positioning of an implant with a length of 12 mm. The implant will be placed with a 2.8 mm of diameter and 20.4 mm of length (with 0.4 mm tip), bur. The metal sleeve will be of 5 mm in length, including the lip of the sleeve and with an internal diameter of 2.89 mm. As a result, the clearance will be 90 μm. The offset is estimated as 8 mm and the total length at 20 mm, since 0.4 mm of the length of the bur is its tip and we do not expect the implant to reach that depth (The osteotomy hole is usually longer than the implant length but the error is calculated by the actual implant length). Under these parameters (total length = 12 + 8 = 20 mm, sleeve length = 5 mm, clearance = 90 μm), we calculate for the maximum errors expected due to the sleeve/drill combination:

Error at the apex = 0.29 mm

Error at the neck = 0.03 mm

And the maximum error of the implant axis deviation according to Table 4 is about 1.26°.

In addition to the equations, we produced in total three tables to present the error at the apex, the error at the neck and the axis deviation for different combinations of parameters (Tables 2, 3 and 4). We tabulated the expected errors at the apex of the implants taking into account the total length (= implant length + offset). That way, we kept our tables as slim and readable as possible. The deviation of the implant axis, in degrees, is also shown in the same table.

The vertical error at the apex of the implant was not tabulated in our study. It was estimated that the maximum vertical error at the apex was not probable to exceed 0.1 mm and therefore most of the cells on the table would be of zero value, after rounding. However, the small theoretical vertical error is in contradiction with actual final implant positions. Lee et al. [16] reported a mean vertical error of 0.935 ± 0.376 mm whilst Vercruyssen et al. [22] reported a mean overall vertical error of 0.9 ± 0.8 mm, concluding that this vertical error was the largest of all the errors possible. It seems that the vertical error is not due to properties of the mechanical components. Other factors such as the vertical sitting of the guide or the roughness of the 3d-printed sleeve may contribute as well. It is of importance that in most systems the length of the osteotomy should be longer than the length of the implant. In the case of in-office 3d printing, this has to be taken into consideration because a virtual osteotomy with the nominal length of the implant will lead to a more clinically shallow final fixture position.

The manufacturing tolerance of the metal sleeves and of the osteotomy drills may need to be included into the consideration of the errors. As an example, the company Blue Sky Bio (Blue Sky Bio, LLC, USA) [23], with as much as 75 different diameters of metal sleeves gives a manufacturing tolerance of its products of ± 50 μm. The clearance value should be estimated taking into account the expected manufacturing tolerances.

Finally, the abrasion of the sleeve, which is usually made of aluminium, caused during the drilling process, needs to be taken into account, especially for longer implants, where the drill engages the sleeve for a longer time. Horwitz et al. [24] found in their in vitro study that multiple uses of the drill and sleeve reduced the accuracy of the system. Cassetta et al. [12] using a modification on the External Hex Safe® (Materialise Dental, Leuven, Belgium) system (Group A) in order to minimise tolerance and reduce friction and damaging of the sleeve by the drill motion showed statistically improved accuracy in a retrospective clinical study. This could be interpreted as the best practice being the use of sleeves for a single time and the drills for the times recommended by the manufacturer. The abrasion of the components due to usage is not incorporated in our study.

Conclusions

The results of this study compute part of the expected maximum differences in the final clinical implant position when a CAD/CAM surgical guide is used. Given this data, the implant surgeon, with an in-office 3d printer, has the equations and the tables to acknowledge the magnitude of the probable errors and to decide the best combination of the sleeve/drill parameters in order to minimise them. Practically, the implantologist can readily decide about the dimensions of the metal sleeve, the clearance between the osteotomy bur and the sleeve and the design of the guide in relation with the distance of the lip of the sleeve to the implant neck (offset), in order to find the best combination based on the available sleeves in the free market, the osteotomy burs he/she already possesses and the clinical situation in hand.

Abbreviations

3d: Three dimensional; CAD: Computer-aided design; CAM: Computer-aided manufacturing; CBCT: Cone beam computed tomography; CI: Confidence interval; CT: Computed tomography; Dicom: Digital imaging and communications in medicine; FDM: Fused deposition modelling; GIS: Guided implant surgery; SLA: Stereolithography apparatus; STL: Surface tessellation language/stereolithography

Authors' contributions

DA conceived the study, developed the C program and did the statistical analyses. GK participated in the study design, revised the study critically for important intellectual content and did the drawings. Both authors read and approved the final manuscript.

Competing interests

Dimitrios Apostolakis and Georgios Kourakis declare that they have no competing interests.

References

1. Sarment DP, Sukovic P, Clinthorne N. Accuracy of implant placement with a stereolithographic surgical guide. Int J Oral and Maxillofac Implants. 2003;18: 571–7.
2. Komiyama A, Klinge B, Hultin M. Treatment outcome of immediately loaded implants installed in edentulous jaws following computer-assisted virtual treatment planning and flapless surgery. Clin Oral Implants Res. 2008;19: 677–85.
3. Flugge T, Derksen W, te Poel J, Hassan B, Nelson K, Wismeijer D. Registration of cone beam computer tomography data and intraoral surface scans—a prerequisite for guided implant surgery with CAD/CAM drilling guides. Clin Oral Implants Res. 2017;9:1113–8.
4. Kalt G, Gehrke P. Transfer precision of three-dimensional implant planning with CT assisted offline navigation. Int J Computerized Dent. 2008;11:213–25.
5. Schneider D, Marquardt P, Zwahlen M, Jung RE. A systematic review on the accuracy and the clinical outcome of computer-guided template-based implant dentistry. Clin Oral Implant Res. 2009;20:73–86.
6. Van de Wiele G, Teughels W, Vercruyssen M, Coucke W, Temmerman A, Quirynen M. The accuracy of guided surgery via mucosa-supported stereolithographic surgical templates in the hands of surgeons with little experience. Clin Oral Implants Res. 2015;26:1489–94.
7. Lee KM, Song JM, Cho JH, Hwang HS. Influence of head motion on the accuracy of 3D reconstruction with cone-beam CT: landmark identification errors in maxillofacial surface model. PLoS One. 2016;11:e0153210.

8. Huotilainen E, Jaanimets R, Valášek J, et al. Inaccuracies in additive manufactured medical skull models caused by the DICOM to STL conversion process. J Craniomaxillofacial Surg. 2014;42:e259–65.
9. Hazeveld A, Huddleston G, Slater J, Ren Y. Accuracy and reproducibility of dental replica models reconstructed by different rapid prototyping techniques. Am J Orthodont Dentofac Orthopaedics. 2014;145:108–15.
10. Gallardo Y, Teixeirada I, Mukai E, Morimoto S, Sesma N, Cordaro L. Accuracy comparison of guided surgery for dental implants according the tissue of support: a systematic review and meta-analysis. Clin Oral Implants Res. 2017; 28:602–12.
11. Van Assche N, Quirynen M. Tolerance within a surgical guide. Clin Oral Implants Res. 2010;21:455–8.
12. Koop R, Vercruyssen M, Vermeulen K, Quirynen M. Tolerance within the sleeve inserts of different surgical guides for guided implant surgery. Clin Oral Implants Res. 2013;24:630–4.
13. Cassetta M, Di Mambro A, Giansanti M, Stefanelli LV, Cavallini C. The intrinsic error of a stereolithographic surgical template in implant guided surgery. Int J Oral Maxillof Surg. 2013;42:264–75.
14. Schneider D, Schober F, Grohmann P, Hammerle CH, Jung RE. In-vitro evaluation of the tolerance of surgical instruments in templates for computer-assisted guided implantology produced by 3-D printing. Clin Oral Implants Res. 2015;26:320–5.
15. Cassetta M, Di Mambro A, Di Giorgio G, Stefanelli LV, Barbato E. The influence of the tolerance between mechanical components on the accuracy of implants inserted with a stereolithographic surgical guide: a retrospective clinical study. Clin Implant Dent Relat Res. 2015;17:580–8.
16. Lee DH, An SY, Hong MH, Jeon KB, Lee KB. Accuracy of a direct drill-guiding system with minimal tolerance of surgical instruments used for implant surgery: a prospective clinical study. J Advanced Prosthodontics. 2016;8:207–11.
17. Tahmaseb A, Wismeijer D, Coucke W, Derksen W. Computer technology applications in surgical implant dentistry: a systematic review. Int J Oral Maxillofac Implants. 2014;29:25–42.
18. D'haese J, Ackhurst J, Wismeijer D, De Bruyn H, Tahmaseb A. Current state of the art of computer-guided implant surgery. Periodontol. 2017;73:121–33.
19. Torres IO, De Luccia N. A simulator for training in endovascular aneurysm repair: the use of three dimensional printers. Eur J Vasc Endovasc Surg. 2017;54:247–53.
20. Dawood A, Marti B, Sauret-Jackson V, Darwood A. 3D printing in dentistry. Br Dent J. 2015;219:521–9.
21. Van Assche N, Vercruyssen M, Coucke W, Teughels W, Jacobs R, Quirynen M. Accuracy of computer-aided implant placement. Clin Oral Implants Res. 2012;23:112–23.
22. Vercruyssen M, Coucke W, Naert I, Jacobs R, Teughels W, Quirynen M. Depth and lateral deviations in guided implant surgery: an RCT comparing guided surgery with mental navigation or the use of a pilot-drill template. Clin Oral Implants Res. 2015;26:1315–132.
23. Bio Tube®: Retrieved from https://blueskybio.com/store/guide-tubes. Accessed 20 Sept 2018.
24. Horwitz J, Zuabi O, Machtei E. Accuracy of a computerized tomography-guided template-assisted implant placement system: an in vitro study. Clin Oral Implants Res. 2009;20:1156–62.

7

Radiographic outcomes following lateral alveolar ridge augmentation using autogenous tooth roots

Puria Parvini[1], Robert Sader[2], Didem Sahin[3], Jürgen Becker[3] and Frank Schwarz[1,3*]

Abstract

Background: To assess and compare the radiographic outcomes following lateral alveolar ridge augmentation using autogenous tooth roots (TR) and autogenous bone (AB) blocks.

Methods: In a total of 30 patients, lateral ridge augmentation was conducted in parallel groups using either (1) healthy autogenous tooth roots (e.g., retained wisdom or impacted teeth) ($n = 15$) or (2) cortical autogenous bone blocks harvested from the retromolar area. Cone-beam computed tomographic (CBCT) scans taken at 26 weeks of submerged healing were analyzed for the basal graft integration (i.e., contact between the graft and the host bone in %) (BI26) and the cross-sectional grafted area (mm^2) (SA26).

Results: Both groups revealed a comparable clinical width of the alveolar ridge at baseline (CWb). Mean BI26 and SA26 values amounted to 69.26 ± 26.01% (median 72.44) and 22.07 ± 12.98 mm^2 (median 18.83) in the TR group and 79.67 ± 15.66% (median 78.85) and 12.42 ± 10.11 mm^2 (median 11.36) in the AB group, respectively. Between-group differences in mean SA26 values were statistically significant ($p = 0.031$). Linear regression analysis failed to reveal any significant correlations between BI26 and CWb/SA26 values in either group.

Conclusions: TR grafts may be associated with improved SA26 values following lateral alveolar ridge augmentation.

Keywords: Clinical study, Alveolar ridge augmentation, Tooth transplantation

Background

Autogenous bone (AB) blocks harvested from intraoral donor sites (i.e., retromandibular, chin) are the most commonly used procedure for lateral alveolar ridge augmentation [1]. However, despite significant horizontal bone gains, cortical bone blocks were noted to undergo an incomplete replacement resorption [2, 3], thus featuring a composition of non-vital residual and newly formed vital bone in the former defect area [4]. Moreover, AB blocks are prone to a rapid degradation and therefore commonly combined with contour augmentation procedures using slowly resorbing particulate grafts and barrier membranes [5].

* Correspondence: f.schwarz@med.uni-frankfurt.de
[1]Department of Oral Surgery and Implantology, Carolinum, Johann Wolfgang Goethe-University, Frankfurt, Germany
[3]Department of Oral Surgery, Universitätsklinikum Düsseldorf, Düsseldorf, Germany
Full list of author information is available at the end of the article

Recent experimental studies have focused on the use of extracted tooth roots (TR) as an alternative scaffold to support bone regeneration at non-self-contained lateral alveolar ridge defects. Various outcome measures based on histological, immunohistochemical, and micro-computed tomographic analyses did not significantly differ between differently conditioned TRs (i.e., healthy, endodontically treated non-infected, periodontally diseased) and retromolar AB grafts [4, 6, 7]. The median bone-to-implant contact (BIC) values at 3 weeks following implant placement ranged from 36.96 to 50.79% in the TR group and from 32.53 to 64.10% in the AB group [4].

These preclinical data have recently been in an initial human case report [8] as well as in a prospective controlled clinical study [9]. In particular, soft tissue healing was uneventful in both TR and AB groups. The crestal ridge width at 26 weeks (CW26) amounted to 10.06 ± 1.85 mm (median 11.0) in the TR group and 9.20 ± 2.09 mm (median 8.50) in the AB group and allowed for a successful implant placement in all patients investigated [9].

The aim of the present analysis was to assess and compare the radiographic outcomes in both groups.

Methods

Study design and participants

This analysis was based on the radiographic (i.e., cone-beam computed tomographic—CBCT) data derived from a prospective controlled clinical monocenter study including a total of 30 patients [9]. Each participant exhibited either a tooth gap or a free-end situation with an inadequate horizontal ridge width and was in need of an implant-supported fixed restoration.

In brief, lateral ridge augmentation was conducted according to a standardized procedure under local anesthesia [8].

One group of patients ($n = 15$; mean age 41.93 years; range 19 to 60 years) exhibited either one or more caries-free partially/fully retained or impacted wisdom teeth without signs of local pathologies (e.g., cysts). TR grafts were separated (i.e., crown decapitation, vertical separation of multi-rooted teeth, preservation of the exposed pulp) from the extracted/surgically removed teeth and adapted in size and shape to match the defect area. At the respective downward aspect of the TR graft, the layer of cementum was carefully removed using a diamond bur to facilitate ankylosis at the recipient site [4].

Due to the absence of any suitable wisdom teeth, another group of patients ($n = 15$; mean age 44.53 years; range 21 to 60 years) was allocated to the harvesting of monocortical block grafts from the linea obliqua. Both TR and AB grafts were rigidly fixed using one to two titanium osteosynthesis screws (1.5 × 9 mm, Medicon, Tuttlingen, Germany) after gently flattening the recipient site using a round carbide bur underwater (i.e., sterile saline) cooling.

Advancement of the mucoperiosteal flaps was achieved using periosteal-releasing incisions. The coronally repositioned flaps were fixed using vertical double sutures to allow for a submerged healing period of 26 weeks (Fig. 1).

All patients had received a perioperative antibiotic (1× amoxicillin 2 g) as well as a peri- and postoperative (2 days) antiphlogistic prophylaxis (prednisolon, total of 40 mg). Analgetics (ibuprofen 600 mg) were provided according to individual needs.

The study outline and the follow-up visits are summarized in Table 1 [9].

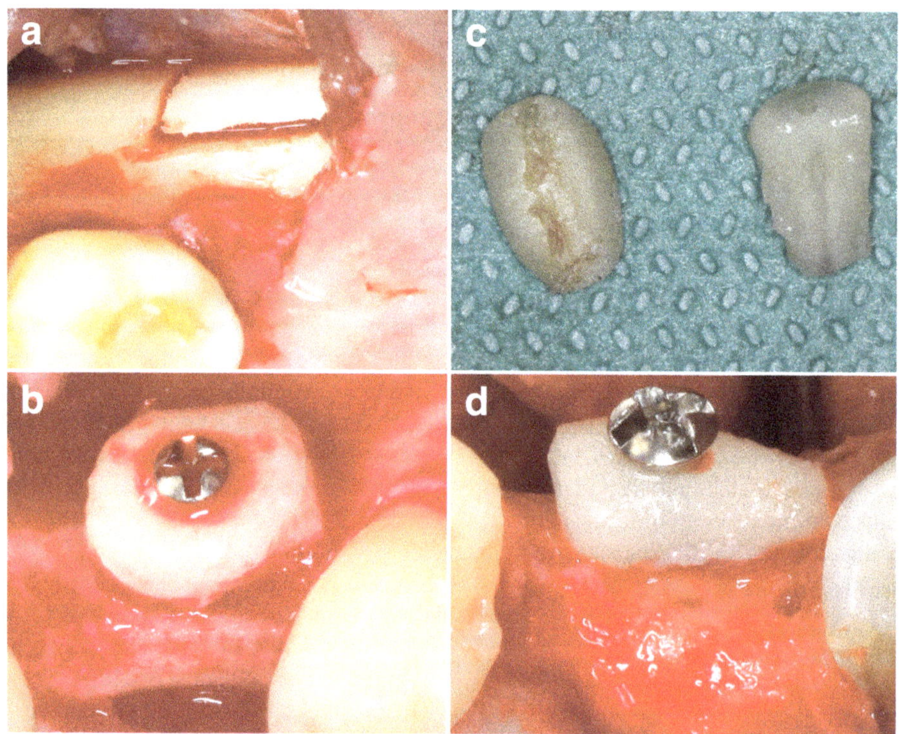

Fig. 1 Lateral ridge augmentation—a surgical procedure in the AB and TR groups. **a** The retromolar area served as a donor site for the harvesting of monocortical bone blocks in the AB group. **b** AB blocks were shaped to match the size and configuration of the defect site and fixed using one central osteosynthesis screw. **c** TR grafts were separated from either partially/fully retained or impacted wisdom teeth. **d** The most suitable specimen was positioned and fixed in a way that the exposed dentin faced the defect area, thus facilitating ankylosis at the recipient site. The crestal perforations were derived from initial attempts to pre-drill the osteosynthesis screw. All sites were left to heal in a submerged position without providing any contour augmentation procedures

Table 1 Study design and follow up visits

Visit 1	Visit 2	Visit 3	Visit 4	Visit 5	Visit 6
Recruitment	Surgery				Re-entry
	D0	D10	W4	W13	W26

D day, *W* week

Ethics, consent, and permissions

Each patient was given a detailed description of the study procedures and signed a consent to participate. The study protocol was approved by the ethics committee (4837R) of the Heinrich Heine University, Düsseldorf, Germany, and registered via the Internet Portal of the German Clinical Trials Register (DRKS00009586).

The present reporting considered the checklist items as proposed in the STROBE statement.

Inclusion and exclusion criteria

The inclusion criteria considered the following conditions: (1) age 18 to 60 years; (2) candidate for lateral ridge augmentation; (3) insufficient bone ridge width associated with a non-contained defect at the recipient site for implant placement, as evidenced intraoperatively; (4) sufficient bone height at the recipient site for implant placement, as evidenced in a preoperative panoramic radiograph; and (5) healthy oral mucosa, at least 3 mm keratinized tissue.

The exclusion criteria included the following conditions: (1) general contraindications for dental and/or surgical treatments; (2) inflammatory and autoimmune disease of the oral cavity; (3) uncontrolled diabetes (HbA1c >7%); (4) history of malignancy requiring chemotherapy or radiotherapy within the past 5 years; (5) previous immunosuppressant, bisphosphonate, or high-dose corticosteroid therapy; (6) smokers; and (7) pregnant or lactating women [9].

Clinical assessments

The clinical width (CW) of the alveolar ridge immediately before the augmentation (CWb) was assessed to the nearest 0.25 mm by means of a caliper. This was positioned at 2 mm below the crest at the most central aspect of the respective defect site, whose vertical plane was marked by the osteosynthesis screw. Measurement of CW was repeated immediately after augmentation (CWa). Graft thickness (GT) was calculated as CWa – CWb.

Radiographic assessments

According to the clinical standard procedure, CBCT scans (25 patients: PaX-i3D Green, Orangedental, Biberach, Germany, at 95 kV, 8.5–9.0 mAs; 5 patients: ProMax3D, Planmeca, Helsinki, Finland, at 90 kV, 5.6–9.0 mAs) using adjusted fields of view (i.e., 5 × 5 and 8 × 5 cm) were taken at 26 weeks for preoperative implant planning at the respective sites.

Images of the coronal planes representing the most central aspect of the respective defect sites were exported and analyzed for the basal graft integration (BI26) and the cross-sectional grafted area (mm^2) (SA26) (ImageJ). In particular, BI26 was measured as a percentage AB/TR to host bone contact along the basal graft extension serving as 100%, respectively (Fig. 2).

All measurements were performed by one previously calibrated investigator.

Sample size calculation and statistical analysis

The sample size calculation considered a standard normal distribution (type I error set at .05; type II error set at .20) and a sigma which was estimated based on the standard deviations observed in a recent preclinical animal study [4]. The clinical width of the alveolar ridge was defined as the primary outcome variable, considering a clinically relevant difference of 2 mm. A sample size of

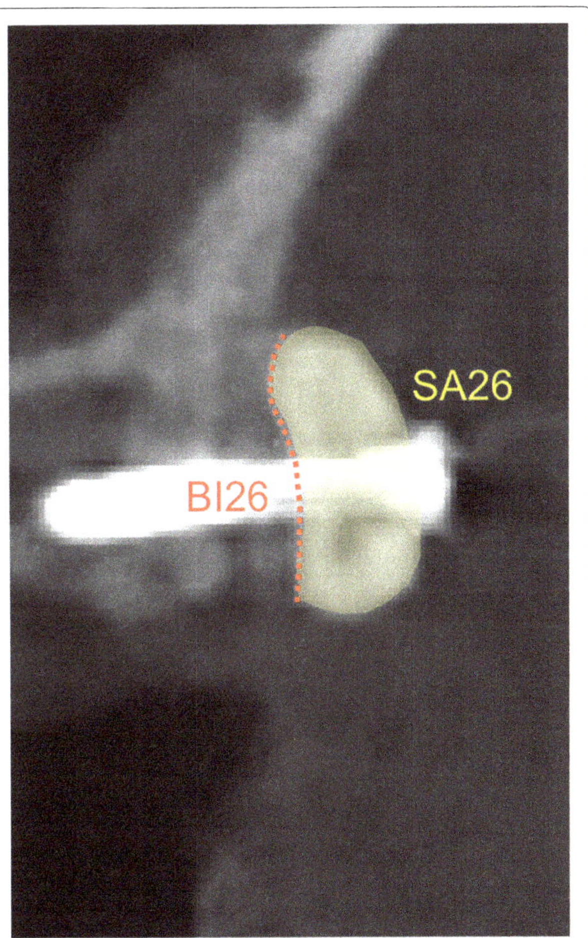

Fig. 2 Radiographic assessments. Images of the coronal planes representing the most central aspect of the respective defect sites were analyzed for the basal graft integration (i.e., contact between the graft and the host bone in %) (BI26) and the cross-sectional grafted area (mm^2) (SA26)

15 patients per group was calculated to achieve a 95% power (Power and Precision, Biostat, Englewood, USA).

The statistical analysis of the pseudonymized data sets was accomplished using a commercially available software program (IBM SPSS Statistics 24.0, IBM Corp., Armonk, NY, USA).

Mean values, standard deviations, medians, 95% confidence intervals (CI), and frequency distributions were calculated for all outcomes assessed. The data rows were examined with the Shapiro-Wilk test for normal distribution. Between-group comparisons were accomplished using the unpaired *t* test. Linear regression analyses were used to depict the relationship between BI26 and CWb as well as SA26 values in both groups. The alpha error was set at 0.05.

Results

Mean CWb and GT values were comparable in both groups and amounted to 4.53 ± 1.54 mm (median 4.50; 95% CI 3.68, 5.38) and 5.66 ± 1.75 mm (median 5.0; 95% CI 4.69, 6.64) in the TR group and 5.26 ± 1.25 mm (median 5.00; 95% CI 4.57, 5.95) and 4.96 ± 1.75 mm (median 5.0; 95% CI 4.24, 5.68) in the AB group, respectively. Between-group differences did not reach statistical significance.

Radiographic performance endpoints

Mean SA26 values were 12.42 ± 10.11 mm^2 (median 11.36; 95% CI 6.82, 18.02) in the AB group and amounted to 22.07 ± 12.98 mm^2 (median 18.83; 95% CI 14.88, 29.26) at the TR-treated sites. The resulting differences between both groups were statistically significant ($p = 0.031$).

Mean BI26 values amounted to 79.67 ± 15.66% (median 78.85; 95% CI 70.99, 88.34) in the AB group and tended to be lower at the TR-treated sites, revealing a mean value of 69.26 ± 26.01% (median 72.44; 95% CI 53.85, 82.66) (Fig. 3). These differences, however, failed to reach statistical significance ($p = 0.157$) (Table 2).

Regression analysis

In both groups investigated, the linear regression analysis failed to reveal any significant correlations between BI26 and CWb (TR: Coef. 1.106; $R^2 = 0.003$; $p = 0.851$; AB: Coef. − 0.410; $R^2 = 0.002$; $p = 0.886$) or BI26 and SA26 (TR: Coef. 0.619; $R^2 = 0.058$; $p = 0.387$; AB: Coef. 0.311; $R^2 = 0.066$; $p = 0.354$) values, respectively (Fig. 4).

Discussion

The present analysis aimed at assessing and comparing CBCT outcomes following lateral alveolar ridge augmentation using TR and AB grafts. After a healing period of 26 weeks, it was observed that TR grafts were associated with significantly higher mean SA26 values when compared with the AB group. A similar tendency was also noted for mean BI26 values; however, this difference did not reach statistical significance.

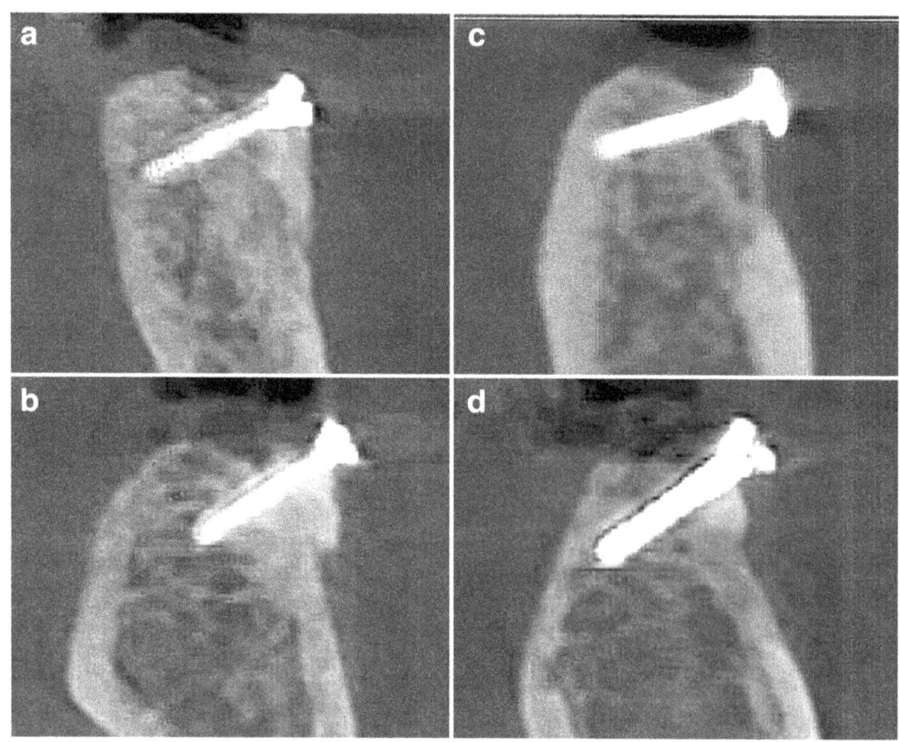

Fig. 3 Representative CBCT outcomes at 26 weeks. **a**, **b** TR graft. **c**, **d** AB graft

Table 2 Secondary performance endpoints (in mm)

	CWb	GT	SA26	BI26
a) TR group ($n = 15$ patients)				
Mean	4.53	5.66	22.07*	69.26
SD	1.54	1.75	12.98	26.01
Median	4.50	5.00	18.83	72.44
95% CI	3.68, 5.38	4.69, 6.64	14.88, 29.26	53.85, 82.66
b) AB group ($n = 15$ patients)				
Mean	5.26	4.96	12.42	79.67
SD	1.25	1.30	10.11	15.66
Median	5.00	5.00	11.36	78.85
95% CI	4.57, 5.95	4.24, 5.68	6.82, 18.02	70.99, 88.34

Comparisons between the groups (unpaired t test): $*p = 0.031$
CWb clinical width of the alveolar ridge immediately before augmentation (D0) (mm), *GT* graft thickness immediately after augmentation (D0) (mm), *SA26* surface area at 26 weeks (W26) (mm^2), *BI26* basal integration at 26 weeks (W26) (%)

When interpreting these results, it must be kept in mind that both groups were associated with comparable CWb and GT values at baseline. However, the clinical re-entry at 26 weeks revealed that mean CW values amounted to 10.06 ± 1.85 mm (median 11.0; 95% CI 9.03, 11.09) in the TR group and 9.20 ± 2.09 mm (median 8.50; 95% CI 8.04, 10.35) in the AB group, respectively. This was associated with a significantly higher gain in ridge width of 5.53 ± 1.88 mm (median 5.00; 95% CI 4.48, 6.57) at TR- over the AB-treated sites (3.93 ± 1.41 mm; median 4.00; 95% CI 3.15, 4.71) [9]. This difference was mainly due to a lower graft resorption in the TR group, which was basically confirmed by the present analysis of SA26 values. Moreover, a recent animal study employing both TR and AB grafts for lateral alveolar ridge augmentation also corroborates, at least in part, the differences in mean SA26 values noted between both groups. In particular, after 12 weeks of healing, the histomorphometrical analysis of the augmented area (AA) at the TR-treated sites ranged between 7.55 and 11.20 mm^2, whereas the median values ranged between 6.60 and 8.56 mm^2 at the AB-treated sites [4]. Similar AA values were also noted when assessing the efficacy of TR grafts that were derived from the periodontally diseased teeth, resulting in 11.01 ± 4.37 mm^2 as compared to 8.07 ± 5.64 mm^2 noted in the AB group [6].

However, previous clinical studies suggest that the resorption of AB grafts may be limited by a simultaneous contour augmentation (e.g., application of a bovine-derived xenograft and coverage by a native collagen membrane) [5, 10]. In particular, CBCT analyses at 10 years revealed only a minor superficial resorption of about 7.7%, which corresponded to 0.38 mm [10].

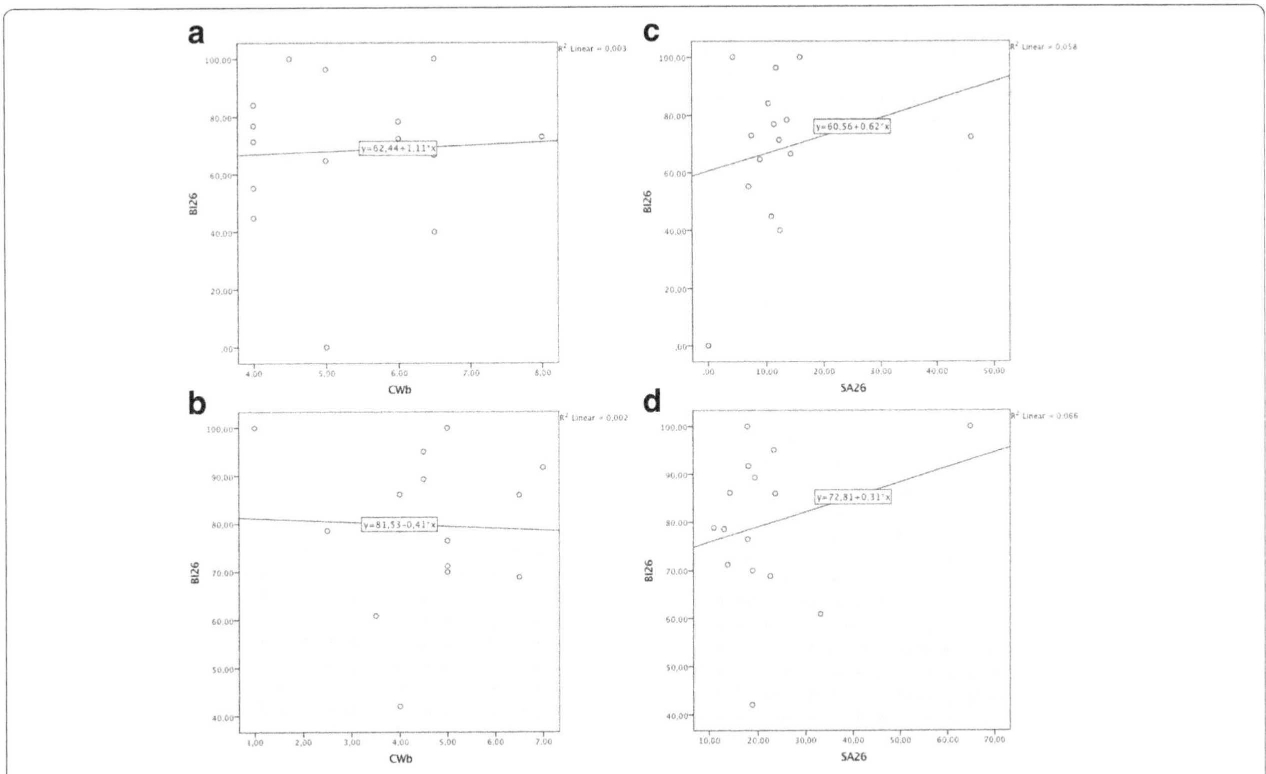

Fig. 4 Linear regression plots to depict the relationship between BI26 and CWb/SA26 values. **a** CWb (TR group). **b** CWb (AB group). **c** SA26 (TR group). **d** SA26 (AB group)

When further analyzing the present data, it was also noted that both TR and AB grafts were associated with comparable BI26 values, thus corroborating the clinical observation of a firm graft connection to the host bone at 26 weeks, which allowed for a proper placement of adequately dimensioned titanium implants at all sites investigated [9]. The regression analysis also revealed that BI26 values were neither related to CWb nor SA26 values. These clinical and radiographic observations are also supported by recent histological analyses pointing to a basal ankylosis and replacement resorption of both TR and AB grafts [4, 6, 7].

Conclusions

In conclusion and within its limitations, the present clinical study revealed that TR grafts may be associated with improved SA26 values following lateral alveolar ridge augmentation.

Funding

The study was funded by a grant of the Deutsche Forschungsgemeinschaft (DFG), Bonn, Germany. The titanium implants were provided by the Institut Straumann, AG, Basel, Switzerland.

Authors' contributions

FS, RS, and JB have made substantial contributions to the study conception, acquisition, and interpretation of data as well as manuscript preparation. PP and DS were involved in the data acquisition, data management, and analysis as well as the statistical analysis. All authors read and approved the final manuscript.

Competing interests

Puria Parvini, Robert Sader, Didem Sahin, Jürgen Becker, and Frank Schwarz declare that they have no competing interests.

Author details

[1]Department of Oral Surgery and Implantology, Carolinum, Johann Wolfgang Goethe-University, Frankfurt, Germany. [2]Department for Oral, Cranio-Maxillofacial and Facial Plastic Surgery, Medical Center of the Goethe University Frankfurt, Frankfurt, Germany. [3]Department of Oral Surgery, Universitätsklinikum Düsseldorf, Düsseldorf, Germany.

References

1. Sanz-Sanchez I, Ortiz-Vigon A, Sanz-Martin I, Figuero E, Sanz M. Effectiveness of lateral bone augmentation on the alveolar crest dimension: a systematic review and meta-analysis. J Dent Res. 2015;94(9 Suppl):128–42.
2. Burchardt H. The biology of bone graft repair. Clin Orthop Relat Res. 1983; 174:28–42.
3. Burchardt H, Enneking WF. Transplantation of bone. Surg Clin North Am. 1978;58(2):403–27.
4. Schwarz F, Golubovic V, Becker K, Mihatovic I. Extracted tooth roots used for lateral alveolar ridge augmentation: a proof-of-concept study. J Clin Periodontol. 2016;43(4):345–53.
5. Cordaro L, Amade DS, Cordaro M. Clinical results of alveolar ridge augmentation with mandibular block bone grafts in partially edentulous patients prior to implant placement. Clin Oral Implants Res. 2002;13(1):103–11.
6. Schwarz F, Golubovic V, Mihatovic I, Becker J. Periodontally diseased tooth roots used for lateral alveolar ridge augmentation. A proof-of-concept study. J Clin Periodontol. 2016;43(9):797–803.
7. Becker K, Drescher D, Hönscheid R, Golubovic V, Mihatovic I, Schwarz F. Biomechanical, micro-computed tomographic and immunohistochemical analysis of early osseous integration at titanium implants placed following lateral ridge augmentation using extracted tooth roots. Clin Oral Implants Res. 2017;28(3):334–40.
8. Schwarz F, Schmucker A, Becker J. Initial case report of an extracted tooth root used for lateral alveolar ridge augmentation. J Clin Periodontol. 2016; 43(11):985–9.
9. Schwarz F, Hazar D, Becker K, Sader R, Becker J. Efficacy of autogenous tooth roots for lateral alveolar ridge augmentation and staged implant placement. A prospective controlled clinical study. J Clin Periodontol. 2018; https://doi.org/10.1111/jcpe.12977.
10. Chappuis V, Cavusoglu Y, Buser D, von Arx T. Lateral ridge augmentation using autogenous block grafts and guided bone regeneration: a 10-year prospective case series study. Clin Implant Dent Relat Res. 2017;19(1):85–96.

Retrospective cohort study of a tapered implant with high primary stability in patients with local and systemic risk factors—7-year data

Sotirios Konstantinos Saridakis[1*], Wilfried Wagner[1] and Robert Noelken[1,2]

Abstract

Objectives: This retrospective study examined the mid- to long-term clinical and radiographic performance of a tapered implant in various treatment protocols in patients with local and systemic risk factors (RFs).

Material and methods: Two hundred seven NobelActive implants were inserted in 98 patients in the period from 10/2008 to 02/2015. The subdivision of the cohort was defined by local ($n = 40$), systemic ($n = 6$), local and systemic ($n = 8$), or without any RFs ($n = 44$) to analyze implant survival and marginal bone levels.

Results: Fifteen implants failed within the follow-up period. The mean follow-up period of the remaining implants was 34 months (range 12 to 77 months). The cumulative survival rate according to Kaplan-Meier was 91.5%. The survival rate for 93 implants in 45 patients with no RFs was 94.8% whereas it was 94% for 83 implants in 48 patients with local RFs ($p = 0.618$), 81.3% for 14 implants in 6 patients with systemic RFs ($p = 0.173$), and 76.5% for 17 implants in 6 patients with local and systemic risk factors ($p = 0.006$). The interproximal marginal bone level was -0.49 ± 0.83 mm at the mesial aspect and -0.51 ± 0.82 mm at the distal aspect in relation to implant shoulder level and showed no relevant difference in the various risk factor groups.

Conclusions: It can be assumed that the negative effects of the local or/and systemic risk factors were partially compensated by the primary stability and grade of osseointegration of the NobelActive implant.

Clinical relevance: The use of this system in patients with risk factors and immediate loading procedures.

Keywords: Local risk factors, Systemic risk factors, Immediate implant placement, Immediate provisionalization, Long-term results, Implant design, Primary stability

Introduction

Based on published demographic data, the median age of the world population constantly increases [1]. This has led to an increase in the number of dental implants inserted in senior individuals with local and systemic risk factors [2]. Nevertheless, despite numerous studies having been conducted on this topic, the results remain controversial, almost 50 years after the first dental implant placement, and there remains no consensus regarding the factors influencing success rates in implant dentistry.

In the presence of diabetes, there is a delayed wound healing [3], especially in patients with poor glycemic control [4]. In both experimental [5] and clinical [6] studies, a reduced osseointegration was noticed, which may have led to an increased risk of failure. Other studies [7] have alluded to the impact of radiation exposure and its side effects like xerostomia and mucositis, which may have also increased the risk for implant failure. It is believed that the irradiated hypocellular, hypovascular, and hypoxic tissues are the main cause of failures in dental implant osseointegration. Moreover, in patients who are undergoing or who earlier received treatment

* Correspondence: ksaridak@gmail.com
[1]Department of Oral and Maxillofacial Surgery – Plastic Surgery, University Medical Center, Johannes Gutenberg University of Mainz, Augustusplatz 2, 55131 Mainz, Germany
Full list of author information is available at the end of the article

with cortisone or chemotherapy, implant placement might lead to loss of osseointegration [8].

In addition to systemic factors, there are also several local factors that may affect implant survival. Any factor or condition that may potentially lead to loss of primary stability should be considered as a risk for implant survival and must be detected and treated early. Such factors are the presence of severe, untreated periodontitis [9, 10], prior endodontic [11] or implant treatment at the placement site [12], previous trauma [13], alveolar clefts [14], and any other factors causing large bony defects.

Despite the existing risk factors, dental implants continue to gain popularity, and in recent years, there is an increasing demand for immediate loading and provisionalization combined with high esthetic expectations. There are several techniques and systems developed, and it can be considered that implant survival rates, although they are directly correlated to variable biological factors, approach those of traditional techniques [15]. The overall treatment time is reduced, which generally increases patient satisfaction [16].

Primary stability is a prerequisite for successful osseointegration and remains the most significant factor for the survival of dental implants [16]. Therefore, current research focuses on amelioration of existing augmentation techniques and materials or on the development of new implants with self-tapping properties for improving bone contact as well for increasing primary stability.

The aim of this clinical study was to evaluate implant survival and marginal bone level in patients with or without local and/or systemic risk factors treated with NobelActive (Nobel Biocare, Zurich, Switzerland) implants after a 2- to 7-year follow-up.

Material and methods

Patients

One hundred and ten patients were invited for follow-up evaluation. All patients were treated in the period from 10/2008 to 02/2015 in the Clinic of Oral and Maxillofacial Surgery, University Medical Center Mainz. Inclusion criteria were as follows: implant placement of a NobelActive implant, study subjects over 18 years old, residual bone dimension in the edentulous region of at least 5 mm in height and 4 mm in width, placement torque of at least 35 Ncm, non-smokers, and a follow-up period of least 1 year after implant placement. Exclusion criterion was treatment with bisphosphonates.

From a total of 110 invited patients, 98 patients showed up for a follow-up evaluation of the clinical and radiological status of the implants and fulfilled the abovementioned criteria. Twelve patients were dropped out because of sudden death ($n = 1$), moved to another place ($n = 4$) and were incompliant and did not appear for the follow-up ($n = 7$). The rest 98 patients included into the study were stratified into different groups according to risk factors (RFs) (local, systematic, both of them, or without risk factor), implant region, implant diameter, implant length, time of implant placement, and time of implant restoration.

Systematic risk factors included poorly controlled diabetes (HbA1c > 7%), irradiation (range; 58–64 Gy), chemotherapy ("EURO-E.W.I.N.G.99"—consisted of vincristin, ifosfamid, doxorubicin, and etoposid in one patient after resection of a sarcoma in the upper jaw), long-term therapy with corticosteroids (≥ 7.5 mg of prednisone equivalent per day during at least 90 days consecutive) [17, 18], and presence of Marfan syndrome. Local risk factors included history of severe [19, 20] periodontitis (clinical attachment loss > 5 mm)—which was not active at the time of implant placement—unsuccessful endodontic treatment with periapical pathology, implant placement in cases with moderate or severe bone defects (> 4 mm need for augmentation according to the Cologne Classification of alveolar ridge defects [21]), and replacement after removal of a previous implant (Table 1). Other co-existent diseases that do not influence the implant survival were not considered systemic risk factors.

These patients received a total of 207 NobelActive implants (Nobel Biocare, Zurich, Switzerland) placed by two experienced surgeons. Between November 2011 and February 2015, 188 implants were placed in the maxilla, and 19 implants in the mandible. All implant placement procedures were conducted at the Department of Oral and Maxillofacial Surgery of the University Medical Center, Mainz, Germany. Fifty-four implants were placed immediately after extraction, and 153 implants were placed after osseous consolidation of the extraction sockets.

Additional simultaneous bone grafting procedures, all of which were done using autologous bone, were required at 113 implant sites; another 24 sites required

Table 1 Distribution of patients with local and systemic risk factors

Systemic RF	No. of implants ($n = 31$)	No. of patients ($n = 14$)	Local RF	No. of implants ($n = 100$)	No. of patients ($n = 54$)
Diabetes	8	5	Infection	30	15
Radio(chemo) therapy	17	6	Bone defect	49	14
Cortisone medication	2	2	Implant removal	31	25
Marfan syndrome	4	1			
Total	*31*	*14*		*100*	54

soft tissue augmentation with subepithelial connective tissue grafts.

Sixty-five implants were provisionalized immediately. After a healing time of at least 3 months, the final restoration was delivered. One hundred thirty implants received single-tooth restoration with a crown, 26 were loaded by an implant bridge, 19 were loaded by an implant bridge with a distal cantilever, and 32 implants were used to anchor a removable denture.

The reason for tooth removal was an endodontic failure in 38, a perio-endodontic lesion in 16, a large cyst in 11, a trauma in 24, and severe periodontitis in 56 sites. In 31 sites, a failed implant had to be removed, and in 31 sites, a pronounced bone defect was present.

The study type is a solely retrospective analysis of data obtained during follow-up in a cohort of patients treated with a CE-certified implant in a University Medical Center. Since the product is already approved in accordance with the German Medical Devices Act, additional ethics approval was not required for treatment. The study was conducted according to the principles stated in the Helsinki Declaration. Informed consent was obtained from the patient prior to any examination that was carried out for study purposes.

Surgical technique and restoration

The cornerstones of the surgical procedure were:

- Preservation of all alveolar socket walls via longitudinal extraction after periotomy avoiding oro-vestibular luxation.
- Meticulous cleaning of the extraction site.
- Placement of rather long implants that allow for a high level of primary stability.
- Implant dimensions were as follows: implant length 8.5 mm, 24 implants; 10 mm, 6 implants; 11.5 mm, 64 implants; 13 mm, 80 implants; 15 mm, 31 implants; and 18 mm, 2 implants. Implant diameters were as follows: 3.0 mm, 25 implants; 3.5 mm, 84 implants; 4.3 mm, 90 implants; and 5 mm, 8 implants.
- If required, simultaneous reconstruction of the facial bony lamella via autologous bone chips harvested at the mandibular ramus.
- Immediate restoration by temporary crown or bridgework either by individual chairside contouring and adjustment of acrylic resin denture teeth or by lab-fabricated restorations (in case of multiple teeth); all provisional restorations were delivered on the day of implant placement and adjusted to clear all contacts in centric occlusion and during eccentric movements.
- Final restoration was delivered after 3 to 6 months.

Follow-up and definition of outcome variables

Patients were examined clinically and radiographically at the time of implant placement and at least 12 months after implant placement. The primary outcome variable was the implant survival rate.

The secondary outcome parameter was the marginal bone level, which was determined using digital sequential periapical radiographs (XIOS XG Supreme, Dentsply Sirona, Bensheim). To ensure reproducibility between the examinations, radiographs were taken with paralleling technique using commercially available film holders (Dentsply/Rinn, Elgin, IL, USA). Specifically, the vertical distance between the implant shoulder and the bone level (mesial and distal) at the implant was measured. The distance was recorded to the nearest 0.1 mm using $\times 7$ magnification. Attachment levels apical to the implant shoulder were designated as negative values.

Statistical analysis

Survival probabilities were estimated by the Kaplan-Meier method on a "per implant" basis [14]. The endpoint of interest was implant failure. To compare the survival distribution of two samples (no RF, local RF, systemic RF, local and systemic RF; maxilla vs. mandible; different implant diameters and lengths; immediate vs. delayed placement; immediate restoration and immediate provisionalization vs. other treatment concepts; with or without bone grafting), the log-rank test was used.

Subpopulations within the study group (immediate vs. delayed placement) were compared using the Wilcoxon-Mann-Whitney non-parametric U test. The reported p values were two sided. All calculations were carried out using SPSS for Mac, Version 22 (SPSS Inc., Chicago, IL, USA).

Results

Ninety-eight patients with 207 implants complied with the treatment protocol attended the follow-up.

Implant survival

During the follow-up period, 15 implants failed in 12 patients. Age and gender were not correlated with a lower implant survival. The implant losses occurred in a time range between 0.5 and 39 months following implant placement (mean 7.3 ± 11.1 months). The reasons for implant failure were loss of osseointegration ($n = 11$), peri-implantitis ($n = 2$), occlusal trauma ($n = 1$), and mechanical complication ($n = 1$). From these 15 failures, 6 implants failed after delivery of the final prosthetic restoration while 9 implants failed without being prosthetically restored. The majority of failures ($n = 13$) occurred during the first year after placement (Table 2).

Cumulative survival rates (SRs) were 91.5% for all implants (Fig. 1). The remaining 194 implants in 88 patients

Table 2 Clinical parameters and reason for implant failures of 15 implants in 12 patients

Region	Systemic RF	Local RF	Immediate procedure	Bone grafting	Time of failure (months)	Reason
26	No	Periodontitis	Immediate restoration	No	5	Screw fracture
15	Marfan syndrome	No	No	Yes	39	Peri-implantitis
14	No	No	No	No	1	Loss of osseointegration
22	No	Defect	Immediate placement	Yes	3	Loss of osseointegration
15	No	Former impl. removal	Immediate placement	Yes	10	Loss of osseointegration
22	No	Defect	No	Yes	3	Loss of osseointegration
24	No	Periodontitis	Immediate placement/restoration	Yes	28	Peri-implantitis
12	Radiochemotherapy	Defect	No	Yes	3	Loss of osseointegration
13	Radiochemotherapy	Defect	No	Yes	3	Loss of osseointegration
22	Radiochemotherapy	Defect	No	Yes	3	Loss of osseointegration
23	Radiochemotherapy	Defect	No	Yes	3	Loss of osseointegration
23	No	No	Immediate placement/restoration	Yes	4	Loss of osseointegration
22	Diabetes	No	Immediate restoration	No	1	Occlusal trauma
12	No	Defect	Immediate placement	Yes	1	Loss of osseointegration
32	No	No	No	No	1	Loss of osseointegration

were evaluated 12 to 77 months (mean 33.9 ± 14.7 months) following implant placement. Two more implants in 2 patients failed in this period.

The survival rate for 93 implants in 45 patients with no RFs was 94.8% whereas it was 94% for 83 implants in 48 patients with only local RFs (log rank, $p = 0.618$), 81.3% for 14 implants in 6 patients with only systemic RFs ($p = 0{,}173$), and 76.5% for 17 implants in 6 patients with both local and systemic risk factors ($p = 0.006$) (Fig. 2). The survival rate of implants in patients with no RFs compared to those with local and systemic RFs displayed a significant difference.

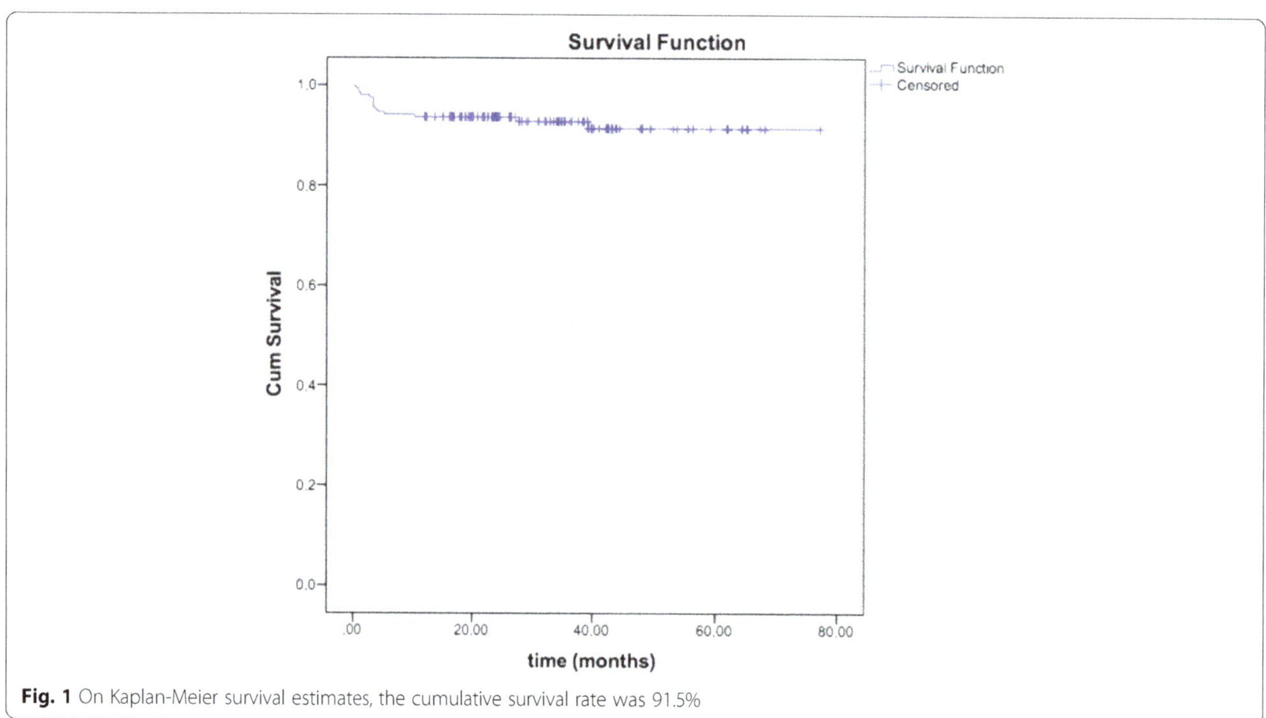

Fig. 1 On Kaplan-Meier survival estimates, the cumulative survival rate was 91.5%

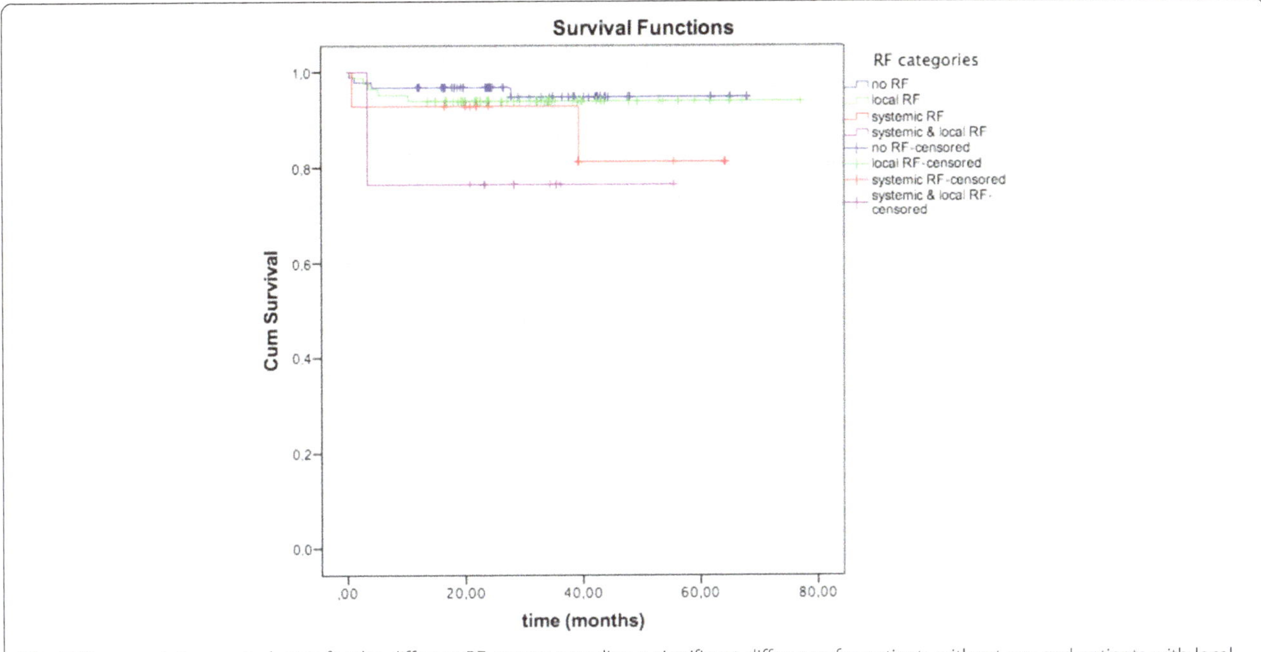

Fig. 2 The cumulative survival rates for the different RF groups revealing a significant difference for patients without any and patients with local and systemic RFs (log rank, $p = 0.006$)

The implant survival was 91.3% in maxilla ($n = 188$) while it was 94.7% in mandible ($n = 19$) (log rank, $p = 0.788$). One hundred twenty-two implants were placed in the anterior region, 65 in the premolar region, and 20 in the molar region. From the total of 15 implant removals (SR 92.7%), 11 (SR 90.98%) occurred in the anterior region, 3 (SR 95.38%) in the premolar region, and 1 (SR 95.0%) in the molar region, so no significant difference was found regarding implant survival rate between the regions (log rank, $p = 0.478$). The implant diameter and length did not show any difference in survival rate. Delayed implant placement ($n = 153$, 91.9%) did not reveal a significant higher survival rate than implants placed immediately into extraction sites ($n = 54$, 90%) ($p = 0.603$). Delayed loaded implants ($n = 142$, 93%) did not show a significant higher survival rate than immediately provisionalized implants ($n = 65$, 89.3%) ($p = 0.935$). The treatment concept of immediate implant placement and immediate provisionalization (IPP, $n = 30$) did not have a negative impact on implant survival (IPP 92.1%, all other implants ($n = 177$) 91.4%, $p = 0.809$). Although the implant survival was lower in the group of implants with simultaneous bone grafting ($n = 113$, 88.1%) compared to those without ($n = 94$, 95.7%), the difference did not reach the level of significance ($p = 0.151$).

Marginal bone levels

Regarding the implant shoulder level, the average interproximal marginal bone level was − 0.49 ± 0.83 mm (range, 0 to − 3.3 mm) at the mesial aspect and − 0.51 ± 0.82 mm (range, 0 to − 3.9 mm) at the distal aspect of the implants.

When the marginal bone level was considered as a function of time, there was no strict correlation between the marginal bone status and the length of the follow-up period ($r = 0.025$, $p = 0.764$; Spearman rank correlation coefficient), suggesting that bone levels remained, by and large, stable during the observation period.

No relevant difference of marginal bone level was noticed for implants in the different risk factor groups (no RF − 0.53 ± 0.82, local RF − 0.50 ± 0.67, systemic RF − 0.63 ± 0.64, local and systemic RF − 0.17 ± 0.23).

The marginal bone level for implants inserted immediately (− 0.46 ± 0.68 mm) or delayed (− 0.52 ± 0.75 mm) did not show a difference ($p = 0.676$).

Discussion

Most implant studies deal only with local risk factors, although the existence of systemic risk factors plays a significant role to the implant survival. We use the NobelActive dental implant in this study in order to investigate if this promising implant with the special design could achieve better survival rates in difficult situations with several risk factors. The present study revealed no statistically significant difference in the survival rate of implants between patients with systemic RFs and healthy controls. The only statistically significant difference concerned implants of patients with both systemic and local RFs ($p = 0.006$).

Despite the heterogeneity of the studies, it appears that diabetes (both types) [22, 23] is related to delayed wound healing [24], alterations in early bone healing due to poor glycemic control [25], and marginal bone loss [26, 27]. Moreover, greater failure rates were found in patients who had diabetes for longer time periods [28]. Other studies, however, did not find a difference in survival rates between diabetics and healthy patients [29, 30].

Our study included a patient after resection of an Ewing sarcoma in the left maxilla who was treated with dental implants 2 years after the hemimaxillectomy and 1 year after the completion of the combined radiochemotherapy in order to achieve an oral rehabilitation. 3 months after the insertion of six implants; four of them should be removed because of lack of osseointegration. At the moment of the implant placement as well as at the moment of the implant removals, there was no recurrence of the sarcoma. Studies comparing patients that had undergone radiation treatments and non-irradiated controls have found similarly ambiguous results [31]. Ihde et al. [32] exhibited a two to three times greater failure rate in irradiated bone compared to non-irradiated. Curi et al. showed that mode of radiation therapy delivery ($p = 0.005$) had a statistically significant influence on implant survival [33].

In one patient with three implants and long intake of corticosteroids against rheumatoid arthritis (7.5 mg prednisolone per day for at least 2 years), no complication was detected in our study. Long-term use of corticosteroids can also lead to implant failures, according to Wood and Vermilyea [34] by modifying the patient's response to bacterial infection [35], but at the present time, there is no important consideration for avoiding implant placement in those patients [36].

One implant removal was also performed on a patient with Marfan syndrome. While there are no reports in the literature regarding implant placement in patients with Marfan syndrome [37], analytical studies of bone mineral density reported adult patients demonstrated a high risk for developing osteoporosis [38]. Implant failures in postmenopausal women with osteoporosis [39] can lead to an assumption that this category of patients might be in higher risk for implant loss.

Our study showed no statistically significant difference between groups with local RFs such as periodontitis or implant placement in areas with a previous endodontic treatment and without any RFs. Hultin et al. [40] reported that a local specific inflammatory reaction related to the presence of bacteria occurs around the implants leading to marginal bone loss and infection (peri-implantitis) and that its incidence is four times higher in patients with history of chronic periodontitis than in patients who have never manifested periodontal disease. Moreover, patients without history of periodontitis present an average of 96.5% of implant survival in comparison to 90.5% of survival in individuals with history of periodontitis [40, 41]. Similar findings [42] were observed by the development of a retrograde peri-implantitis and how it affects the implant either from an adjacent tooth or from remaining infected periapical tissue in the prior position of the tooth [13]. The incidence of retrograde peri-implantitis was 7.8% in a study of 128 implants placed in areas adjacent to the teeth that had received endodontic treatment [43]. The mechanism of this procedure is considered multifaceted [15].

The survival rate for 93 implants in 45 patients with no RFs was 94.8%. Moraschini et al. [44] have exhibited in their systematic review, based on 7711 implants, similar SRs with cumulative mean values of 94.6%. Moreover, in the subcohort of our study, by 44 of the above 93, implants were performed immediate procedures (25 immediate implantations, 35 immediate restorations, 16 both of them) so the survival rate could be also correlated with studies tasking with immediate procedures as well [45–47].

Very encouraging results came out by a secondary implant placement in areas of previous removed implants. Only one implant was lost out of a total of 31, which translates to a survival rate of 96.8%. According to studies by Grossmann and Levin [12] and Greenstein and Cavallaro [48], survival rates ranged between 50 and 100%.

The timing of implant placement and prosthetic restoration showed no statistically significant influence in our study. A meta-analysis of Hartog et al. [41] showed a survival rate of 95.5% and no difference between immediate, immediate-delayed, and delayed implant placement in the esthetic zone. Schropp et al. [49] used CBCT technology to test the remaining vestibular bone in conventional implant placements and immediate procedures and came to no statistically significant differences regarding bone preservation. Esposito et al. [46] demonstrated an increased risk of implant failure in patients after immediate implant placement (9%) when compared to delayed implant placement (2%). In our study, we found no significant difference between delayed implant placement ($n = 153$, 91.9%) and immediate implant placement ($n = 54$, 90%) ($p = 0.603$). Finally, Rocci et al. [47] presented the results of a study looking at a 9-year follow-up of Brånemark implants with a survival rate of immediately loaded implants of 92.2% that was very similar to the results of this study.

We found no difference of survival rate between implants with and without augmentation procedures. The relative lower implant survival rate of implants with augmentation procedures ($n = 113$, 88.1%) compared to those without ($n = 94$, 95.7%) can be explained from the fact that the sites needed augmentation showed a significant bone loss that maybe cannot be compensated from the augmentation procedure.

A major weakness of the study is the relative small size of the group with systemic RFs (14 implants by 6 patients) as well as of the group with systematic and local RFs (17 implants by 6 patients). Because of the relative small size of the sample, this study can provide the basis for further investigations based on larger patient samples.

Conclusions

This study was based on the recruitment of a quite heterogeneous group of patients treated with NobelActive implants, for the purpose of investigating the influence of local and systemic risk factors on implant survival and marginal bone levels. It can be considered that the presence of local or systemic risk factors does not influence implant survival whereas the combination of local and systemic risk factors reveals significantly lower implant survival.

Acknowledgements

Not applicable

Funding

The work was supported by the Clinic of Oral and Maxillofacial Surgery, University Medical Center, Mainz.

Authors' contributions

SKS has participated in the preoperative planning of the implantations, in the operations, and in the follow-up of the patients. This article contains data of the dissertation of SKS which was published in the Medical University of Mainz on 22.03.2016. WW has participated in the preoperative planning of the implantations, in the operations, and in the follow-up of the patients and was the supervisor of the above dissertation. RN has participated in the preoperative planning of the implantations, in the operations, and in the follow-up of the patients and was the supervisor of this article. All authors read and approved the final manuscript.

Competing interests

Sotirios Konstantinos Saridakis, Wilfried Wagner, and Robert Noelken declare that they have no competing interests.

Author details

[1]Department of Oral and Maxillofacial Surgery – Plastic Surgery, University Medical Center, Johannes Gutenberg University of Mainz, Augustusplatz 2, 55131 Mainz, Germany. [2]Private Practice for Oral Surgery, Lindau/Lake Constance, Germany.

References

1. U.S. Census Bureau, 2012 Population Estimates and 2014 National Projections. [Zitiert:18.12.2014]. https://www.census.gov/data/tables/2014/demo/popproj/2014-summary-tables.html.
2. Ikebe K, Wada M, Kagawa R, Maeda Y. Is old age a risk factor for dental implants? Jpn Dent Sci Rev. 2009;45:59–64.
3. Hu SC, Lan CE. High-glucose environment disturbs the physiologic functions of keratinocytes: focusing on diabetic wound healing. J Dermatol Sci.2016;84(2):121–27.
4. Liddelow G, Klineberg I. Patient-related risk factors for implant therapy. A critique of pertinent literature. Aust Dent J. 2011;56(4):417–26.
5. Schlegel KA, Prechtl C, Möst T, Seidl C, Lutz R, von Wilmowsky C. Osseointegration of SLActive implants in diabetic pigs. Clin Oral Implants Res. 2013;24(2):128–34.
6. Moy PK, Medina D, Shetty V, Aghaloo TL. Dental implant failure rates and associated risk factors. Int J Oral Maxillofac Implants. 2005;20:569–77.
7. Shugaa-Addin B, Al-Shamiri H-M, Al-Maweri S, Tarakji B. The effect of radiotherapy on survival of dental implants in head and neck cancer patients. J Clin Exp Dent. 2016;8(2):e194–200.
8. Alsaadi G, Quirynen M, Komárek A, van Steenberghe D. Impact of local and systemic factors on the incidence of oral implant failures, up to abutment connection. J Clin Periodontol. 2007;34(7):610–7 Epub 2007.
9. Casado PL, Pereira MC, Duarte ME, Granjeiro JM. History of chronic periodontitis is a high risk indicator for peri-implant disease. Braz Dent J. 2013;24(2):136–41.
10. Wen X, Liu R, Li G, Deng M, Liu L, Zeng XT, Nie X. History of periodontitis as a risk factor for a long-term survival of dental implants: a metaanalysis. Int J Oral Maxillofac Implants. 2014;29(6):1271–80.
11. Chaffee NR, Lowden K, Tiffee JC, Cooper LF. Periapical abscess formation and resolution adjacent to dental implants: a clinical report. J Pros- thet Dent. 2001;85:109–12.
12. Grossmann Y, Levin L. Success and survival of single dental implants placed in sites of previously failed implants. J Periodontol. 2007;78(9):1670–4.
13. Romanos G, Stuart F, Costa-Martins S, Meitner S, Tarnow D. Implant periapical lesions: etiology and treatment options. J Oral Implantol. 2011;XXXVII(1):53–63.
14. Kramer FJ, Baethge C, Swennen G, Bremer B, Schwestka-Polly R, Dempf R. Dental implants in patients with orofacial clefts: a long-term follow-up study. Int JOral Maxillofac Surg. 2005;34:715–21.
15. Ortega-Martinez J, Perez-Pascual T, Mareque-Bueno S, Hernandez-Alfaro F, Ferres-Padro E. Immediate implants following tooth extraction. A systemic review. Med Oral Patol Oral Cir Bucal. 2012;17(2):e251–61.
16. Lioubavina-Hack N, Lang NP, Karring T. Significance of primary stability for osseointegration of dental implants. Clin Oral Implants Res. 2006;17(3):244–50.
17. Couvaras L, Trijau S, Lamotte GD, et al. AB1141 prevalence of long-term steroid therapy: French data. Ann Rheum Dis. 2017;76:1454.
18. Rice JB, White AG, Scarpati LM, Wan G, Nelson WW. Long-term systemic corticosteroid exposure: a systematic literature review. Clin Ther. 2017;39(11): 2216–29.
19. Wiebe CB, Putnins EE. The periodontal disease classification system of the American Academy of periodontology - an update. J Can Dent Assoc. 2000; 66:594–7.
20. Highfield J. Diagnosis and classification of periodontal disease. Aust Dent J. 2009 Sep;54(Suppl 1):S11–26.
21. Kölner Defektklassifikation CCARD (Cologne Classification of Alveolar Ridge Defect) für Regelfallversorgungen bei Knochenaugmentation: 8.European Congress of European Association of Dental Implantologists; 2013. https://www.bdizedi.org/bdiz/web.nsf/gfx/guidelines_Konsensus-Leitfaden-2013_engl.pdf/$file/guidelines_Konsensus-Leitfaden-2013_engl.pdf.
22. Olson JW, Shernoff AF, Tarlow JL, Colwell JA, Scheetz JP, Bingham SF. Dental endosseous implant assessments in a type 2 diabetic population: a prospective study. Int J Oral Maxillofac Implants. 2000;15(6):811–8.
23. Hurst D. Evidence unclear on whether type I or II diabetes increases the risk of implant failure. Evid Based Dent. 2014;15(4):102–3.
24. Devlin H, Garland H, Sloan P. Healing of tooth extraction sockets in experimental diabetes mellitus. J Oral Maxillofac Surg. 1996;54:1087–91.
25. Oates TW Jr, Galloway P, Alexander P, Vargas Green A, Huynh-Ba G, Feine J, McMahan CA. The effects of elevated hemoglobin A(1c) in patients with type 2 diabetes mellitus on dental implants: Survival and stability at one year. J Am Dent Assoc. 2014;145(12):1218–26.
26. Morris HF, Ochi S, Winkler S. Implant survival in patients with type 2 diabetes: placement to 36 months. Ann Periodontol. 2000;5:157–65.
27. Chrcanovic BR, Albrektsson T, Wennerberg A. Diabetes and oral implant failure: a systematic review. J Dent Res. 2014;93(9):859–67.
28. Balshi TJ, Wolfinger GJ. Dental implants in the diabetic patient: a retrospective study. Implant Dent. 1999;8:355–9.
29. Fiorellini JP, Chen PK, Nevins M, Nevins ML. A retrospective study of dental implants in diabetic patients. Int J Periodontics Restorative Dent. 2000;20(4): 366–73.
30. Busenlechner D, Fürhauser R, Haas R, Watzek G, Mailath G, Pommer B. Long-term implant success at the Academy for Oral Implantology: 8-year follow-up and risk factor analysis. J Periodontal Implant Sci. 2014;44:102–8.
31. Esposito M, Worthington HV. Interventions for replacing missing teeth: hyperbaric oxygen therapy for irradiated patients who require dental implants. Cochrane Database Syst Rev. 2013;9:CD003603.
32. Ihde S, Kopp S, Gundlach K, Konstantinovic VS. Effects of radiation therapy on craniofacial and dental implants: a review of the literature. Oral Surg Oral Med Oral Pathol Oral Radiol Endod. 2009;107:56–65.
33. Curi MM, Condezo AFB, Ribeiro KDCB, Cardoso CL. Long-term success of dental implants in patients with head and neck cancer after radiation therapy. Int J Oral Maxillofac Surg. 2018;47(6):783–8.
34. Wood MR, Vermilyea SG. A review of selected dental literature on evidence-based treatment planning for dental implants: report of the Committee on Research in Fixed Prosthodontics of the Academy of Fixed Prosthodontics.

J Prosthet Dent. 2004;92(5):447–62.
35. Cranin AN. Endosteal implants in a patient with corticosteroid dependence. J Oral Implantol. 1991;17(4):414–7.
36. Fujimoto T, Niimi A, Sawai T, Ueda M. Effects of steroid-induced osteoporosis on osseointegration of titanium implants. Int J Oral Maxillofac Implants. 1998;13(2):183–9.
37. Hayward C, Brock DJ. Fibrillin-1 mutations in Marfan syndrome and other type-1 fibrillinopathies. Hum Mutat. 1997;10(6):415–23.
38. Giampietro P, Peterson M, Schneider R, Davis J, Burke S, Boachie-Adjei O, Mueller C, Raggio C. Bone mineral density determinations by dual-energy x-ray absorptiometry in the management of patients with Marfan syndrome - some factors which affect the measurement. HSSJ. 2007;3:89–92.
39. August M, Chung K, Chang Y, Glowacki J. Influence of estrogen status on endosseous implant osseointegration. J Oral Maxillofac Surg. 2001;59:1285–9.
40. Hultin M, Gustafsson A, Hallstrom H, Johansson LA, Ekfeldt A, Klinge B. Microbiological findings and host response in patients with periimplantitis. Clin Oral Implants Res. 2002;13:349–58.
41. Heitz-Mayfield LJA. Peri-implant diseases: diagnosis and risk indicators. J Clin Periodontol. 2008;35:292–304.
42. Safii S, Palmer R, Wilson RF. Risk of implant failure and marginal bone loss in subjects with a history of periodontitis: a systematic review and meta-analysis. Clin Implant Dent Relat Res. 2010;12(3):165–74.
43. Zhoun W, Hann C, Li D, Li Y, Song Y, Zhao Y. Endodontic treatment of teeth induces retrograde peri-implantitis. Clin Oral Impl Res. 2009;20:1326–32.
44. Moraschini V, Poubel LA, Ferreira VF, Barboza Edos S. Evaluation of survival and success rates of dental implants reported in longitudinal studies with a follow-up period of at least 10 years: a systematic review. Int J Oral Maxillofac Surg. 2015;44(3):377–88. https://doi.org/10.1016/j.ijom.2014.10.023.
45. Den Hartog L, Slater JJ, Vissink A, Meijer HJ, Raghoebar GM. Treatment outcome of immediate, early and conventional single-tooth implants in the aesthetic zone: a systematic review to survival, bone level, soft-tissue, aesthetics and patient satisfaction. J Clin Periodontol. 2008;35(12):1073–86.
46. Esposito M, Cannizzaro G, Bozzoli P, Checchi L, Ferri V, Landriani S, Leone M, Todisco M, Torchio C, Testori T, Galli F, Felice P. Effectiveness of prophylactic antibiotics at placement of dental implants: a pragmatic multicentre placebo-controlled randomised clinical trial. Eur J Oral Implantol. 2010;3(2):135–43.
47. Rocci A, Rocci M, Rocci C, Scoccia A, Gargari M, Martignoni M, Gottlow J, Sennerby L. Immediate loading of Brånemark system TiUnite and machined-surface implants in the posterior mandible, part II: a randomized open-ended 9-year follow-up clinical trial. Int J Oral Maxillofac Implants. 2013;28(3):891–5.
48. Greenstein G, Cavallaro J. Failed dental implants: diagnosis, removal and survival of reimplantations. J Am Dent Assoc. 2014;145(8):835–42.
49. Schropp L, Isidor F, Kostopoulos L, Wenzel A. Patient experience of, and satisfaction with, delayed-immediate vs delayed single-tooth implant placement. Clin Oral Implants Res. 2004;15:498–503.

9

In vitro comparison of two titanium dental implant surface treatments: 3M™ESPE™ MDIs versus Ankylos®

Jagjit Singh Dhaliwal[1,2†], Juliana Marulanda[1†], Jingjing Li[3], Sharifa Alebrahim[1], Jocelyne Sheila Feine[1] and Monzur Murshed[1,3,4*]

Abstract

Background: An ideal implant should have a surface that is conducive to osseointegration. In vitro cell culture studies using disks made of same materials and surface as of implants may provide useful information on the events occurring at the implant-tissue interface. In the current study, we tested the hypothesis that there is no difference in the proliferation and differentiation capacities of osteoblastic cells when cultured on titanium disks mimicking the surface of 3M™ESPE™ MDIs or standard (Ankylos®) implants.

Methods: Cells were grown on disks made of the same materials and with same surface texture as those of the original implants. Disks were sterilized and coated with 2% gelatin solution prior to the cell culture experiments. C2C12 pluripotent cells treated with 300 ng/ml bone morphogenetic protein 2 BMP-2 and a stably transfected C2C12 cell line expressing BMP2 were used as models for osteogenic cells. The Hoechst 33258-stained nuclei were counted to assay cell proliferation, while alkaline phosphatase (ALPL) immunostaining was performed to investigate osteogenic differentiation. MC3T3-E1 cells were cultured as model osteoblasts. The cells were differentiated and assayed for proliferation and metabolic activities by Hoechst 33258 staining and Alamar blue reduction assays, respectively. Additionally, cultures were stained by calcein to investigate their mineral deposition properties.

Results: Electron microscopy showed greater degree of roughness on the MDI surfaces. Nuclear counting showed significantly higher number of C2C12 cells on the MDI surface. Although immunostaining detected higher number of ALPL-positive cells, it was not significant when normalized by cell numbers. The number of MC3T3-E1 cells was also higher on the MDI surface, and accordingly, these cultures showed higher Alamar blue reduction. Finally, calcein staining revealed that the MC3T3-E1 cells grown on MDI surfaces deposited more minerals.

Conclusions: Although both implant surfaces are conducive for osteoblastic cell attachment, proliferation, and extracellular matrix mineralization, cell proliferation is higher on MDI surfaces, which may in turn facilitate osseointegration via increased ECM mineralization.

Keywords: Cell culture, Osteoblasts, Implant surface

* Correspondence: monzur.murshed@mcgill.ca
†Equal contributors
[1]Faculty of Dentistry, McGill University, Montreal, Quebec, Canada
[3]Faculty of Medicine, McGill University, Montreal, Quebec, Canada
Full list of author information is available at the end of the article

Background

Prosthetic devices are often used as surrogates for missing skeletal and dental elements. These devices are in close contact with the surrounding tissues, and their functionality and stability are critically dependent on the successful integration within the tissue's extracellular matrix (ECM). The surface of the implanted device directly interacts with cell and extracellular milieu and influences their biological activities affecting the healing of the implant site after the surgery, tissue regeneration, and the formation of an organic interface with cells and ECM proteins.

Dental implants are commonly used to replace missing teeth, and the long-term success of these implants depends on their proper integration with the mineralized bone, a process commonly known as osseointegration [1].

It has been a long-standing challenge to achieve successful osseointegration of implants in older population with poor bone mass and low bone turnover rates. Therefore, an ideal implant should have a surface which is conducive to osseointegration regardless of the implant site, bone quality, and bone quantity. A large body of literature recommends the use of mini dental implants for stabilization of removable partial and complete dentures in selected situations [2].The 3M™ESPE™ mini dental implant (MDI) system makes use of a self-tapping threaded screw design and needs a minimal surgical intervention. Also, small-size implants have been widely used for orthodontic anchorage [3–5], single tooth replacements [6, 7], fixing the surgical guides for definitive implant placement [8], and as transitional implants for the support of interim removable prosthesis during the healing phase of final fixtures [9, 10]. The MDIs have several advantages over the regular implants used for overdentures such as, simpler surgical protocol and minimally invasive surgery, and they can often be loaded immediately [6]. This helps in reducing postoperative distress to the patient and minimizing resorption of the bone during healing [11]. It has been shown that bone healing around immediately loaded transitional implants is not disturbed and causes no bone loss, which represents a solution for patients who have ridge deficiency and who cannot have surgery for medical reasons [12, 13]. Mini dental implants are also cost-effective, and the price of one MDI is 3.5 times lower than that of a standard size mandibular implant [14].

Despite the advantages of the MDI, evidence on their potential for osseointegration and long-term success is lacking. [15–18]. Newer implant systems entering the market must be studied first in vitro and then in vivo with animal models followed by human studies to demonstrate their osseointegration capability.

Modifications of implant surface properties have been shown to have a positive influence on the successful osseointegration of an implant [19–22]. Surface properties such as roughness, topography, and chemistry are strongly related to the biocompatibility of implants [23]. Thus, modulation of these properties can be useful means to improve implant osseointegration in patients with poor bone quality. The most common treatments used for implant surface modifications are acid etching and sandblasting [24–27]. Implants with moderate surface coarseness demonstrate a better bone response than a smoother or rougher surface [28–30]. When an implant is placed in the bone, a series of cell and matrix events takes place. These mainly include host response to the implant material and behavior of the implant in the host tissue, which culminates in an intimate deposition of a new bone on the implant surface [31].

The immediate event after implantation is adsorption of proteins which may facilitate cell attachment [31]. Various studies show that direct osteoblast-implant interactions are critical for proper osseointegration. Cell culture models using osteoblastic cells are being commonly used to study bone-biomaterial interface [32].

In the current study, we examined the proliferation and differentiation characteristics of differentiated C2C12 cells and MC3T3-E1 preosteoblasts on surfaces mimicking the 3M™ESPE™ MDI (test group) and Ankylos® implants. The Ankylos® implant surface was used for comparison as it is a well-established and widely characterized standard implant.

The surfaces of 3M™ESPE™ MDIs are treated to impart roughness which includes sandblasting with aluminum oxide particles, followed by cleaning and passivation with an oxidizing acid [33]. The Ankylos® implant has the FRIADENT plus surface (Dentsply Implants, Mannheim, Germany). It is formed by sandblasting in a temperature-controlled process and acid etching (hydrochloric, sulfuric, hydrofluoric, and oxalic acid) followed by a proprietary neutralizing technique [34]. Considering that both surfaces were sandblasted and acid-treated, we hypothesize that there is no difference in the proliferation and differentiation capacity of osteoblastic cells when cultured on 3M™ESPE™ MDIs and standard implants.

Methods

Implant disks

Titanium disks made up with the same materials and surface characteristics as those with the original implants were obtained from the respective manufacturers. Two types of disks were used; the small disks represented 3M™ESPE™ MDI implants, while the large disks represented Ankylos®, Dentsply Friadent implants. A total of 10 disks of each brand were used for the study.

Cell culture and in vitro mineralization

Disks were sterilized and coated with 2% gelatin solution to facilitate the attachment of cells. MC3T3-E1 and C2C12 cells were purchased from ATCC (Manassas, VA, USA). Recombinant human bone morphogenetic protein 2 BMP-2 was purchased from GenScript (Piscataway, NJ, USA). MC3T3-E1 and C2C12 cells were cultured in alpha-MEM (Invitrogen, Carlsbad, CA, USA) and DMEM (Invitrogen, Carlsbad, CA, USA), respectively. Culture media were supplemented with 10% FBS (PAA, Etobocoke, Ontario, Canada) and 100 U/ml penicillin–streptomycin (Invitrogen, Carlsbad, CA, USA). Cells were grown at 37 °C under 5% CO2 in a humidified incubator. Mineralization of MC3T3-E1 cultures was induced by addition of ascorbic acid (50 μg/ml) and sodium phosphate (4 mM) to the culture medium for 12 days.

Calcein staining

Cells were fixed with 4% paraformaldehyde. 0.25% calcein (Sigma-Aldrich, Saint Louis, MO, USA), and 2% $NaHCO_3$ solution prepared in 0.15 M NaCl was added to the fixed cells and incubated for 5 min at room temperature. After washing once in PBS, H33258 nuclear staining was performed, washed twice in PBS and images were taken using an inverted fluorescence microscope (EVOS FL, Thermo Fisher Scientific).

Alamar blue

In order to examine cellular viability/metabolic activity, Alamar blue solution (Resazurin sodium salt, Sigma-Aldrich, Saint Louis, MO, USA) was directly added to the medium to 100 μM final concentration. The reduction of Alamar blue was measured at 560 nm (reference wavelength 610 nm) after 5-h incubation at 37 °C using a microplate reader (Infinite 200, Tecan).

Generation of BMP2 expressing C2C12 cells

C2C12 cells were electroporated together with 0.4 μg of a BMP-2 expression vector (a kind gift from Dr. Katagiri) and 0.1 μg of pCMV-Tag, which expresses a neomycin-resistance gene. Culture medium was supplemented with 300 μg/ml of G418 (Fisher, Pittsburgh, PA, USA) for 9 days. Clones were picked, amplified, and screened by alkaline phosphatase (ALPL; a downstream target for BMP-2 signaling) staining [35].

Zymography and Western blotting

Protein samples from the transfected cells were prepared in 1× SDS gel-loading buffer (Laemmli buffer) without adding β-mercaptoethanol and quantified using the Pierce™ Coomassie Plus Assay kit (Thermo Scientific, Rockford, IL, USA). Without heat denaturation, equal amount of protein samples (50 μg) were loaded on a 10% SDS-polyacrylamide gel. After electrophoresis, the gel was incubated in NBT/BCIP (Roche, Mannheim, Germany) staining solution until the bands corresponding to ALPL were clearly visible. Same protein extracts upon heat denaturation in the presence of β-mercaptoethanol were used for Western blotting. The primary antibody used for the analysis was anti-actin (Sigma-Aldrich, Saint Louis, MO, USA). An anti-actin antibody raised in rabbit anti-actin (Sigma-Aldrich, Saint Louis, MO, USA). The secondary antibody was anti-rabbit HRP-IgG (Cell Signaling Technology, Beverly, MA, USA).

Cell proliferation

Nuclear staining was done by H33258 (Sigma-Aldrich, Saint Louis, MO, USA). After washing in PBS, cells grown on the implants were imaged using an inverted fluorescent microscope (EVOS FL, Thermo Fisher Scientific) and cell nuclei were counted.

Alkaline phosphatase immunostaining and assay

BMP-2-transfected C2C12 cells were fixed in 4% PFA for 15 min, and then blocked with 5% bovine serum albumin (Fisher, Pittsburgh, PA, USA) in Tris buffered saline-0.025%Triton for 30 min at room temperature, followed by overnight incubation with an anti-mouse alkaline phosphatase antibody (R&D systems, Minneapolis, MN, USA). Detection was done by Dylight 488 rabbit anti-goat secondary antibody (Jackson ImmunoResearch, West Grove, PA, USA) with 1-h incubation at room temperature. Fluorescence imaging was performed using an inverted microscope (EVOS FL, Thermo Fisher Scientific). ALPL assay using p-nitrophenyl phosphate was performed as described before [35].

Scanning electron microscopy

For scanning electron microscopy (SEM), cleaned and sterilized disks in self-sealed pouches were received as such from the respective manufacturers. The disks were carefully mounted on stubs, sputter-coated, and viewed with Carl Zeiss AG-EVO® 40-series scanning electron microscope.

Statistical analysis

Statistical significance of the differences between the groups was determined using Student's *t* test. The statistical power was calculated using the Biomath online software (http://www.biomath.info/power/index.html). We analyzed 10 samples for each group (alpha error 0.05), which resulted in a statistical power of 92%.

Blinding of the investigators

While performing the experiments, JM (first co-author) was not aware of the sources/manufacturers of the disks, which were identified by their size (small and large) only. At the end of the analyses, each disk's manufacturer was revealed to her by JSD (first co-author).

Results

Ring culture technique

The variable sizes of the implant disks obtained from two different manufacturers demanded an innovative culture system to ensure equal surface areas on both disks for the cell culture experiments. We achieved this by attaching constant diameter (5 mm) plastic cylinders to the disk surface. Disks were sterilized with absolute alcohol, and polystyrene cloning cylinders (Sigma) were attached onto the disks using vacuum grease. The enclosed surfaces on the disks were then coated with sterile 2% gelatin solution (Fig. 1).

Increased surface roughness in the 3M™ESPE™ MDIs

Scanning electron microscopy was used in a secondary electron mode under 10-kV acceleration voltage for producing the images to observe the surface topography, and it showed an increased surface roughness in the 3M™ESPE™ MDIs as compared with Ankylos® (Fig. 2).

Increased proliferation of C2C12 cells grown on 3M™ESPE™ MDI disks

We first examined the proliferation of C2C12 cells treated with BMP-2, a pro-osteogenic cytokine, or without BMP-2 treatment on both types of disks. Ten thousand C2C12 cells were plated, and on the following day, the medium was supplemented with 300 ng/ml of BMP-2. Cells were grown for 3 days, stained with the nuclear stain H33258, and imaged using fluorescence microscopy. Counting of cell nuclei revealed an increased proliferation of the C2C12 cells grown on 3M™ESPE™ MDI disks under both conditions, when treated with BMP-2 or without any treatment (Fig. 3).

Disk type does not affect osteogenic differentiation

C2C12 myoblastic cells were transfected with BMP-2. These cells express high levels of ALPL when compared with the control (untransfected) group (Fig. 4a). ALPL zymography showed a more intense band indicating very high expression of functional ALPL protein in the stably transfected cells (Fig. 4b). The transfected cells were then seeded onto each type of disks (15,000 cells/disk) and were cultured for 3 days. Immunostaining using a goat anti-mouse ALPL antibody revealed a significantly higher number of ALPL-positive cells on the 3M™ESPE™ MDI disks in comparison to those on the Ankylos® disks. Interestingly, when the number of ALPL-positive cells was normalized to the total cell number, no differences were observed. This finding suggests that the increase of ALPL-positive cells was not due to an increased cell differentiation, but because of an increased cell proliferation (Fig. 4c).

Increased proliferation of MC3T3-E1 cells and extracellular matrix mineralization on 3M™ESPE™ MDI disks

Pre-osteoblastic MC3T3-E1 cells were plated on each implant disk (40,000 cells/disk) and were differentiated with mineralization medium for 12 days. Quantification of cells after nuclear staining by H33258 revealed an increased number of cells on the 3M™ESPE™ MDI disks (Fig. 5a). Measurement of cell viability by the reduction of Alamar blue® after 3 days of culture of MC3T3-E1 cells further supported an increase of cell proliferation on the 3M™ESPE™ MDI disks (Fig. 5b).

In order to assess the ability of the system to promote ECM mineralization, MC3T3-E1 cells were plated at equal densities on each disk type and were grown in the presence of differentiation medium for 12 days. Calcein (binds to calcium salts) staining demonstrated an increased mineral deposition on the surface of the 3M™ESPE™ MDI disks when compared with that on the Ankylos® disks. Increased cell proliferation in the 3M™ESPE™ MDI disks cultures may explain the increase in ECM mineralization (Fig. 5c).

Discussion

In the current study, we used an in vitro cell culture system to evaluate the biocompatibility of two implant materials with different surface topography. Our objective was to establish the osseointegration potential of MDIs versus an established regular implant. Disks prepared from the implant material were coated with gelatin to grow cells,

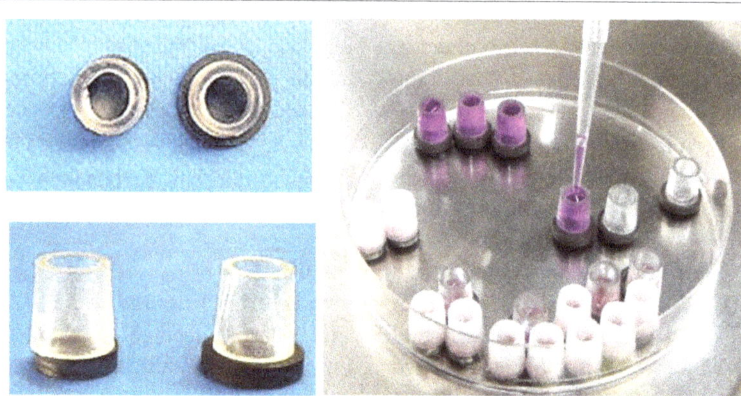

Fig. 1 Preparation of specimens. Small disks represent 3M™ESPE™ MDI implants, and large disks represent Ankylos® implants. Note that the attachment of polystyrene rings ensures the area of culture remains constant regardless of the disk size

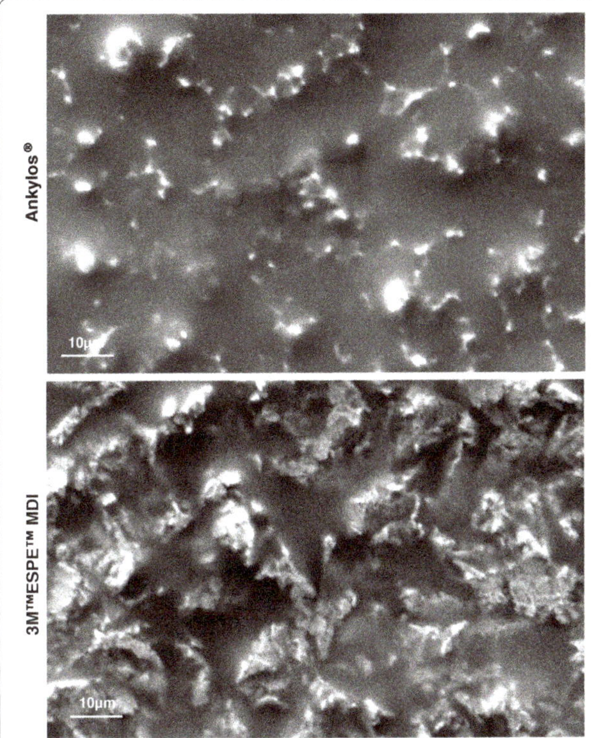

Fig. 2 Implant surface characterization under SEM. Increased surface roughness in the 3M™ESPE™ MDI dental implants when compared to Ankylos® implants

and proliferation and osteogenic differentiation parameters were evaluated. Considering that the disks obtained from two different sources varied in diameter, we attached 5-mm silicon rings to the surface of both types of disks in order to standardize the culture area. The use of vacuum grease created a leak-proof culture well that enabled us to grow and treat cells for the required period of time. Also, it was possible to use a limited number of disks as the system was easy to clean, disinfect, and reuse.

As cells were grown on metallic surfaces, it was not possible to detect them using light microscopy. This is why we used florescence microscopy to examine the cells and their functional properties once the experiment was complete. Considering that we were unable to routinely examine the live cells on the disks during the culture period, we grew the same number of cells under identical conditions on a plastic cell culture dish enclosed by the same type of culture rings. These cells were evaluated daily using an inverted light microscope, and based on the cell density and the amount of mineral precipitation in this latter culture, we decided to terminate the experiments with the cells grown on the disks.

Two different cell lines were used in our in vitro system: C2C12 and MC3T3-E1 cells. Both of these cell lines were developed from mouse tissues. C2C12 cells are myogenic, but retain the potential to express osteogenic markers under appropriate signaling events. Because of

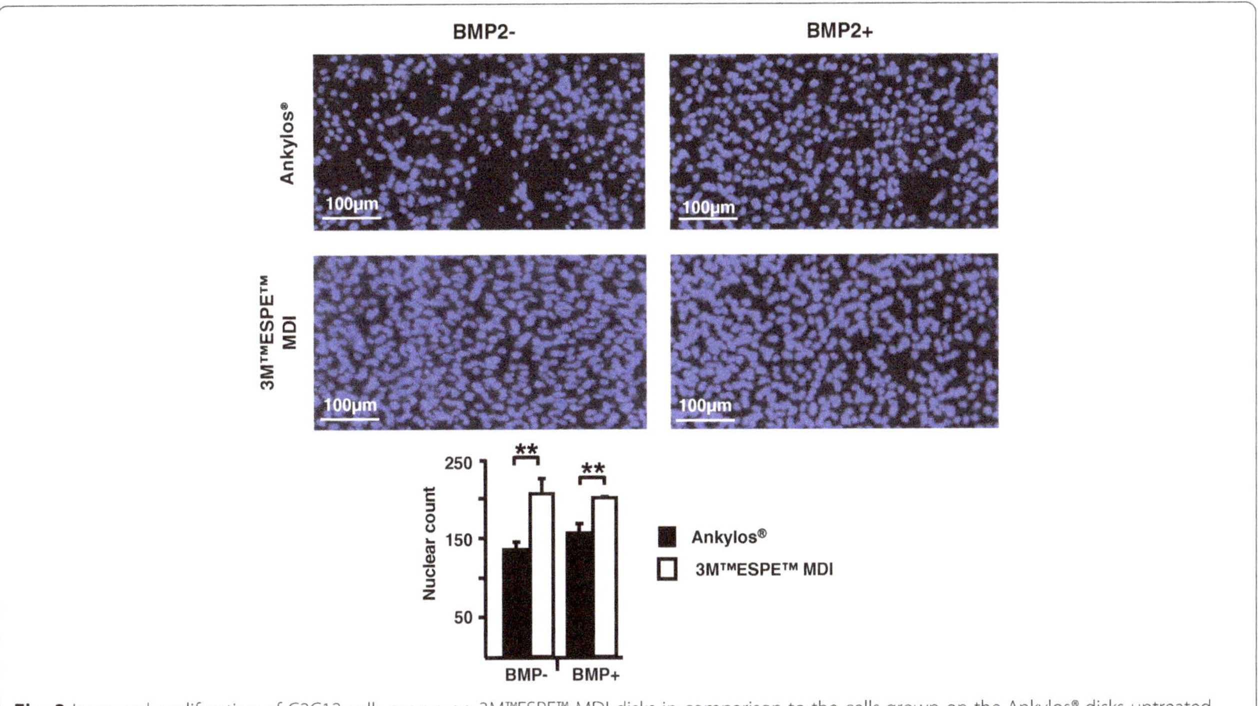

Fig. 3 Increased proliferation of C2C12 cells grown on 3M™ESPE™ MDI disks in comparison to the cells grown on the Ankylos® disks untreated and treated with bone morphogenetic protein-BMP-2

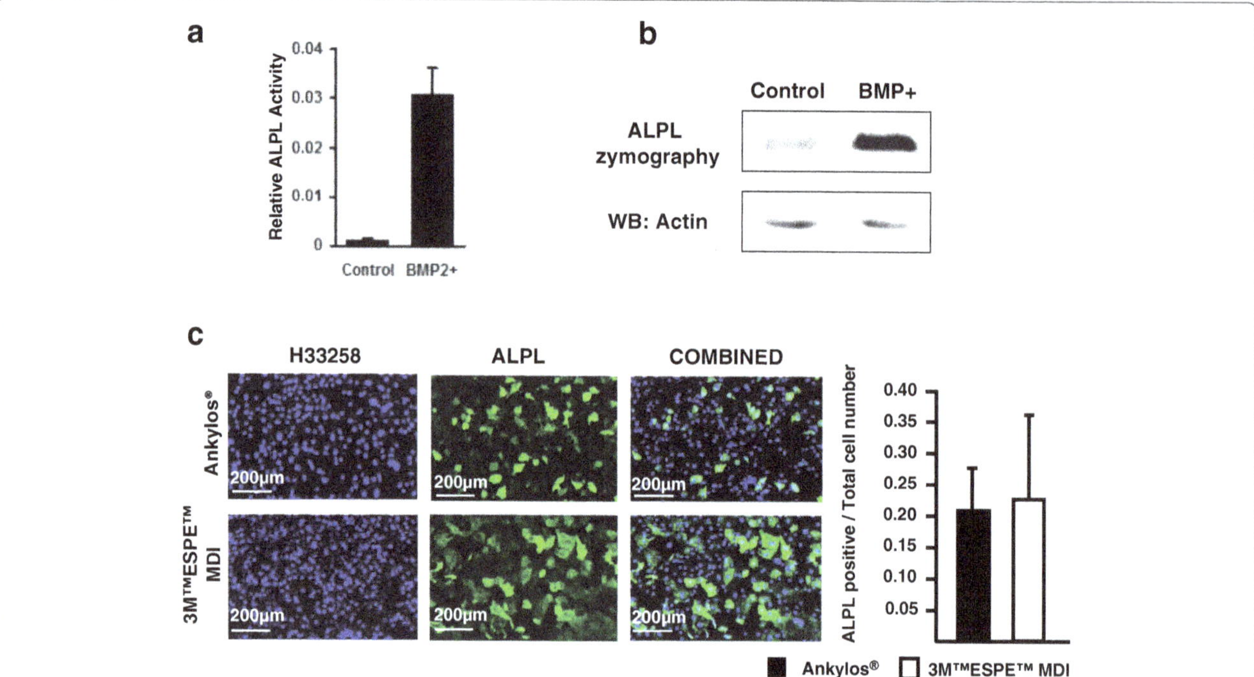

Fig. 4 **a** C2C12 cells (control) and pBMP-2-transfected C2C12 cells were seeded on a 24-well plate (50,000 cell/well) and cultured in DMEM medium for 48 h. ALPL assay showing upregulated ALPL activity in the BMP-2-transfected C2C12 cells. **b** Cell extracts of C2C12 cells and pBMP-2-transfected cells were run on a 10% SDS-PAGE under non-denaturing conditions. The gel was then stained with NBT/BCIP solution (upper panel). Western bloting of actin showing the equal protein loading on the gel (*lower panel*). **c** Increased proliferation of C2C12 cells transfected with BMP-2 as well as ALPL activity when seeded on 3M™ESPE™ MDI disks. However, when the number of ALPL-positive cells is normalized to the total cell number, no differences are observed

their pluripotency, these cells have been considered as a type of mesenchymal stem cells. It has been shown that when treated with BMPs, these cells readily upregulate many key osteoblast markers including RUNX2, OSX, osteocalcin, and alkaline phosphatase (ALPL) [35]. In the current study, we used C2C12 cells that were treated with BMP-2 or stably transfected with a BMP-2 expression vector.

MC3T3-E1 cells have been extensively used in numerous cell culture experiments as a model for osteoblasts [36]. Under differentiating conditions, e.g., in the presence of ascorbic acid and β-glycerol phosphate, these cells upregulate the osteogenic markers and, more importantly, promote the deposition of calcium phosphate minerals within and around the collagen-rich extracellular matrix (ECM). In comparison to BMP2-treated C2C12 cells, MC3T3-E1 cells are considered to be at a more advanced stage of differentiation towards the osteogenic lineage [35].

Our cell culture system was compatible with both cell types as evident by the outcome of various functional studies, which include cell adherence, synthesis of alkaline phosphatase, and mineralization of the ECM. However, there was a clear difference in the degree of biocompatibility between the two types of implant surfaces; the 3M™ESPE™ MDI showed higher cell numbers and increased deposition of calcium phosphate minerals in comparison to Ankylos®.

The MDI surface was treated with sandblasting and passivation with an oxidizing acid [33] whereas Ankylos® surface was sandblasted and acid etched [34]. The scanning electron microscopic images showed rougher surface in MDIs in comparison to Ankylos®. The blasting process causes a moderate roughness (1–2 micron) to the implants [33].

The surface chemistry and topography of biomaterials seem to play an important role in the success or failure upon placement in a biological environment [37]. It has been established that alterations on the surface topography enhance the bone implant contact and biomechanical interaction of the interface during early implantation periods [37].

MacDonald et al. have shown that wettability, i.e., hydrophilic surfaces support cell interactions and biological fluids better than the hydrophobic surfaces [38]. It has also been shown that roughening the titanium surface improves hydrophilicity [38]. In addition, many authors have stated that rougher surfaces promote differentiation, growth and attachment of bone cells, and higher production of growth factors and augment mineralization [39–43]. However, an in vitro study has demonstrated that osteoblastic cells

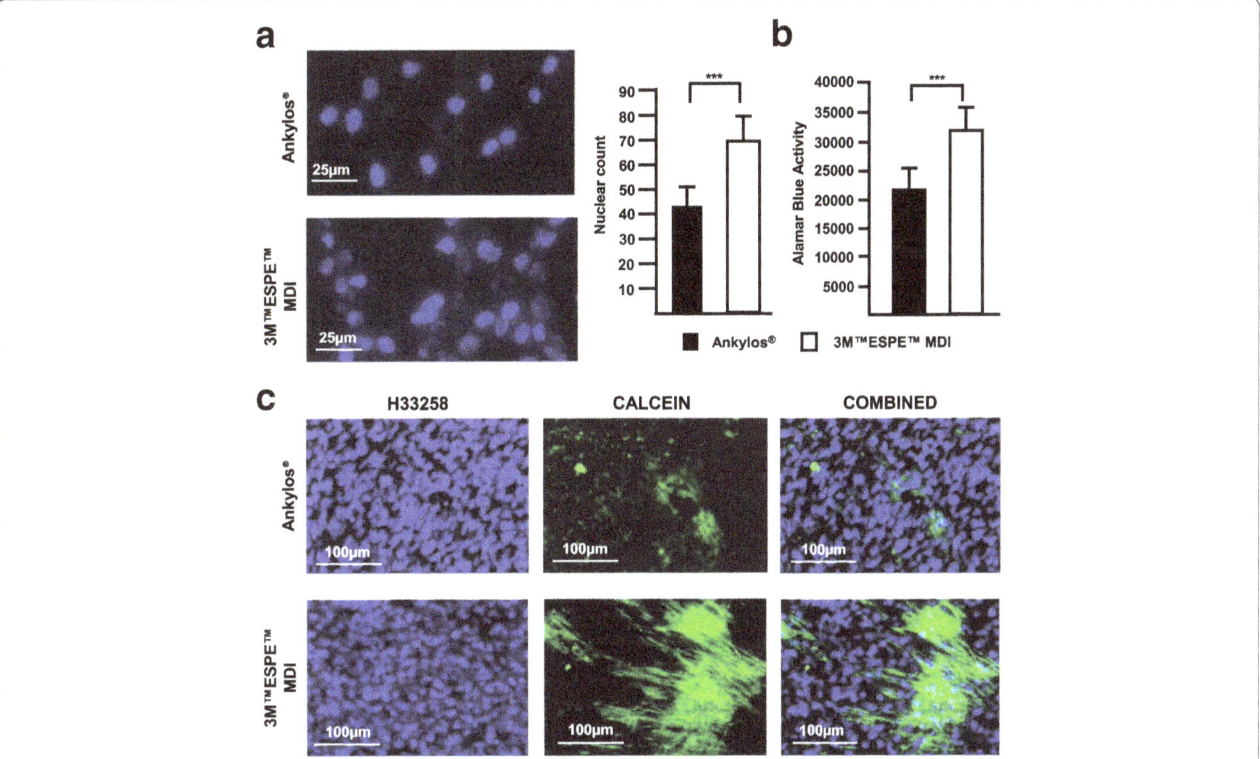

Fig. 5 **a** Florescence microscopy showing H33258-stained MC3T3-E1 cells on Ankylos® and 3M™ESPE™ MDI disks. Although equal numbers of cells were plated, after 12 days of culture, more cells were detected on the 3M™ESPE™ MDI disks. **b** Increased Alamar blue® reduction in MC3T3-E1 cells seeded on 3M™ESPE™ MDI disks when compared to cells cultured on Ankylos®. **c** Increased mineral deposition in the MC3T3-E1 cultures on the 3M™ESPE™ MDI disks in comparison to those on the Ankylos® disks as detected by calcein staining

attach, spread, and proliferate faster on smooth surfaces than on rough surfaces [44].

ALPL is a late osteogenic marker, which is essential for normal bone mineralization. ALPL-deficient osteoblasts fail to mineralize in culture. Considering that there was no significant difference in the relative ALPL activity in cells grown on two surfaces, it is unlikely that the surface property of the disks affected cell differentiation. This observation does not support the findings of Davies that BMPs, alkaline phosphatase and osteocalcin, the important markers of osteogenic differentiation and bone tissue formation, were express at higher levels on rougher surfaces [45]. In addition to surface topography, surface chemistry is also a very strong variable [46, 47]. Therefore, the different surface chemistry of the implant materials used by Davies and our group might have contributed to this discrepancy. Regardless, there is a general agreement that roughening the implant surface greater than the degree seen by machining only leads to a stronger bone formation as shown in a systematic review [48].

Our data suggest that the increased cell number is the primary reason why cultures grown on 3M™ESPE™ MDI deposited more minerals in comparison to those grown on Ankylos®. Taken together, we reject the null hypothesis, since our data demonstrates that MDIs have a superior surface quality that promotes cell proliferation, facilitating osseointegration. However, this needs to be tested in vivo.

Conclusions

Our results demonstrate that both implant surfaces are conducive for osteoblastic cell attachment, proliferation, and mineralization. However, 3M™ESPE™ MDI surface shows more pronounced effects on cell proliferation, which may in turn facilitate better osseointegration by enhancing ECM mineralization. Our ongoing research will provide further information on how implant surfaces may affect cell behavior at the implant-tissue interface.

Acknowledgements

The authors would like to thank Prof. Georgios Romanos, School of Dental Medicine, Dept. of Periodontology, Stony Brook University, Stony Brook, NY, USA, for his contribution to the study. We would also like to thank 3M ESPE and Dentsply Friadent for providing the implant disks. This work is a part of the thesis submitted by JD for attaining a PhD degree at the Faculty of Dentistry, McGill University, Montreal, Canada.

Funding
The funding was received from 3M ESPE for a larger study to establish the osseointegration potential of the 3M™ESPE™ MDI for building a scientific evidence. Authors had no commercial interest involved. The comparator implant disks were obtained from Dentsply Friadent for research and comparison purpose only.

Authors' contributions
JM carried out the cell cultures experiments, analyzed the data, and drafted the manuscript. JSD conceived the study and drafted the manuscript. SA established the in vitro culture system. JL generated and characterized the BMP-2-transfected cell line. JSF participated in designing the study. MM provided lab support, designed and coordinated the study, analyzed the data, and drafted the final version of the manuscript. All authors read and approved the final manuscript.

Competing interests
Jagjit Singh Dhaliwal, Juliana Marulanda, JingJing Li, Sharifa Alebrahim, Jocelyne S. Feine, and Monzur Murshed declare that they have no competing interests in the manuscript.

Author details
[1]Faculty of Dentistry, McGill University, Montreal, Quebec, Canada. [2]PAPRSB, Institute of Health Sciences, Universiti Brunei Darussalam, Jalan Tungku Link, Gadong BE1410, Brunei Darussalam. [3]Faculty of Medicine, McGill University, Montreal, Quebec, Canada. [4]Shriners Hospital for Children, Montreal, Quebec H4A 0A9, Canada.

References

1. Branemark PI, Hansson BO, Adell R, Breine U, Lindstrom J, Hallen O, et al. Osseointegrated implants in the treatment of the edentulous jaw. Experience from a 10-year period. Scand J Plast Reconstr Surg Suppl. 1977;16:1–132.
2. Bulard RA, Vance JB. Multi-clinic evaluation using mini-dental implants for long-term denture stabilization: a preliminary biometric evaluation. Compend Contin Educ Dent. 2005;26(12):892–7.
3. Buchter A, Wiechmann D, Koerdt S, Wiesmann HP, Piffko J, Meyer U. Load-related implant reaction of mini-implants used for orthodontic anchorage. Clin Oral Implants Res. 2005;16(4):473–9.
4. Fritz U, Diedrich P, Kinzinger G, Al-Said M. The anchorage quality of mini-implants towards translatory and extrusive forces. J Orofac Orthop. 2003;64(4):293–304.
5. Hong RK, Heo JM, Ha YK. Lever-arm and mini-implant system for anterior torque control during retraction in lingual orthodontic treatment. Angle Orthod. 2005;75(1):129–41.
6. Mazor Z, Steigmann M, Leshem R, Peleg M. Mini-implants to reconstruct missing teeth in severe ridge deficiency and small interdental space: a 5-year case series. Implant Dent. 2004;13(4):336–41.
7. Siddiqui AA, Sosovicka M, Goetz M. Use of mini implants for replacement and immediate loading of 2 single-tooth restorations: a clinical case report. J Oral Implantol. 2006;32(2):82–6.
8. Yeh S, Monaco EA, Buhite RJ. Using transitional implants as fixation screws to stabilize a surgical template for accurate implant placement: a clinical report. J Prosthet Dent. 2005;93(6):509–13.
9. Kwon KR, Sachdeo A, Weber HP. Achieving immediate function with provisional prostheses after implant placement: a clinical report. J Prosthet Dent. 2005;93(6):514–7.
10. Ohkubo C, Kobayashi M, Suzuki Y, Sato J, Hosoi T, Kurtz KS. Evaluation of transitional implant stabilized overdentures: a case series report. J Oral Rehabil. 2006;33(6):416–22.
11. Campelo LD, Camara JR. Flapless implant surgery: a 10-year clinical retrospective analysis. Int J Oral Maxillofac Implants. 2002;17(2):271–6.
12. Ahn MR, An KM, Choi JH, Sohn DS. Immediate loading with mini dental implants in the fully edentulous mandible. Implant Dent. 2004;13(4):367–72.
13. Dilek OC, Tezulas E. Treatment of a narrow, single tooth edentulous area with mini-dental implants: a clinical report. Oral Surg Oral Med Oral Pathol Oral Radiol Endod. 2007;103(2):e22–5.
14. Griffitts TM, Collins CP, Collins PC. Mini dental implants: an adjunct for retention, stability, and comfort for the edentulous patient. Oral Surg Oral Med Oral Pathol Oral Radiol Endod. 2005;100(5):e81–4.
15. Cooper LF, Zhou Y, Takebe J, Guo J, Abron A, Holmen A, et al. Fluoride modification effects on osteoblast behavior and bone formation at TiO2 grit-blasted c.p. titanium endosseous implants. Biomaterials. 2006;27(6):926–36.
16. Bachle M, Kohal RJ. A systematic review of the influence of different titanium surfaces on proliferation, differentiation and protein synthesis of osteoblast-like MG63 cells. Clin Oral Implants Res. 2004;15(6):683–92.
17. Marinucci L, Balloni S, Becchetti E, Belcastro S, Guerra M, Calvitti M, et al. Effect of titanium surface roughness on human osteoblast proliferation and gene expression in vitro. Int J Oral Maxillofac Implants. 2006;21(5):719–25.
18. Sader MS, Balduino A, Soares Gde A, Borojevic R. Effect of three distinct treatments of titanium surface on osteoblast attachment, proliferation, and differentiation. Clin Oral Implants Res. 2005;16(6):667–75.
19. Le Guehennec L, Soueidan A, Layrolle P, Amouriq Y. Surface treatments of titanium dental implants for rapid osseointegration. Dent Mater. 2007;23(7):844–54.
20. Sennerby L, Meredith N. Resonance frequency analysis: measuring implant stability and osseointegration. Compend Contin Educ Dent. 1998;19(5):493–8. 500, 2 ; quiz 4.
21. Weinstein RL, Francetti L, Sironi R. An analysis of the diagnostic criteria in assessing peri-implant tissues. A critical analysis of the literature. Minerva Stomatol. 1996;45(5):219–26.
22. Zreiqat H, Valenzuela SM, Nissan BB, Roest R, Knabe C, Radlanski RJ, et al. The effect of surface chemistry modification of titanium alloy on signalling pathways in human osteoblasts. Biomaterials. 2005;26(36):7579–86.
23. Boyan BD, Hummert TW, Dean DD, Schwartz Z. Role of material surfaces in regulating bone and cartilage cell response. Biomaterials. 1996;17(2):137–46.
24. Buser D, Broggini N, Wieland M, Schenk RK, Denzer AJ, Cochran DL, et al. Enhanced bone apposition to a chemically modified SLA titanium surface. J Dent Res. 2004;83(7):529–33.
25. Buser D, Nydegger T, Oxland T, Cochran DL, Schenk RK, Hirt HP, et al. Interface shear strength of titanium implants with a sandblasted and acid-etched surface: a biomechanical study in the maxilla of miniature pigs. J Biomed Mater Res. 1999;45(2):75–83.
26. Li D, Ferguson SJ, Beutler T, Cochran DL, Sittig C, Hirt HP, et al. Biomechanical comparison of the sandblasted and acid-etched and the machined and acid-etched titanium surface for dental implants. J Biomed Mater Res. 2002;60(2):325–32.
27. Zhang F, Yang GL, He FM, Zhang LJ, Zhao SF. Cell response of titanium implant with a roughened surface containing titanium hydride: an in vitro study. J Oral Maxillofac Surg. 2010;68(5):1131–9.
28. Albrektsson T, Wennerberg A. Oral implant surfaces: part 1—review focusing on topographic and chemical properties of different surfaces and in vivo responses to them. Int J Prosthodont. 2004;17(5):536–43.
29. Ivanoff CJ, Widmark G, Johansson C, Wennerberg A. Histologic evaluation of bone response to oxidized and turned titanium micro-implants in human jawbone. Int J Oral Maxillofac Implants. 2003;18(3):341–8.
30. Sul YT, Johansson C, Wennerberg A, Cho LR, Chang BS, Albrektsson T. Optimum surface properties of oxidized implants for reinforcement of osseointegration: surface chemistry, oxide thickness, porosity, roughness, and crystal structure. Int J Oral Maxillofac Implants. 2005;20(3):349–59.
31. Puleo DA, Nanci A. Understanding and controlling the bone-implant interface. Biomaterials. 1999;20(23-24):2311–21.
32. Cooper LF. Biologic determinants of bone formation for osseointegration: clues for future clinical improvements. J Prosthet Dent. 1998;80(4):439–49.
33. ESPE M. 3M ESPE MDI Mini Dental Implants [Technical Data Sheet] St. Paul, MN: 3M ESPE Dental Products. 2012. Available at: tinyurlcom/pz3brkq.
34. Rupp F, Scheideler L, Rehbein D, Axmann D, Geis-Gerstorfer J. Roughness induced dynamic changes of wettability of acid etched titanium implant modifications. Biomaterials. 2004;25(7-8):1429–38.
35. Li J, Khavandgar Z, Lin SH, Murshed M. Lithium chloride attenuates BMP-2 signaling and inhibits osteogenic differentiation through a novel WNT/GSK3- independent mechanism. Bone. 2011;48(2):321–31.

36. Sudo H, Kodama HA, Amagai Y, Yamamoto S, Kasai S. In vitro differentiation and calcification in a new clonal osteogenic cell line derived from newborn mouse calvaria. J Cell Biol. 1983;96(1):191–8.
37. Novaes Jr AB, de Souza SL, de Barros RR, Pereira KK, Iezzi G, Piattelli A. Influence of implant surfaces on osseointegration. Braz Dent J. 2010;21(6):471–81.
38. MacDonald DE, Markovic B, Allen M, Somasundaran P, Boskey AL. Surface analysis of human plasma fibronectin adsorbed to commercially pure titanium materials. J Biomed Mater Res. 1998;41(1):120–30.
39. Cooper LF, Masuda T, Yliheikkila PK, Felton DA. Generalizations regarding the process and phenomenon of osseointegration. Part II. In vitro studies. Int J Oral Maxillofac Implants. 1998;13(2):163–74.
40. Anselme K, Ponche A, Bigerelle M. Relative influence of surface topography and surface chemistry on cell response to bone implant materials. Part 2: biological aspects. Proc Inst Mech Eng H. 2010;224(12):1487–507.
41. Keller JC, Schneider GB, Stanford CM, Kellogg B. Effects of implant microtopography on osteoblast cell attachment. Implant Dent. 2003;12(2):175–81.
42. Mustafa K, Wroblewski J, Hultenby K, Lopez BS, Arvidson K. Effects of titanium surfaces blasted with TiO2 particles on the initial attachment of cells derived from human mandibular bone. A scanning electron microscopic and histomorphometric analysis. Clin Oral Implants Res. 2000;11(2):116–28.
43. Sinha RK, Morris F, Shah SA, Tuan RS. Surface composition of orthopaedic implant metals regulates cell attachment, spreading, and cytoskeletal organization of primary human osteoblasts in vitro. Clin Orthop Relat Res. 1994;305:258–72.
44. Anselme K, Bigerelle M. Topography effects of pure titanium substrates on human osteoblast long-term adhesion. Acta Biomater. 2005;1(2):211–22.
45. Davies JE. Mechanisms of endosseous integration. Int J Prosthodont. 1998;11(5):391–401.
46. Morra M, Cassinelli C, Bruzzone G, Carpi A, Di Santi G, Giardino R, et al. Surface chemistry effects of topographic modification of titanium dental implant surfaces: 1. Surface analysis. Int J Oral Maxillofac Implants. 2003;18(1):40–5.
47. Cassinelli C, Morra M, Bruzzone G, Carpi A, Di Santi G, Giardino R, et al. Surface chemistry effects of topographic modification of titanium dental implant surfaces: 2. In vitro experiments. Int J Oral Maxillofac Implants. 2003;18(1):46–52.
48. Wennerberg A, Albrektsson T. Effects of titanium surface topography on bone integration: a systematic review. Clin Oral Implants Res. 2009;20 Suppl 4:172–84.

Diagnostic ability of limited volume cone beam computed tomography with small voxel size in identifying the superior and inferior walls of the mandibular canal

Hiroko Ishii[1], Akemi Tetsumura[1*], Yoshikazu Nomura[1], Shin Nakamura[1], Masako Akiyama[2] and Tohru Kurabayashi[1]

Abstract

Background: The aim of this study was to evaluate the visibility of the superior and inferior walls of the mandibular canal separately using limited volume cone beam computed tomography (CBCT) with small voxel size.

Methods: CBCT cross-sectional images of 86 patients obtained by 3D Accuitomo FPD and reconstructed with a voxel size of 0.08 mm were used for the evaluation. A 30-mm range of the mandible just distal to the mental foramen was divided into three equal areas (areas 1, 2, and 3, from anterior to posterior). Each area contained 10 cross-sectional images. Two observers evaluated the visibility of the superior and inferior walls of the mandibular canal on each of the cross-sectional images in these three areas. The visibility ratio in each area was determined as the number of cross-sectional images with a visible wall divided by 10.

Results: In all areas, the visibility ratio of the superior wall was significantly lower than that of the inferior wall. As for variance among the three areas, the ratio was highest in the most posterior area (area 3) and tended to decrease gradually towards the mental foramen for both walls. Cases in which more than two thirds of the superior wall could be identified (visibility ratio of 0.7 or more) in areas 1, 2, and 3 were 44, 62, and 66%, respectively.

Conclusions: The superior wall was significantly more poorly visualized than the inferior wall in all areas examined. The visibility of the superior wall on CBCT images was limited even when a limited volume device with small voxel size was used.

Keywords: CBCT, Mandibular canal, Dental implants

Background

The mandibular canal is an important anatomical structure that contains the neurovascular bundle, i.e., the inferior alveolar nerve and artery. The location of the mandibular canal must be correctly identified prior to dental implant surgery to avoid complications including intraoperative and postoperative hemorrhage and neurosensory loss. Cone beam computed tomography (CBCT) is considered the imaging modality of choice for this purpose [1, 2] and is widely used for dental implant treatment planning. Several studies have evaluated the visibility of the mandibular canal on CBCT images [3–8]. However, the results varied widely, around 50–90%, among the studies. Further, no study has evaluated the superior and inferior walls of the canal separately by CBCT, although the location of the former is more important than that of the latter.

Another issue that should be noted for CBCT is the large variability in spatial resolution among devices. High-resolution devices offer the smallest voxel sizes, as small as 0.08 mm or even less [9, 10]. However, the previous studies all evaluated CBCT images having voxel sizes of 0.2 mm or more [3–8], which does not sufficiently reflect the diagnostic advantage of CBCT in demonstrating fine structures. Thus,

* Correspondence: akemi.orad@tmd.ac.jp
[1]Department of Oral and Maxillofacial Radiology, Graduate School of Medical and Dental Sciences, Tokyo Medical and Dental University, 1-5-45, Yushima, Bunkyo-ku, Tokyo, Japan
Full list of author information is available at the end of the article

further study is necessary to evaluate the diagnostic ability of CBCT in identifying the mandibular canal.

The purpose of our study was to evaluate the visibility of the superior and inferior walls of the mandibular canal using limited-volume CBCT with a small voxel size.

Methods

This study was approved by an institutional review board of our university (D2016-061).

Patients

Among the patients whose mandibles were examined by CBCT at our dental hospital between April 2012 and August 2016, 96 patients who fulfilled the following two conditions were selected.

On CBCT imaging:

- The smallest field of view (FOV) of the device, 40 × 40 mm, was used.
- The mental foramen and the mandibular body over a range of 30 mm or more just distal to the foramen were imaged.

Of those, 10 patients were excluded because the mandibular canals were affected by lesions on the images. The remaining 86 patients (31 male and 55 female; mean age, 55 years; age range, 19–79 years) were included in this study. The reasons for the CBCT study were to assess a dental lesion in 56 (periapical lesion in 51, root fracture in 4, and periodontal disease in 1) and treatment planning for dental implants in 30 patients.

Imaging

CBCT images were obtained using 3D Accuitomo FPD (Morita Corp., Kyoto, Japan) operated at tube voltage of 87–90 kV, tube current of 5–8 mA, and scan time of 9 or 18 s. In all cases, the smallest FOV, 40 × 40 mm, was used and the images were reconstructed with a voxel size of 0.08 mm.

Evaluation of images

Using OsiriX software version 3.8.1 (http://www.osirix-viewer.com), cross-sectional CBCT images of the mandible with 1-mm thickness and at 1-mm intervals were reformatted. After the mental foramen was localized, cross-sectional images in a range of 30 mm just distal to the foramen were used for the evaluation. The range was divided into three areas, each of which was 10 mm in length. These were designated as area 1, area 2, and area 3, from anterior to posterior. Each area contained 10 cross-sectional images (Fig. 1).

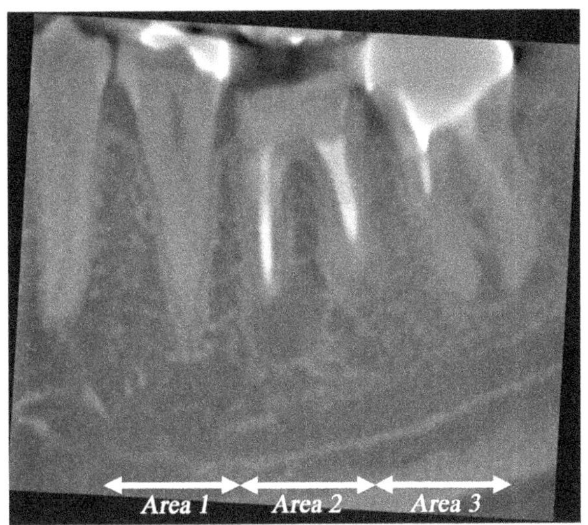

Fig. 1 Cross-sectional images in the range of 30 mm just distal to the mental foramen were used for evaluation. The range was divided into three areas, each of which was 10 mm in length, designated as area 1, area 2, and area 3, from anterior to posterior. (The mental foramen was identified on another section and was not visualized on this image)

Two observers (A.T. and H.I., with over 20 years' and 3 years' experience as oral radiologists, respectively) independently evaluated the images in a darkened room for the presence or absence of visualization of the superior and inferior walls of the mandibular canal in each of the 10 cross-sectional images in all three areas (Fig. 2). For the purpose of calibration, training was held using typical images prior to the evaluation. Each observer was blind to the other's results. When disagreement existed between the two observers, another observer (T.K., with over 30 years' experience as oral radiologist) made a final judgment. After the evaluation, the visibility ratio of the superior and inferior walls in each area was determined as follows:

$$\text{Visibility ratio} \\ = \text{number of cross-sectional images with visible wall}/10$$

The ratio ranged from 0 to 1.

Sample size

Sample size was determined using the free software G* Power 3.1 [11]. We evaluated 30 patients, and the effect size was calculated from the mean, standard deviation, and correlation. Wilcoxon signed-rank sum test was chosen, and the significance level was set to 0.05. The result showed that a sample size of 26 to 75 patients would provide a power of at least 0.8 for the difference between the superior and inferior walls. For the difference between areas, 27 to 48 patients were needed to provide a power of at least 0.8. Thus, the sample size in our study, 86 patients, was considered sufficient.

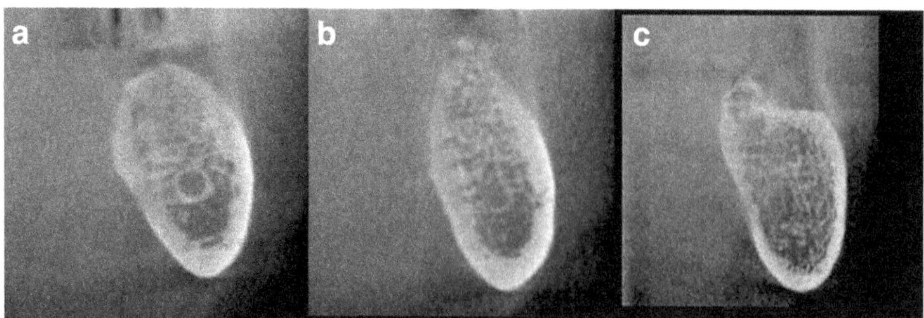

Fig. 2 Visibilities of the superior and inferior walls of the mandibular canal. **a** Both walls are visible. **b** Only the inferior wall is visible. **c** Neither of the walls is visible

Statistical analysis

Interobserver agreement was evaluated by weighted κ-statistics. A κ-value of 0–0.2 was considered poor agreement, 0.2–0.4 fair agreement, 0.4–0.6 moderate agreement, 0.6–0.8 substantial agreement, and 0.8–1.0 almost perfect agreement [12].

To compare the visibility ratio between the superior and inferior walls in each area, the Wilcoxon signed-rank test was used. Further, to compare the visibility ratio of each wall among the three areas, post hoc comparisons with Scheffe's test to make multiple comparisons following Friedman's test were used. Analysis was performed with statistical software, Ekuseru-Toukei 2008, v. 1.10 (Social Survey Research Information Co., Ltd., Tokyo, Japan). A p value of < 0.05 was considered statistically significant.

Results

Interobserver agreement was substantial or almost perfect agreement (Table 1).

The mean values of the visibility ratio of the superior and inferior walls in each area are shown in Table 2 and Fig. 3. In all areas, the ratio of the superior wall was significantly lower than that of the inferior wall ($p = 0.0000$). As for variance among the three areas, the ratio was highest in the most posterior area (area 3) and tended to decrease gradually towards the mental foramen for both walls. For the superior wall, the ratio of area 1 was significantly lower than that of area 3 ($p = 0.0006$). In contrast, for the inferior wall, significant differences were found between area 1 and area 2 ($p = 0.0001$), area 1 and area 3 ($p = 0.0000$), and area 2 and area 3 ($p = 0.0132$). A representative case is shown in Fig. 4.

Table 1 κ-values for interobserver agreement

Mandibular canal wall	Area 1	Area 2	Area 3
Superior wall	0.7795	0.7744	0.7380
Inferior wall	0.8433	0.8815	0.8887

Table 3 shows the frequency of cases with visibility ratios of 0.7 or greater (i.e., more than two thirds of the wall was visible) in each area. Cases in which more than two thirds of the superior wall could be identified on CBCT images in areas 1, 2, and 3 were 44, 62 and 66%, respectively.

Discussion

It is very important to know the location of the mandibular canal prior to dental implant surgery to avoid surgical complications including vascular trauma or nerve damage.

CBCT is widely accepted to be the imaging method of choice for obtaining this information [1, 2]. However, it is well known that the mandibular canal cannot usually be identified over its entire course even when CBCT is used. Shokri et al. [3] reported that CBCT could demonstrate both sides of the mandibular canal in 87.5% of cases. In contrast, Miles et al. [4] evaluated 360 CBCT cross-sectional images of the premolar and molar regions and reported that the mandibular canal was only visualized in just over half of the images (56%). So, the diagnostic ability of CBCT in identifying the mandibular canal differs widely among studies. Further, localizing the superior wall of the canal is more important than the inferior wall because information about the distance from the former to the alveolar crest is essential for dental implant surgery treatment planning [13]. However, to the best of our knowledge, no study has evaluated visualization of the two walls separately using CBCT.

Another concern regarding CBCT is the large variability in spatial resolution among devices. High-resolution scanners offer the smallest voxel sizes, which are as small as 0.08 mm or even less [9]. Although voxel size may not be identical to spatial resolution, a smaller voxel size generally provides better resolution [9, 10, 14, 15]. However, all of the previous studies that evaluated

Table 2 Mean visibility ratio ± SD

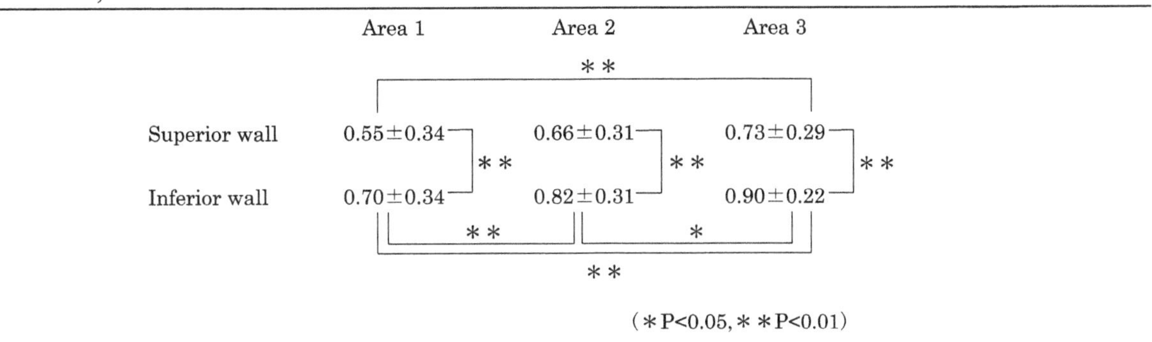

	Area 1	Area 2	Area 3
Superior wall	0.55±0.34	0.66±0.31	0.73±0.29
Inferior wall	0.70±0.34	0.82±0.31	0.90±0.22
Superior vs. inferior wall	**	**	**

Superior wall: Area 1 vs Area 3 **; Inferior wall: Area 1 vs Area 2 **, Area 2 vs Area 3 *, Area 1 vs Area 3 **

(*P<0.05, **P<0.01)

visibility of the mandibular canal by CBCT used large FOV protocols in which images were reconstructed with voxel sizes of 0.2 mm or greater [3–8]. These studies thus did not sufficiently reflect the diagnostic advantage of CBCT in demonstrating fine structures. In this study, we used a 3D Accuitomo scanner. We selected the smallest FOV (40 × 40 mm) available in this device, providing a voxel size of 0.08 mm. Pauwels et al. [10] compared the spatial resolutions of 13 CBCT and 1 medical CT devices by line pair test and reported that 3D Accuitomo showed the highest resolution. Similarly, Liang et al. [16] compared the visibility of anatomical structures including trabecular bone, periodontal ligament, and lamina dura among five CBCT and one medical CT and concluded that 3D Accuitomo yielded the best results. According to those studies, 3D Accuitomo is one of the best commercially available CBCT devices with regard to image quality. It was thus suitable for the purpose of our study to evaluate the diagnostic ability of CBCT with high spatial resolution in identifying the mandibular canal.

In this study, we only used CBCT images of the mandible obtained with the smallest FOV, 40 × 40 mm. On those images, the range of 30 mm in length in the mandible just posterior to the mental foramen was divided into three equal areas, each of which was 10 mm in length. They were designated as areas 1, 2, and 3, from anterior to posterior. After that, the visibilities of the superior and inferior walls of the mandibular canal in each area were evaluated separately. Although the location of the mental foramen differs among individuals, it is mostly situated below the second premolar or between the apices of the first and second premolars [17, 18]. Thus, it is considered that areas 1, 2, and 3 in our study nearly corresponded to the second premolar to first molar region, the first molar region, and the second molar region, respectively. Visualization of the superior wall in our study was significantly poorer than that of the inferior wall in all areas. Further, concerning the variance among areas, the visibility ratio was highest in the most posterior area (area 3) and tended to decrease gradually towards the mental foramen for both walls.

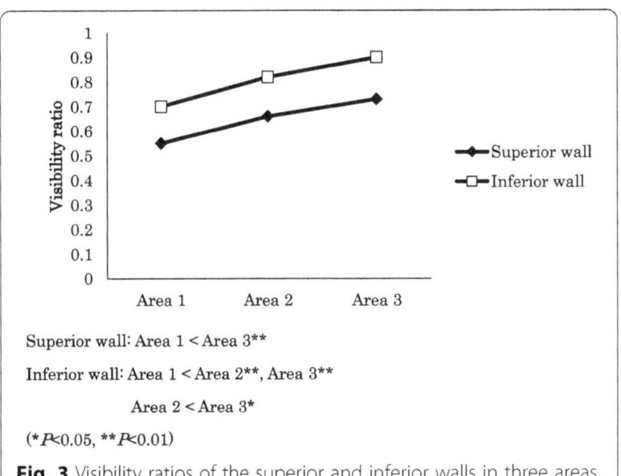

Fig. 3 Visibility ratios of the superior and inferior walls in three areas. The Friedman test and Scheffe's test were used for the statistical analysis

Although there have been no detailed studies using CBCT, poorer visualization of the superior wall compared with the inferior wall has been reported by some studies using conventional radiographs or medical CT images [19–21]. Whether the wall of the mandibular canal is visible or invisible on images largely depends on the presence or absence of corticalization of the wall surrounding the neurovascular bundle. Bertl et al. [22] performed histomorphological observation of the mandibular canal wall using thin sections of the first molar region of the mandible from 50 cadavers. They identified corticalization of the cranial (superior) and caudal (inferior) wall in 65% and 81%, respectively. Although they only observed the first molar area, their results may be considered consistent with ours of poorer visibility of the superior wall on CBCT images. The presence of nerves and vessels rising to the lower teeth from the mandibular canal may partly explain the lower corticalization rate of the superior wall [23, 24]. Further, the presence or absence of corticalization of the canal wall may be correlated with the trabecular bone volume or density [22, 25]. However, quantitative evaluation of the

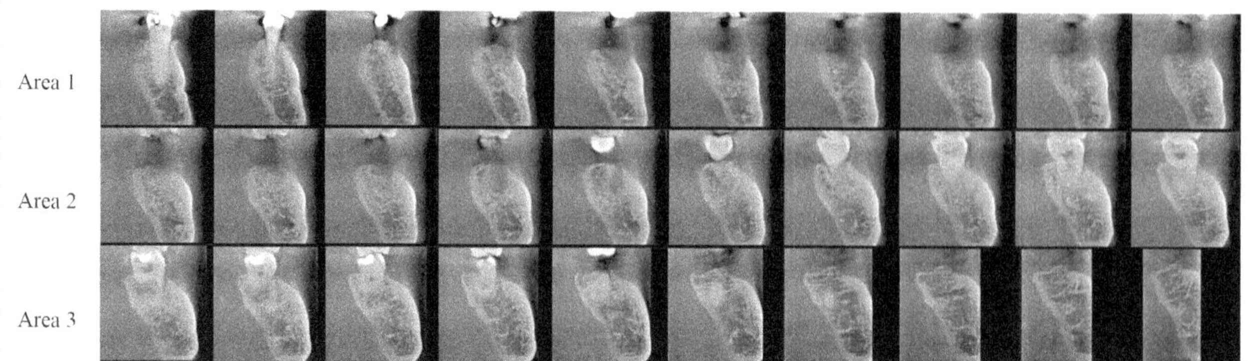

Fig. 4 Cross-sectional images of areas 1–3 of a 39-year-old female. The visibility ratios for the superior wall in areas 1, 2, and 3 were 0.2, 0.9, and 0.9, respectively, whereas those of the inferior wall were 0.7, 0.9, and 1.0, respectively

trabecular bone was difficult in our study using CBCT images. On the other hand, concerning the variance in the visibility of the mandibular canal based on antero-posterior location, several studies using CBCT reported that the mandibular canal can be more easily identified in the posterior region compared with the anterior region [3, 5–8]. An anatomical study using cadavers has reported similar results [23]. Our study evaluated the superior and inferior walls separately, with similar results, although a significant difference was only found between area 3 and area 1 for the superior wall.

Jung and Cho [6] reported that the mandibular canal was clearly visible in 50% of CBCT images in the first molar and in 58% in the second molar region. Similarly, Oliveira-Santos et al. [5] reported that it was visible in 63, 66, and 67% of second premolar, first molar, and second molar regions, respectively. As described above, these studies did not discriminate between the superior and the inferior walls. In our study, cases in which more than two thirds of the superior wall was identified on CBCT images (visibility ratio of 0.7 or more) in areas 1, 2, and 3 were 44, 62, and 66%, respectively (Table 3). It may be difficult to compare the results of our study with those of previous studies because of marked differences of evaluation methods. However, we consider that our results indicate nearly the maximum visibility of the mandibular canal when using CBCT, because we used a limited volume CBCT device with inherent small voxel size, as described above.

Because of poor visualization of the superior wall of the mandibular canal, some ingenuity may be necessary when using CBCT for treatment planning of dental implant surgery. The simplest method is to utilize the average diameter of the mandibular canal. Koivisto et al. [26] evaluated CBCT images and reported that the average diameter of the right and the left mandibular canal in the premolar/molar region was 2.91 and 3.03 mm, respectively. Utilizing these data, the approximate location of the superior wall can be estimated in cases in which the inferior wall was visible. As another method to localize the mandibular canal on CT, the use of panoramic views in addition to cross-sectional views has been recommended [27]. Probably, the imaging modality with the highest visibility of the mandibular canal is high-resolution MRI with small voxel size. Deepho et al. [28] recently reported that 3D-VIBE images at 3T MRI with voxel size of 0.8 mm clearly demonstrated the mandibular canal in 144 out of 147 areas of 62 mandibles. However, MRI has not become a routine imaging technique for dental implant treatment because of its low availability and high cost.

Table 3 Frequency of cases with visibility ratio of 0.7 or more

	Number of cases		
Mandibular canal wall	Area 1	Area 2	Area 3
Superior wall	38 (44%)	53 (62%)	57 (66%)
Inferior wall	57 (66%)	68 (79%)	77 (90%)

Our study had some limitations that should be addressed. First, in our study, antero-posterior location of the mandibular canal was defined by the distance from the mental foramen. Tooth positions could not be used as a reference, because premolars and molars were totally or partially missing in considerable number of the cases. Although areas 1–3 were considered mostly to correspond to the area from the second premolar to second molar, it might not be true for some cases due to anatomical variations for the position of the mental foramen. Second, we did not evaluate the difference of the visibility of the mandibular canal by age or gender. According to the study by Miles et al. [4], the visibility was significantly lower in females than in males. It was also affected by age depending on the location. Although we applied power analysis to determine the sample size, the sample size was not sufficient for such analysis. Third, we could not confirm the actual positions of the mandibular canal walls because we used CBCT images of clinical cases. Thus, it might be possible that a few cases with misinterpretation were included in our data.

Conclusions

In conclusion, we evaluated the visibility of the mandibular canal walls on limited volume CBCT images with a small voxel size. Evaluation was performed in the range of 30 mm in length just posterior to the mental foramen, which was divided into three equal areas (areas 1, 2, and 3, from anterior to posterior). The superior wall was significantly more poorly visualized than the inferior wall in all areas. Cases in which more than two thirds of the superior wall was identified on CBCT images in areas 1, 2, and 3 were 44, 62 and 66%, respectively.

Abbreviations

CBCT: Cone beam computed tomography; FOV: Field of view

Authors' contributions

HI contributed to the protocol preparation, case selection, data analysis, and preparation of the manuscript. AT contributed to the protocol preparation, case selection, data analysis, and preparation of the manuscript. YN contributed to the protocol preparation. SN contributed to the protocol preparation and preparation of the manuscript. MA contributed to the data analysis. TK contributed to the protocol preparation, data analysis, and preparation of the manuscript and guidance of the study. All authors read and approved the final manuscript.

Competing interests

Hiroko Ishii, Akemi Tetsumura, Yoshikazu Nomura, Shin Nakamura, Masako Akiyama, and Tohru Kurabayashi declare that they have no competing interests.

Author details

[1]Department of Oral and Maxillofacial Radiology, Graduate School of Medical and Dental Sciences, Tokyo Medical and Dental University, 1-5-45, Yushima, Bunkyo-ku, Tokyo, Japan. [2]URA, Research Administration Division, Tokyo Medical and Dental University, 1-5-45, Yushima, Bunkyo-ku, Tokyo, Japan.

References

1. Tyndall DA, Price JB, Tetradis S, Ganz SD, Hildebolt C, Scarfe WC. Position statement of the American Academy of Oral and Maxillofacial Radiology on selection criteria for the use of radiology in dental implantology with emphasis on cone beam computed tomography. Oral Surg Oral Med Oral Pathol Oral Radiol. 2012;113:817–26.
2. Weckx A, Agbaje JO, Sun Y, Jacobs R, Politis C. Visualization techniques of the inferior alveolar nerve (IAN): a narrative review. Surg Radiol Anat. 2016;38:55–63.
3. Shokri A, Shakibaei Z, Langaroodi AJ, Safaei M. Evaluation of the mandibular canal visibility on cone-beam computed tomography images of the mandible. J Craniofac Surg. 2014;25:e273–7.
4. Miles MS, Parks ET, Eckert GJ, Blanchard SB. Comparative evaluation of mandibular canal visibility on cross-sectional cone-beam CT images: a retrospective study. Dentomaxillofac Radiol. 2016;45:20150296.
5. Oliveira-Santos C, Cappelozza ALÁ, Dezzoti MSG, Fischer CM, Poleti ML, Rubira-bullen IRF. Visibility of the mandibular canal on CBCT crosssectional images. J Appl Oral Sci. 2011;19:240–3.
6. Jung YH, Cho BH. Radiographic evaluation of the course and visibility of the mandibular canal. Imaging Sci Dent. 2014;44:273–8.
7. Angelopoulos C, Thomas S, Hechler S, Parissis N, Hlavacek M. Comparison between digital panoramic radiography and cone-beam computed tomography for the identification of the mandibular canal as part of presurgical dental implant assessment. J Oral Maxillofac Surg. 2008;66: 2130–5.
8. de Oliveira-Santos C, Souza PH, de Azambuja Berti-Couto S, Stinkens L, Moyaert K, Rubira-Bullen IR, Jacobs R. Assessment of variations of the mandibular canal through cone beam computed tomography. Clin Oral Investig. 2012;16:387–93.
9. Brüllmann D, Schulze RK. Spatial resolution in CBCT machines for dental/ maxillofacial applications—what do we know today? Dentomaxillofac Radiol. 2015;44:20140204.
10. Pauwels R, Beinsberger J, Stamatakis H, Tsiklakis K, Walker A, Bosmans H, Bogaerts R, Jacobs R, Horner K; SEDENTEXCT Project Consortium. Comparison of spatial and contrast resolution for cone-beam computed tomography scanners. Oral Surg Oral Med Oral Pathol Oral Radiol 2012; 114: 127-135.
11. Faul F, Erdfelder E, Lang A-G, Buchner A. G*Power 3: a flexible statistical power analysis program for the social, behavioral, and biomedical sciences. Behav Res Methods. 2007;39:175–91.
12. Kundel HL, Polansky M. Measurement of observer agreement. Radiology. 2003;228:303–8.
13. Alhassani AA, AlGhamdi AS. Inferior alveolar nerve injury in implant dentistry: diagnosis, causes, prevention, and management. J Oral Implantol. 2010;36:401–7.
14. Waltrick KB, Nunes de Abreu Junior MJ, Corrêa M, Zastrow MD, Dutra VD. Accuracy of linear measurements and visibility of the mandibular canal of cone-beam computed tomography images with different voxel sizes: an in vitro study. J Periodontol. 2013;84:68–77.
15. Hassan BA, Payam J, Juyanda B, van der Stelt P, Wesselink PR. Influence of scan setting selections on root canal visibility with cone beam CT. Dentomaxillofac Radiol. 2012;41:645–8.
16. Liang X, Jacobs R, Hassan B, Li L, Pauwels R, Corpas L, Souza PC, Martens W, Shahbazian M, Alonso A, Lambrichts I. A comparative evaluation of cone beam computed tomography (CBCT) and multi-slice CT (MSCT) Part I. on subjective image quality. Eur J Radiol. 2010;75:265–9.
17. Greenstein G, Tarnow D. The mental foramen and nerve: clinical and anatomical factors related to dental implant placement: a literature review. J Periodontol. 2006;77:1933–43.
18. de Oliveira Júnior MR, Saud AL, Fonseca DR, De-Ary-Pires B, Pires-Neto MA, de Ary-Pires R. Morphometrical analysis of the human mandibular canal: a CT investigation. Surg Radiol Anat. 2011;33:345–52.
19. Denio D, Torabinejad M, Bakland LK. Anatomical relationship of the mandibular canal to its surrounding structures in mature mandibles. J Endod. 1992;18:161–5.
20. Kamrun N, Tetsumura A, Nomura Y, Yamaguchi S, Baba O, Nakamura S, Watanabe H, Kurabayashi T. Visualization of the superior and inferior borders of the mandibular canal: a comparative study using digital panoramic radiographs and cross-sectional computed tomography images. Oral Surg Oral Med Oral Pathol Oral Radiol. 2013;115:550–7.
21. Kubilius M, Kubilius R, Varinauskas V, Žalinkevičius R, Tözüm TF, Juodžbalys G. Descriptive study of mandibular canal visibility: morphometric and densitometric analysis for digital panoramic radiographs. Dentomaxillofac Radiol. 2016;45:20160079.
22. Bertl K, Heimel P, Reich KM, Schwarze UY, Ulm C. A histomorphometric analysis of the nature of the mandibular canal in the anterior molar region. Clin Oral Investig. 2014;18:41–7.
23. Starkie C, Stewart D. The intra-mandibular course of the inferior dental nerve. J Anat. 1931;65:319–23.
24. Carter RB, Keen EN. The intramandibular course of the inferior alveolar nerve. J Anat. 1971;108:433–40.
25. Naitoh M, Katsumata A, Kubota Y, Hayashi M, Ariji E. Relationship between cancellous bone density and mandibular canal depiction. Implant Dent. 2009;18:112–8.
26. Koivisto T, Chiona D, Milroy LL, McClanahan SB, Ahmad M, Bowles WR. Mandibular canal location: cone-beam computed tomography examination. J Endod. 2016;42:1018–21.
27. Takahashi A, Watanabe H, Kamiyama Y, Honda E, Sumi Y, Kurabayashi T. Localizing the mandibular canal on dental CT reformatted images: usefulness of panoramic views. Surg Radiol Anat. 2013;35:803–9.
28. Deepho C, Watanabe H, Kotaki S, Sakamoto J, Sumi Y, Kurabayashi T. Utility of fusion volumetric images from computed tomography and magnetic resonance imaging for localizing the mandibular canal. Dentomaxillofac Radiol. 2017;46:20160383.

11

The use of a biphasic calcium phosphate in a maxillary sinus floor elevation procedure: a clinical, radiological, histological, and histomorphometric evaluation with 9- and 12-month healing times

W. F. Bouwman[1,5], N. Bravenboer[2], J. W. F. H. Frenken[3], C. M. ten Bruggenkate[1,4] and E. A. J. M. Schulten[1*]

Abstract

Background: This study evaluates the clinical, radiological, histological, and histomorphometric aspects of a fully synthetic biphasic calcium phosphate (BCP) (60% hydroxyapatite and 40% ß-tricalcium phosphate), used in a human maxillary sinus floor elevation (MSFE) procedure with 9- and 12-month healing time.

Methods: A unilateral MSFE procedure, using 100% BCP, was performed in two series of five patients with healing times of 9 and 12 months respectively. Clinical and radiological parameters were measured up to 5 years postoperatively. Biopsy retrieval was carried out during dental implants placement. Histology and histomorphometry were performed on 5-μm sections of undecalcified bone biopsies.

Results: The MSFE procedure with BCP showed uneventful healing in all cases. All dental implants appeared to be well osseointegrated after 3 months. Radiological evaluation showed less than 1 mm tissue height loss from MSFE to the 5-year follow-up examination. No signs of inflammation were detected on histological examination. Newly formed mineralized tissue was found cranially from the native bone. The BCP particles were surrounded by connective tissue, osteoid islands, and newly formed bone. Mineralized bone tissue was in intimate contact with the BCP particles. After 12 months, remnants of BCP were still present. The newly formed bone had a trabecular structure. Bone maturation was demonstrated by the presence of lamellar bone. Histomorphometric analysis showed at 9 and 12 months respectively an average vital bone volume/total volume of 35.2 and 28.2%, bone surface/total volume of 4.2 mm^2/mm^3 and 8.3 mm^2/mm^3, trabecular thickness of 224.7 and 66.7 μm, osteoid volume/bone volume of 8.8 and 3.4%, osteoid surface/bone surface (OS/BS) of 42.4 and 8.2%, and osteoid thickness of 93.9 and 13.6 μm.

Conclusions: MFSE with BCP resulted in new bone formation within the augmented sinus floor and allowed the osseointegration of dental implants in both groups. From a histological and histomorphometric perspective, a 9-month healing time for this type of BCP may be the optimal time for placement of dental implants.

Keywords: Biphasic calcium phosphate, Bone substitute, Sinus augmentation, Sinus floor elevation

* Correspondence: eajm.schulten@vumc.nl
[1]Department of Oral and Maxillofacial Surgery/Oral Pathology, VU University Medical Center/Academic Centre for Dentistry Amsterdam (ACTA), P.O. Box 7057, 1007 MB Amsterdam, The Netherlands
Full list of author information is available at the end of the article

Background

Maxillary sinus floor elevation (MSFE) is a surgical procedure to enhance the bone height in the posterior maxilla with graft material, allowing dental implant placement (later or at the same time) [1, 2]. This pre-implant procedure is predictable and results in a dental implant survival of more than 93.8% 3 years after dental implant placement [3]. According to Pjetursson [4] in his systematic review on success of implants inserted in combination with sinus floor elevation, the implant survival increases to 98.3% after 3 years when compared to non-augmented jawbone.

Autogenous bone is still the gold standard, because of its osteoconductive and osteoinductive properties, due to the possible osteogenic capacity [5–10]. Moreover, the bone morphogenic proteins, present in autogenous bone grafts, can attract osteogenic cells from the surrounding tissues, in their turn containing other growth factors essential for the process of bone graft incorporation [4].

As the maxillary tuberosity, mandibular retromolar or chin region do not always supply enough bone graft volume, bone grafts can also be harvested from the anterior iliac crest, the tibia, the rib, and the calvarian bone. However, these harvesting procedures have disadvantages, such as prolonged operating time, donor site morbidity, hospitalization [9, 11–13], sensory disturbances [14], and unpredictable resorption rate of the bone grafts [5, 15]. Donor site morbidity may be a major reason to question the use of autogenous bone [16]. Therefore, several types and properties of bone substitutes (alloplast, xenograft, allograft, and mixtures of various materials) have been developed [16, 17] to overcome the disadvantages mentioned above.

Calcium phosphates, such as hydroxyapatite (HA), β-tricalcium phosphate (β-TCP), or biphasic calcium phosphate (BCP), a mixture of HA and β-TCP, are osteoconductive as they resemble the chemical composition of natural bone [18, 19]. Calcium phosphates are biocompatible and do not induce a sustained foreign body response or toxic reaction [20]. At a physiological pH, calcium phosphates are the least soluble of the naturally occurring calcium phosphates, which makes them relatively resistant to resorption [21–23].

β-TCP is a biocompatible osteoconductive calcium phosphate that may provide a scaffold for potential bony ingrowth [24]. β-TCP resorbs rather quickly but not necessarily at the same rate as new bone formation [25–27]. Most research focused on either using the relative unresorbable HA as a scaffold or β-TCP as a degradable component [19, 24–26, 28, 29]. Zerbo et al. [30] concluded that due to the absence of osteoinductive properties of TCP, the rate of bone formation was delayed in comparison with autogenous bone grafts. It would be beneficial for the patient to reduce the interval between the MSFE procedure and dental implant placement to accelerate the process of integration of the grafted material. BCP, in a combination of 60% HA and 40% β-tricalcium phosphate, demonstrated new bone formation in both animals and humans [24, 31–33]. This biphasic calcium phosphate (BCP) appeared to be a suitable graft material for vertical augmentation of the posterior maxilla by means of an MSFE procedure and dental implants placement in a study with a healing time of 6 months [16, 27, 34].The process of bone substitution may not be completed after 6 months of follow-up [27, 35]. Even though clinically, the tissue seems stable enough for dental implant placement, the high bone formation, especially in the newly formed bone areas, indicates that after 6 months, bone cells are still actively replacing BCP in vital bone tissue. To date, no long-term follow-up has been reported on the use of a synthetic BCP, consisting of 60% HA and 40% β-TCP, which may elucidate the degradation properties of BCP material. One may have to consider that more time is necessary to achieve a new bone balance. The aim of this study is to evaluate the clinical, radiological, histological, and histomorphometric aspects of a synthetic BCP (Straumann® Bone Ceramic, Institut Straumann AG, Basel Switzerland) that was used in a MSFE procedure with 9- and 12-month healing times.

Methods

Study population

In this study, 10 consecutive healthy patients were selected for a unilateral MSFE procedure. Five patients received dental implants 9 months after MSFE and five patients underwent dental implant surgery 12 months after MSFE. In the 9-month group (three men and two women), the average age was 56.6 years (range 40 to 64 years); in the 12-month group (one man and four women), the average age was 58.2 years (range 51 to 67 years). All patients were partially edentulous in the posterior maxilla without the need for onlay bone grafting of the alveolar crest to achieve an adequate alveolar ridge. A minimal native bone height of 4 mm (calculated from measurements on a preoperative panoramic radiograph) was preferred in both study groups. All selected patients were non-smokers, showed no systemic disease, and were not drug users.

The study was performed in accordance with the principles of the Declaration of Helsinki. Since the study involved CE-marked devices (calcium phosphates) being used for their intended purpose (use as carrier material for bone augmentation in sinus floor elevation procedures) and the harvested material can be regarded as surgical waste, no specific regulatory approval from a medical ethical committee was required. Patients provided written consent before the study-related procedures were undertaken. The biopsies were retrieved during dental implant surgery by means of trephine drills, implicating the tissue in the hollow drill is considered surgical waste. For the patient, this is not an additional invasive procedure. The different healing times did not have a negative impact on the patients.

Maxillary sinus floor elevation procedure

Ten patients were scheduled for a unilateral two-stage MSFE top-hinge door lateral window technique procedure, as described by Tatum [2]. All 10 patients were treated in an outpatient procedure under local anesthesia. Perioperatively, all patients received an antibiotic profylaxis, consisting of amoxicillin 500 mg four times daily for 7 days, starting 1 day before the MSFE procedure. An oral rinse with chloorhexidine-digluconate 0.12%, three times, 10 cm^3 daily for 1 min for 2 weeks was prescribed, as part of the standard protocol for an MSFE procedure.

A midcrestal incision was made with vertical release incisions at the canine and tuberosity region. A full-thickness mucoperiosteal flap was elevated. The lateral maxillary sinus wall was prepared using a diamond burr with copious irrigation with sterile isotonic saline, regarding the contour of the maxillary sinus as observed on the preoperative panoramic radiograph. A bony top-hinge trap-door was mobilized and turned inward and upward into a horizontal position in the maxillary sinus, together with the carefully elevated Schneiderian membrane. The area created between the lifted lid and the sinus floor was filled only with BCP (Straumann® Bone Ceramic). The BCP was 100% crystalline, highly pure, and had a porosity of 90%. The pores were 100 to 500 μm in diameter. No membrane was used to cover the lateral window [36]. Primary wound closure was performed with Gore-Tex® sutures (W.L. Gore & Associates, Newark, DE, USA). Immediately after the procedure, a panoramic radiograph was made. Postoperative examination and removal of the sutures were performed 10 to 14 days after the MSFE procedure.

Dental implant surgery and biopsy retrieval

After 9-month (five patients) and 12-month (five patients) healing times, a crestal incision was made with small mesial and distal buccal vertical release incisions. Subsequently, a full-thickness mucoperiostal flap was raised. The alveolar ridge was inspected for suitable implant placement, and the former lateral window area was inspected for tissue condition. Implant preparations were made, and biopsies were obtained from the grafted area at planned dental implant positions using trephine drills with an external diameter of 3.5 mm and internal diameter of 2.5 mm (Straumann® trephine drill) with copious irrigation of sterile saline. In the 10 patients, 22 standard plus, regular neck, soft tissue level Straumann® SLA dental implants with a diameter of 4.1 mm and a length of 10 or 12 mm were placed (Fig. 1). The implants were left to integrate in a non-submerged unloaded fashion. Soft tissue closure was performed with Gore-Tex® sutures. A postoperative radiological examination (panoramic radiograph) was taken directly after dental implantation. Sutures were removed after 10 to 14 days and, if needed, provisional prosthetics were adapted to the new situation. Attention was paid to prevent premature loading of the dental implants. The patients were instructed to avoid loading of the posterior maxilla upon which the operation had been conducted until the 3-month

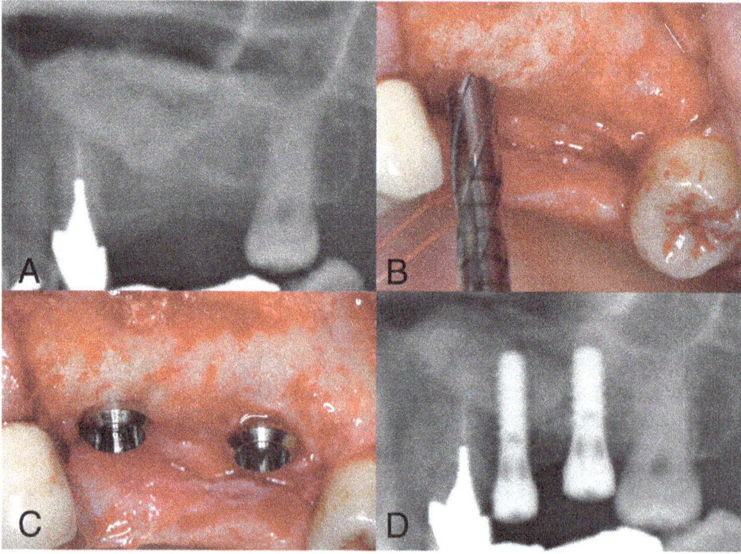

Fig. 1 Images of patient # 5 (9-month healing time). **a.** Radiograph of the left maxillary sinus: situation 9 months after the maxillary sinus floor elevation procedure. **b.** With a trephine drill, the implant osteotomy is made and the biopsy is obtained. **c.** Clinical situation after placing two Straumann® SLA implants in the left posterior maxilla. **d.** Radiograph of two Straumann® SLA implants in the left posterior maxilla

integration time of the dental implants had passed and the fixed superstructures were fabricated and placed.

Clinical evaluation

All 22 inserted dental implants were clinically tested for good primary stability. Osseointegration at abutment connection was tested with a 35-Ncm torque. One experienced oral and maxillofacial surgeon (CB) carried out all follow-up examinations.

Radiological evaluation

Panoramic radiographs were made at patient's intake (T0); immediately after the MSFE procedure (T1); immediately after dental implant placement (T2); 1 year after dental implant placement (T3); and 5 years after dental implant placement (T4). On the panoramic radiographs, changes in tissue height (mm) of the grafted area were measured at the implant site on the following time points: T0, T1, T2, T3, and T4. An average magnification of ×1.25 was taken into account to calculate true tissue heights.

Qualitative histological and quantitative histomorphometric analysis

Bone biopsies were obtained during implant surgery as previously described [37]. Trephines were split and opened in order to secure the orientation of the biopsies. The biopsies were fixed overnight in 4% phosphate-buffered formaldehyde and transferred to alcohol 70% [38]. After dehydration, the bone specimens were embedded without prior decalcification in methylmethacrylate supplemented with 20% dibuthylphtalaat and 0.008 g/ml Lucidol. The biopsies were cut into 5-μm longitudinal sections (Polycut S., Leica microtome type sm2500s, Leica, Wetzlar, Germany). Bone mass indices and osteoid surface were measured in Goldner's trichrome stained sections [39]. Tartrate-resistant acid phosphate (TRAP) staining was performed to visualize osteoclasts. Measurements were performed semi-automatically using a digitizer and image analysis software (Osteomeasure, Atlanta, GA, USA). In this study, the Von Kossa staining was used to verify remnant particles of BCP (Straumann® Bone Ceramic). BCP particles were detected semi-quantitatively by three independent observers and classified into quartiles (<25% of BCP, >25% and <50% of BCP, >50 <75% of BCP, >75% of BCP). Nomenclature was used according to the American Society for Bone and Mineral Research (ASBMR) nomenclature committee [40].

Since it was impossible to discriminate between resident and augmented bone, histomorphometric measurements were performed over the total section of the biopsy, including native and newly formed bone. The parameters were measured in consecutive fields of a complete section, in four 150-μm separated sections throughout the biopsy, covering a total measured area of 60 mm^2. The specimens were examined for the following parameters:

Parameters evaluating vital bone mass/bone structure:

1: Vital bone volume (BV): percentage of the grafted section that is vital bone tissue (%)

2: Bone surface (BS): BS expressed as a fraction of the total vital bone volume (mm^2/mm^3)

3: Thickness of bone trabeculae (Tb.Th) (μm)

Parameters evaluating bone turnover:

1: Osteoid volume (OV): fraction of the vital bone tissue section that is osteoid (%)

2: Osteoid surface (OS): osteoid-covered surfaces expressed as the fraction of the total BS (%) to measure new vital bone formation

3: Osteoid thickness (O.Th) (μm)

4: Number of osteoclasts (N.Oc) per mm^2 total area

Statistical analysis

Because of the observational nature of this study and the limited number of biopsies, only descriptive statistics are presented. Results are expressed as mean standard deviation.

Results

Clinical evaluation

None of the 10 patients showed postoperative inflammation or infection after the MSFE procedure nor during surgical re-entry for dental implant placement. When opening the area for dental implant insertion, the grafted area proved to be well vascularized and the tissue at the site of the former trap-door location was slightly flexible and had a fibrous aspect. Between the periosteum and the bone graft area, adhesions were seen. Macroscopically, no voids or presence of purulent discharge were observed. Although a demarcation was observed between the grafted area and the original bone of the alveolar process, there was continuity between the grafted area and the native bone. There was no jiggling of the drill, even though bone substitute particles could still be recognized in the tissue specimen retrieved. All particles appeared well integrated in newly formed tissue. These findings were consistent in all 10 patients. In total, 22 Straumann® SLA solid screw (standard plus regular neck, soft tissue level) dental implants with a diameter of 4.1 mm and a length of 10 or 12 mm were placed. Primary stability was achieved with all dental implants. All dental implants osseointegrated well and could be loaded with fixed prostheses 3 months after implant surgery. No dental implants were lost during 5-year follow-up.

Radiological evaluation

The increase in height of the grafted area achieved by the MSFE procedure was on an average of 7.5 mm (SD ±2.8) in the 9-month group (Table 1) and 9.3 mm (SD ±3.1) in

Table 1 Alveolar tissue height measurements on panoramic radiographs (in true mm) in the 9-month group

Patient	Gender/age	Implant site	T0	T1	Increase	T2	T3	T4
1	F/54	15	5.4	15.2	9.8	14.0	13.6	13.2
1	F/54	16	5.7	14.3	8.6	14.6	13.0	13.5
2	M/62	16	5.5	15.1	9.6	13.2	12.4	12.4
3	F/64	15	7.0	15.2	8.2	13.4	12.8	12.2
4	M/63	26	6.0	11.7	5.7	14.7	14.8	14.6
4	M/63	27	10.0	11.3	1.3	14.8	13.5	13.4
5	M/40	26	4.1	12.3	8.2	12.4	12.0	12.5
5	M/40	27	7.3	16.3	9.0	15.5	14.3	13.8
Mean	56.6		6.4	13.9	7.5	14.1	13.3	13.2
SD			1.7	1.9	2.8	1.0	0.9	0.8

Age in years at biopsy retrieval; hard tissue height corrected for magnification (×1.25) on panoramic radiograph
M male, *F* female, *T0* (native bone height) preoperative alveolar bone height, *T1* directly after MSFE procedure, *T2* immediately after dental implant placement, *T3* 1 year after dental implant placement, *T4* 5 years after dental implant placement

the 12-month group (Table 2). The measured tissue height appeared to be stable between 1 and 5 years in the 9-month group (Fig. 2) and the 12-month group (Fig. 3).

Qualitative histological evaluation

The histological evaluation was performed on the complete section, comprising native bone, newly formed bone, and residual graft material. The BCP particles were surrounded by connective tissue, osteoid islands, and newly formed bone. From the residual bone in all specimens, new bone formation was detected following the scaffold of the bone substitute, starting in cranial direction. This newly formed bone consisted of woven bone as well as lamellar bone and appeared as vital bone tissue containing osteoblasts, osteoid covering the border, and osteocytes inside bone lacunae. Cranially, near the lifted trap-door, some osteoid islands with osteogenic activity were detected.

Table 2 Radiological results (alveolar tissue height measurements in true mm) in the 12-month group

Patient	Gender/age	Implant site	T0	T1	Increase	T2	T3	T4
1	F/53	15	6.3	17.6	11.3	18.7	17.4	17.4
1	F/53	16	2.5	17.6	15.1	17.9	16.4	15.9
1	F/53	17	1.3	15.5	14.2	13.7	12.8	12.6
2	F/53	26	8.8	17.2	8.4	16.7	16.1	17.0
2	F/53	27	7.9	13.1	5.2	11.3	12.0	11.9
3	F/67	14	4.2	13.4	9.2	14.1	14.0	14.0
3	F/67	15	4.1	11.0	6.9	9.9	12.7	12.8
3	F/67	16	5.6	9.9	4.3	9.0	11.4	11.0
4	M/67	14	2.5	13.9	11.4	13.8	13.3	14.1
4	M/67	15	3.0	12.2	9.2	12.5	11.2	11.8
4	M/67	17	4.3	10.7	6.4	10.5	10.1	10.3
5	F/51	24	5.5	13.7	8.2	14.0	13.8	14.4
5	F/51	25	2.5	13.0	10.5	14.6	13.6	13.2
5	F/51	26	3.6	14.1	10.5	14.0	13.2	13.4
Mean	58.2		4.4	13.8	9.3	13.6	13.4	13.5
SD			2.0	2.3	3.1	3.8	2.0	2.1

Age in years at biopsy retrieval; hard tissue height corrected for magnification (×1.25) on panoramic radiograph
M male, *F* female, *T0* (native bone height) preoperative alveolar bone height, *T1* after MSFE procedure, *T2* immediately after dental implant placement, *T3* 1 year after dental implant placement, *T4* 5 years after dental implant placement

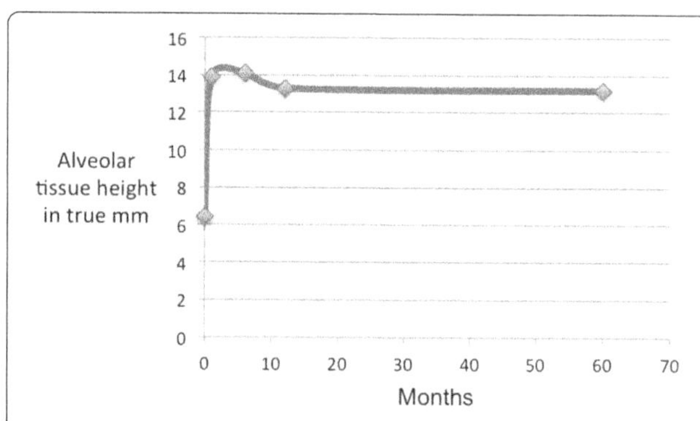

Fig. 2 Aveolar tissue height (in true mm) over a 5-year period in the 9-month group

Histological observations did not show inflammatory cells in the tissue adjacent to the bone substitute particles. Bone marrow-like tissue, which included blood vessels, was observed in between the bone trabeculae (Fig. 4). Reinforcement by lamellar bone was shown in some areas after 9 and 12 months (Figs. 5 and 6). No Howship's lacunae could be detected on the characteristic outlines of the substitute particles. Fragments of the substitute particles were present in the sections of the 9-month group and the 12-month group, as confirmed by Von Kossa staining. Regardless of the histological process, the contours of the bone substitute remnants were clearly detectable which enabled analyses.

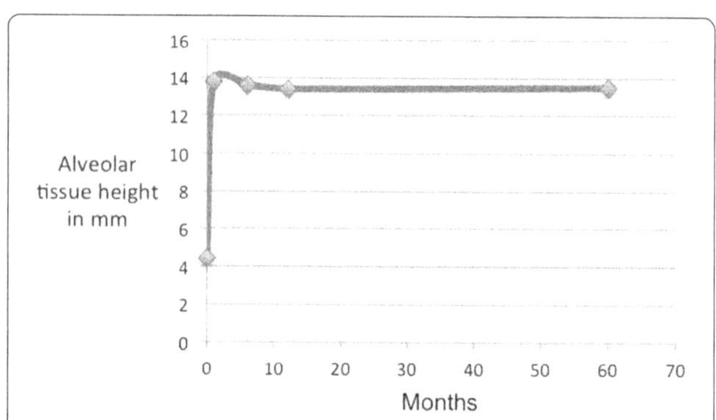

Fig. 3 Alveolar tissue height (in true mm) over a 5-year period in the 12-month group

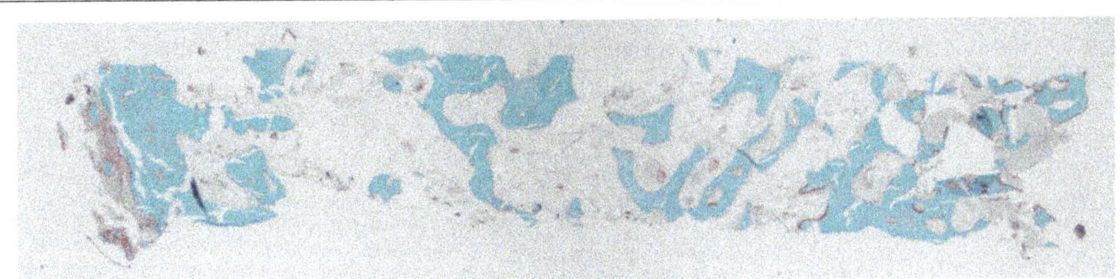

Fig. 4 Patient # 1 (12-month healing time): overview of a typical example of a bone biopsy stained with Goldner trichrome staining (magnification ×10)

Quantitative histomorphometric evaluation

In the 9-month group, the average vital bone volume was 35.2% of the total biopsy volume (SD ±9.5) of which 8.8% (SD ±3.8) was osteoid. The osteoid surface covered 42.4% (SD ±12.1) of the bone surface. The BS covered 4.2 mm^2/mm^3 (SD ±1.9). In the total area for the 12-month group, the average vital bone volume was 28.2% of the total biopsy volume (SD ±3.2) of which 3.4% (SD ±2.5) was osteoid. The osteoid surface covered 8.2% (SD ±5.3) of the bone surface. The BS covered 8.3 mm^2/mm^3 (SD ±1.3). In conclusion, vital bone volume and bone turnover decreased in the 12-month group compared to the 9-month group. An overview of the individual histomorphometric findings is listed in Tables 3 and 4.

Discussion

This study presents the clinical, radiological, histological and histomorphometric results on the use of a biphasic calcium phosphate (Straumann® bone ceramic) in a MSFE procedure with healing times of 9 and 12 months. During the clinical evaluation, it appeared that both 9-month and 12-month healing times resulted in integration of the grafted BCP with the original maxillary bone (sinus floor), which was stable enough to ensure successful dental implant placement. It should be mentioned that in this study, a minimal native alveolar bone height of 4 mm was preferred, ensuring a certain primary stability of the dental implants placed. An adequate and stable tissue height in the grafted area was observed radiologically in a 5-year follow-up in all patients in both 9-month and 12-month healing time groups.

Radiological observations show very stable results in different healing times, in a previous 6-month study [27] and after 9- and 12-month healing times in the present study. However, this does not reveal the actual vital bone height available for attachment to the dental implant surfacc. This can only be measured by histological investigations. Reviews show that the loss of dental implants with an intra-osseous length of 8 mm or more, placed in native bone, is minimal [4]. Previously, the histomorphometrical and histological evaluation, 6 months after an MSFE procedure, using Straumann® bone ceramic was reported with a 1-year follow-up. At that time, no loss of dental implants was reported. In the present study, none of the implants in the 9- and 12-month groups were lost. Histological investigation showed that mineralized bone tissue was observed to be in intimate contact with the bone substitute particles, indicating that the graft

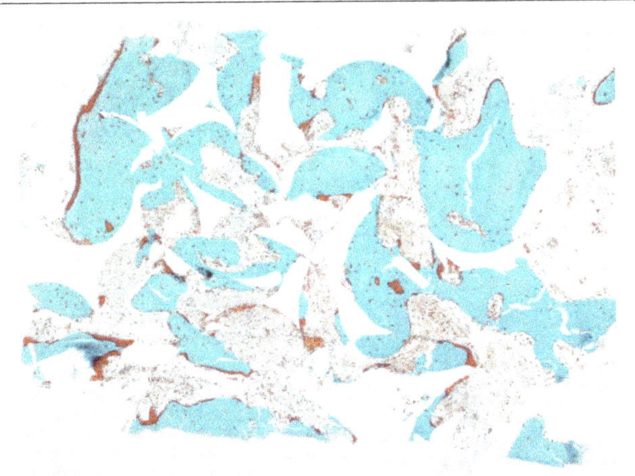

Fig. 5 Patient # 4 (9-month healing time): increased bone formation following the shape of the grafted particles stained with Goldner trichrome staining (magnification ×100)

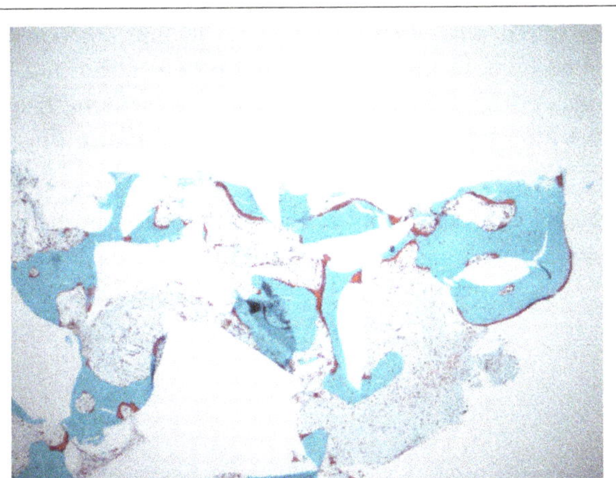

Fig. 6 Patient # 1 (12-month healing time): increased bone formation following the shape of the grafted particles that are still present (magnification ×100)

Table 3 Histomorphometric evaluation of the biopsies after a 9-month healing time

Patient (*N*)	Gender/age	Retrieval location	BV/TV (%)	BS/TV (mm^2/mm^3)	Tb.Th (μm)	OV/BV (%)	OS/BS (%)	O.Th (μm)	N.Oc/Tar ($1/mm^2$)
1	F/54	15	51.3	2.3	461.3	5.4	43.4	28.3	0.8
2	M/62	16	30.4	2.2	278.6	13.3	53.3	331.8	2.0
3	F/64	15	29.3	4.6	121.7	8.5	50.0	10.2	2.5
4	M/63	27	36.3	5.8	168.8	4.7	22.3	18.8	2.3
5	M/40	26	28.5	6.2	93.0	12.0	43.0	80.2	5.0
Mean			35.2	4.2	224.7	8.8	42.4	93.9	2.5
SD			9.5	1.9	150.0	3.8	12.1	135.8	1.5

Not intact biopsies were excluded from histomorphometric examination. Age in years at biopsy retrieval
M male, *F* female, *BV/TV* vital bone volume/total volume, *BS/TV* bone surface/total volume, *Tb.Th* trabeculae thickness, *OV/BV* osteoid volume/vital bone volume, *OS/BS* osteoid surface/bone surface, *O.Th* osteoid thickness, *N.Oc/Tar* number of osteoclasts in total area

material possesses osteoconductive properties [27] (which is in agreement with other observations) [16, 24, 34]. This positive effect might be explained by its chemical composition. BCP materials have shown bone formation simultaneously with material degradation [24, 25]. BCP exhibited moderate signs of substitute degradation in humans not only after 6 months, as previously reported by Frenken et al. [27]. The present study still observed remnants of BCP after 9 and 12 months which suggests that the ossification rate is not the same as the resorption rate of the BCP. Because osteoclasts were detected next to the characteristic outlines of the substitute particles, it is suggested that BCP is resorbed by osteoclasts. The high bone formation in the newly formed bone area indicates that after 12 months, bone cells are still actively forming new bone matrix, thereby absorbing and replacing BCP in vital bone tissue.

In the cranial part of the biopsy, some osteoid islands with osteogenic activity were detected, possibly caused by osteoinductive properties from the lifted bony trapdoor. In the present study, histomorphometric analyses revealed that the vital bone volume was higher in the 9-month healing time group than in the 12-month healing time group, while one would expect to find more newly formed bone in time as more of the bone substitute resorbs. As the mean original native alveolar bone height is 6.4 mm in the 9-month group and 4.4 mm in the 12-month group and augmented portion of the 12-month group (9.3 mm) is higher than the 9-month group (7.5 mm), this may have a negative impact on the relatively smaller portion of the bone volume of the total biopsy in the 12-month group. This is a limitation of the present study.

However, the average 2 mm of difference in the native bone height between the 9- and 12-month groups does not fully explain the difference in BT/TV that was found between the two groups. Furthermore, the thickness of the bone trabeculae decreased suggesting that at 12 months, bone turnover returns to a relatively normal bone remodeling status, indicative of a new balance in bone tissue. However, woven bone (data not shown) and the remnants of the BCP were still present at 12 months, contradicting this hypothesis. Nevertheless, from a histological and histomorphometric perspective in the present study, a 9-month healing time may be the optimal time for the placement of dental implants. Although the sample size of the two groups is small, multiple dental implant placements deliver sufficient data for evaluation. The 12-month period from MSFE to implant placement(s) is considered to be a long time. Most patients are not willing to wait that long, which makes these bone samples very scarce and therefore valuable for long-term observations. The implication of the small sample size is that this study has an

Table 4 Histomorphometric evaluation of the biopsies after a 12-month healing time

Patient (*N*)	Gender/age	Retrieval location	BV/TV (%)	BS/TV (mm^2/mm^3)	Tb.Th (μm)	OV/BV (%)	OS/BS (%)	O.Th (μm)
1	F/53	16	25.5	6.9	74.1	1.7	5.2	12.8
2	F/53	25	30.8	9.2	66.8	1.1	3.1	12.7
2	F/53	26	29.3	9.5	61.5	4.2	9.2	14.7
3	M/67	17	24.0	7.5	64.4	6.6	15.2	14.0
Mean			28.2	8.3	66.7	3.4	8.2	13.6
SD			3.2	1.3	5.4	2.5	5.3	1

Not intact biopsies were excluded from histomorphometric examination. Age in years at biopsy retrieval
M male, *F* female, *BV/TV* vital bone volume/total volume, *BS/TV* bone surface/total volume, *Tb.Th* trabeculae thickness, *OV/BV* osteoid volume/vital bone volume, *OS/BS* osteoid surface/bone surface, *O.Th* osteoid thickness, *NOc/BPm* not measured as an insignificant number of osteoclasts were available

observational nature and, therefore, only descriptive statistics are presented.

Conclusions

Based on clinical, radiological, histological, and histomorphometric analysis, this study confirms the suitability of BCP for vertical augmentation of the posterior maxilla by means of an MSFE procedure, allowing dental implant placement after 9 and 12 months healing times. Yet, complete degradation of the BCP particles does not occur within a 12-month healing time. From a histological and histomorphometric perspective, a 9-month healing time for this type of BCP may be the optimal time for the placement of dental implants.

Authors' contributions

WB contributed to the data acquisition, data analysis, and writing of the manuscript. BS and CB contributed to the design of the study and critical reading of the manuscript and have given final approval of the manuscript. NB contributed to the design of the study, data analysis, and critical reading of the manuscript. JF contributed to the data acquisition. All authors read and approved the final manuscript.

Competing interests

Authors W.F. Bouwman, N. Bravenboer, J.W.F.H. Frenken, C.M. ten Bruggenkate and E.A.J.M. Schulten state that there are no conflicts of interest, either directly or indirectly.

Author details

[1]Department of Oral and Maxillofacial Surgery/Oral Pathology, VU University Medical Center/Academic Centre for Dentistry Amsterdam (ACTA), P.O. Box 7057, 1007 MB Amsterdam, The Netherlands. [2]Department of Clinical Chemistry, VU University Medical Center, Amsterdam, The Netherlands. [3]Department of Oral and Maxillofacial Surgery, St. Antonius Hospital, Nieuwegein, The Netherlands. [4]Department of Oral and Maxillofacial Surgery, Alrijne Hospital, Leiderdorp, The Netherlands. [5]Department of Oral and Maxillofacial Surgery, The Tergooi Hospital, Blaricum, The Netherlands.

References

1. Boyne PJ, James RA. Grafting of the maxillary sinus floor with autogenous marrow and bone. J Oral Surg. 1980;38:613–6.
2. Tatum H Jr. Maxillary and sinus implant reconstructions. Dent Clin N Am. 1986;30:207–29.
3. Del Fabbro M, Rosano G, Taschieri S. Implant survival rates after maxillary sinus augmentation. Eur J Oral Sci. 2008;116:497–506.
4. Pjetursson BE, Tan WC, Zwahlen M, Lang NP. A systematic review of the success of sinus floor elevation and survival of implants inserted in combination with sinus floor elevation. Part I: lateral approach. J Clin Periodontol. 2008;35:216–40.
5. Burchardt H. The biology of bone graft repair. Clin Orthop Relat Res. 1983; 174:28–42.
6. Jensen OT, Shulman LB, Block MS, Iacono VJ. Report of the sinus consensus conference of 1996. Int J Oral Maxillofac Implants. 1998;13(Suppl):11–45.
7. Tong DC, Rioux K, Drangsholt M, Beirne OR. A review of survival rates for implants placed in grafted maxillary sinuses using meta-analysis. Int J Oral Maxillofac Implants. 1998;13:175–82.
8. van den Bergh JP, ten Bruggenkate CM, Krekeler G, Tuinzing DB. Sinusfloor elevation and grafting with autogenous iliac crest bone. Clin Oral Implants Res. 1998;9:429–35.
9. Klijn RJ, Meijer GJ, Bronkhorst EM, Jansen JA. A meta-analysis of histomorphometric results and graft healing time of various biomaterials compared to autologous bone used as sinus floor augmentation material in humans. Tissue Eng Part B Rev. 2010;16:493–507.
10. Misch CM. Autogenous bone: is it still the gold standard? Implant Dent. 2010;19(5):361.
11. Kalk WW, Raghoebar GM, Jansma J, Boering G. Morbidity from iliac crest bone harvesting. Int J Oral Maxillofac Surg. 1996;54:1424–9.
12. Raghoebar GM, Louwerse C, Kalk WW, Vissink A. Morbidity of chin bone harvesting. Clin Oral Implants Res. 2001;12:503–7.
13. Zijderveld SA, ten Bruggenkate CM, van Den Bergh JP, EAJM S. Fractures of the iliac crest after split-thickness bone grafting for preprosthetic surgery: report of 3 cases and review of the literature. J Oral Maxillofac Surg. 2004;7:781–6.
14. Beirne JC, Barry HJ, Brady FA, Morris VB. Donor site morbidity of the anterior iliac crest following cancellous bone harvest. Int J Oral Maxillofac Surg. 1996; 25:268–71.
15. Vermeeren JIJF, Wismeijer D, van Waas MAJ. One-step reconstruction of the severely resorbed mandible with onlay bone grafts and endosteal implants: a 5-year follow-up. Int J Oral Maxillofac Surg. 1996;2:112–5.
16. Nkenke E, Stelzle F. Clinical outcomes of sinus floor augmentation for implant placement using autogenous bone or bone substitutes: a systematic review. Clin Oral Implants Res. 2009;20(Suppl. 4):124–33.
17. Wheeler SL. Sinus augmentation for dental implants: the use of alloplastic materials. J Oral Maxillofac Surg. 1997;55:1287–93.
18. Nery EB, Lee KK, Czajkowski S, Dooner JJ, Duggan M, Ellinger RF, Henkin JM, Hines R, Miller M, Olson JW. A veterans administration cooperative study of biphasic calcium phosphate ceramic in periodontal osseous defects. J Periodontol. 1990;61:737–44.
19. Zerbo IR, Bronckers AL, de Lange G, Burger EH. Localisation of osteogenic and osteoclastic cells in porous beta-tricalcium phosphate particles used for human maxillary sinus floor elevation. Biomaterials. 2005;26:1445–51.
20. Joosten U, Joist A, Frebel T, Walter M, Langer M. The use of an in situ curing hydroxyapatite cement as an alternative to bone graft following removal of enchondroma of the hand. J Hand Surg Br Eur. 2000;25(3):288–91.
21. Costantino PD, Friedman CD, Jones K, Chow LC, Pelzer HJ, Sisson GAS. Hydroxyapatite cement: I. Basic chemistry and histologic properties. Arch Otolaryngol Head Neck Surg. 1991;117:397–84.
22. Costantino PD, Friedman CD. Synthetic bone graft substitutes. Otolaryngolic Clin North Am. 1994;27:1037–74.
23. Jensen SS, Aaboe M, Pinholt EM, Hjorting-Hansen E, Melsen F, Ruyter IE. Tissue reaction and material characteristics of four bone substitutes. Int J Oral Maxillofac Implants. 1996;11:55–66.
24. Daculsi G, Laboux O, Malard O. Weiss P. Current state of the art of biphasic calcium phosphate bioceramics. J Mater Sci Mater Med 2003;14: 195–200.
25. LeGeros RZ, Lin S, Rohanizadeh R, Mijares D, LeGeros JP. Biphasic calcium phosphate bioceramics: preparation, properties and applications. J Mater Sci Mater Med. 2003;14:201–9.
26. Schopper C, Ziya-Ghazvini F, Goriwoda W, Moser D, Wanschitz F, Spassova E, Lagogiannis G, Auterith A, Ewers R. HA/TCP compounding of a porous CaP biomaterial improves bone formation and scaffold degradation—a long-term histological study. J Biomed Mater Res B Appl Biomater. 2005;74:458–67.
27. Frenken JW, Bouwman WF, Bravenboer N, Zijderveld SA, Schulten EA, ten Bruggenkate CM. The use of Straumann ® Bone Ceramic in a maxillary sinus floor elevation procedure: a clinical, radiological, histological and histomorphometric evaluation with a 6-month healing period. Clin Oral Implants Res. 2010;21:201–8.
28. Bodde EW, Wolke JG, Kowalski RS, Jansen JA. Bone regeneration of porous betatricalcium phosphate (Conduit TCP) and of biphasic calcium phosphate ceramic (Biosel) in trabecular defects in sheep. J Biomed Mater Res. 2007;A 82:711–22.
29. Cordaro L, Bosshardt DD, Palattella P, Rao W, Serino G, Chiapasco M. Maxillary sinus grafting with Bio-Osss or Straumanns Bone Ceramic: histomorphometric results from a randomized controlled multicenter clinical trial. Clin Oral Implants Res. 2008;19:796–803.
30. Zerbo IR, Zijderveld SA, de Boer A, Bronckers AL, de Lange G, ten Bruggenkate CM, Burger EH. Histomorphometry of human sinus floor augmentation using a porous beta-tricalcium phosphate: a prospective study. Clin Oral Implants Res. 2004;15:724–32.
31. Nery EB, LeGeros RZ, Lynch KL, Lee K. Tissue response to biphasic calcium phosphate ceramic with different ratios of HA/beta TCP in periodontal osseous defects. J Periodontol. 1992;63:729–35.

32. Boix D, Gauthier O, Guicheux J, Pilet P, Weiss P, Grimandi G, Daculsi G. Alveolar bone regeneration for immediate implant placement using an injectable bone substitute: an experimental study in dogs. J Periodontol. 2004;75:663–71.
33. Jensen SS, Yeo A, Dard M, Hunziker E, Schenk R. Buser D. Evaluation of a novel biphasic calcium phosphate in standardized bone defects. A histologic and histomorphometric study in the mandibles of minipigs. Clin Oral Implants Res 2007;18: 752–760.
34. Klijn RJ, Hoekstra JWM, Van Den Beucken JJJP, Meijer GJ, Jansen JA. Maxillary sinus augmentation with microstructured tricalcium phosphate ceramic in sheep. Clin Oral Implants Res. 2012;23:274–80.
35. Groeneveld EH, van den Bergh JP, Holzmann P, ten Bruggenkate CM, Tuinzing DB, Burger EH. Mineralization processes in demineralized bone matrix grafts in human maxillary sinus floor elevations. J Biomed Mater Res. 1999;48:393–402.
36. Schulten EAJM, Prins HJ, Overman JR, Helder MN, ten Bruggenkate CM, Klein-Nulend JA. Novel approach revealing the effect of collagenous membrane on osteoconduction in maxillary sinus floor elevation with β-tricalcium phosphate. Eur Cells Mater. 2013;25:215–28.
37. Oostlander AE, Bravenboer N, Sohl E, Holzmann PJ, van der Woude CJ, Dijkstra G, Stokkers PC, Oldenburg B, Netelenbos JC, Hommes DW, van Bodegraven AA, Lips P, Dutch Initiative on Crohn and Colitis (ICC). Histomorphometric analysis reveals reduced bone mass and bone formation in patients with quiescent Crohn's disease. Gastroenterology. 2011;140(1):116–23. Epub 2010 Sep 18
38. Schenk RK, Olah AJ, Herrmann W. Preparation of calcified tissues for light microscopy. In Methods of calcified tissue preparation. Dickson GR, editor. Amsterdam: Elsevier Science Publishers B.V.; 1984;1–56.
39. Romeis B. Trichromfaerbung nach Goldner, Mikroskopische Technik. Muenchen: Urban & Schwarzenberg; 1989.
40. Dempster DW, Compston JE, Drezner MK, Glorieux FH, Kanis JA, Malluche H, Meunier PJ, Ott SM, Recker RR, Parfitt AM. Standardized nomenclature, symbols, and units for bone histomorphometry: a 2012 update of the report of the ASBMR Histomorphometry Nomenclature Committee. Journal of Bone and Mineral Research. 2012;DOI: 10.1002/jbmr.180.

12

Treatment with teriparatide for advanced bisphosphonate-related osteonecrosis of the jaw around dental implants

Yusuke Zushi, Kazuki Takaoka*, Joji Tamaoka, Miho Ueta, Kazuma Noguchi and Hiromitsu Kishimoto

Abstract

We report a case of a 66-year-old severely osteoporotic woman with bisphosphonate-related osteonecrosis of the jaw (BRONJ) around her dental implants, who was treated successfully with teriparatide and sequestrectomy of the mandible. After 5 months of teriparatide therapy, the sequestrum separation had progressed and a sequestrectomy was performed under general anesthesia. Five months after the operation, new bone formation was observed around the bone defect in the region of the sequestrectomy. A repeat computed tomographic image revealed improvement in the bone defect in the mandible. These results suggest that teriparatide provides beneficial effects in the treatment of advanced BRONJ around dental implants.

Keywords: Bisphosphonate-related osteonecrosis of the jaw, Dental implant, Teriparatide

Background

Oral bisphosphonates (BPs) are used to treat osteoporosis, Paget's disease, and osteogenesis imperfecta. They are most widely used for treatment of osteoporosis. BP-related osteonecrosis of the jaw (BRONJ) was first reported by Marx in 2003 [1]. The risk of BRONJ in osteoporotic patients treated with BPs remains low compared with that of oncology patients [2]. Recent studies have indicated that the relative incidence of BRONJ in patients with osteoporosis is higher than previously thought [3]. Madrid and Sanz [4] suggested that the placement of dental implants in patients treated with oral bisphosphonates was not associated with the onset of BRONJ; they found no relationship between the treatment and the survival of implants. However, more recently, an increasing number of peri-implant BRONJ cases have been described [5–9]. Peri-implant BRONJ currently is considered an additional complication related to oral implants, along with nerve injury, bleeding, sinus perforation, implant ingestion/aspiration, peri-implantitis, and mucositis [6].

We present a case of a severely osteoporotic woman with BRONJ around her dental implants, who was treated successfully with teriparatide and sequestrectomy.

Case presentation

A 66-year-old woman was referred to the Oral and Maxillofacial Surgery Clinic at Hyogo College of Medicine Hospital, Japan, in September 2011, for an extraoral fistula and refractory pain of the right mandible associated with a purulent discharge and soft tissue swelling. The patient's osteoporosis was diagnosed in 2005 and treated with 35 mg of alendronate weekly by the family doctor. The patient had a past history of severe osteoporosis, multiple vertebral fractures, and renal failure. She had taken 20 mg of prednisone for 3 months from 2005 for the treatment of IgA nephropathy.

Dental implant treatment in the maxilla and mandible was begun in June 2009 by the family dentist. Five implants (Spline Twist implant, Zimmer Dental, Carlsbad, CA) were placed at the same time in the posterior region of the mandible. The surgical procedure was uneventful, and primary stability of the implants was achieved. In September 2010, at the time of implant reopening for the second surgery, the implants had integrated and the

* Correspondence: ktaka@hyo-med.ac.jp
Department of Oral and Maxillofacial Surgery, Hyogo College of Medicine, 1-1 Mukogawa-cho, Nishinomiya, Hyogo 663-8501, Japan

healing abutments were connected. Provisional maxillary and left mandibular prostheses were cemented onto the abutments.

Nine months after the second surgery in June 2011, the patient started to complain of a painful cheek swelling on the right side of the mandible, associated with gingival bleeding. She was prescribed oral antibiotics by her dentist and underwent occasional antibiotic therapy thereafter.

In September 2011, the patient was referred to our clinic because her symptoms were getting worse. Clinical examination revealed an intraoral fistula on the lingual side of the dental implant replacing the right mandibular first molar, associated with mucosal inflammation and a purulent discharge (Fig. 1a, b). She also had hypoesthesia of the right lower lip. The patient underwent panoramic radiography (Fig. 2a) and computed tomography (CT), which showed bone resorption around the dental implant in the right mandibular first molar area and severe peri-implantitis in the right mandibular molar region. There was no obvious sequestrum separation (Fig. 2b, c). Under a clinical diagnosis of perimandibular inflammation and peri-implantitis, conservative treatment consisting of local irrigation and use of antibiotics was implemented. Meropenem hydrate was given initially, then changed to ampicillin/sulbactam. The inflammatory state improved, and when the symptoms subsided, treatment with clarithromycin was continued. Debridement and removal of the dental implant in the right mandibular first molar area was performed under local anesthesia. Irrigation of the site was continued as part of the treatment regimen.

In November 2011, after a consultation with an osteoporosis expert at the Orthopedic Medicine Clinic of our hospital, alendronate therapy was stopped and subcutaneous teriparatide therapy at a dose of 20 μg per day was started. During the course of the teriparatide therapy, the patient continued to use 0.02% benzalkonium chloride solution for local irrigation.

In April 2012, after 5 months of teriparatide therapy, the sequestrum separation had progressed (Fig. 3), and a sequestrectomy was performed under general anesthesia (Fig. 4). At 5 months after the operation, a CT scan revealed new bone formation around the bone defect in the region of the sequestrectomy, with all symptoms including bone exposure disappearing (Fig. 5). The patient's osteoporosis treatment was continued, and 16 months after the sequestrectomy, further new bone formation was observed (Fig. 6).

Discussion

We describe a case of a patient with a 6-year history of alendronate therapy, in which BRONJ developed around her dental implants. In this patient, the dental implants achieved successful osseointegration, and BRONJ occurred after the second surgery. Several factors could have played a role in the development of BRONJ in this patient. Glucocorticoid therapy is associated with an increased risk of BRONJ. This may be a result of multiple factors including inhibition of osteoblast function and increased osteoblast and osteocyte apoptosis. Other effects of glucocorticoids that may contribute to an increased risk of BRONJ include increased bone resorption, immunosuppression, impaired wound healing, and increased risk of local infection [10]. Patient-related local risk factors include dentoalveolar surgery (e.g., tooth extraction) and pre-existing inflammatory dental disease, such as periodontal disease or periapical pathology [11]. Although BPs tend to accumulate in sites of active bone remodeling, such as the jaws, the surgical trauma to the alveolar bone during implant surgery could have further stimulated the postoperative accumulation of the drug in the implant site. The localized interference of BPs on bone turnover may have influenced the peri-implant bone resistance to oral bacteria in the long term, thus increasing the risk of peri-implantitis. Once infection of the implanted bone site is established, BPs further accumulate because of the increased bone turnover; the onsite activation of bisphosphonates will hamper the healing capacity of bone, leading to bone necrosis and sequestration [5].

Nevertheless, the role of the dental implant procedure as a BRONJ pathogenetic factor [12–15] is still unclear.

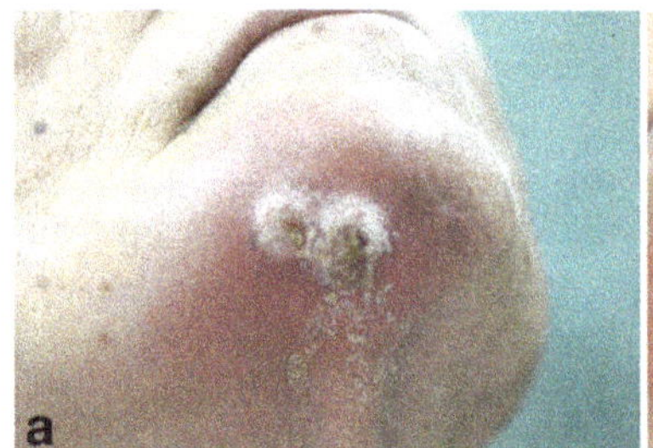

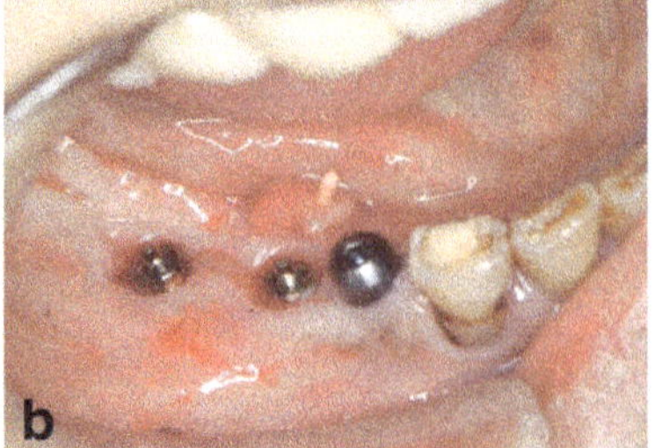

Fig. 1 **a** Extraoral photograph showing an extraoral fistula in the right mandibular region. **b** Intraoral photograph showing an intraoral fistula on the lingual side of the distal dental implants associated with mucosal inflammation and a purulent discharge

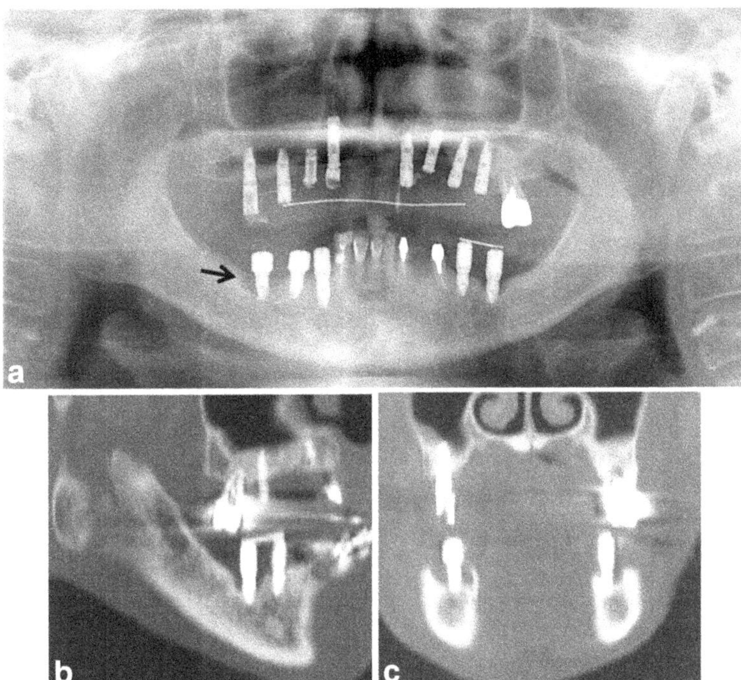

Fig. 2 a Panoramic radiograph showing marked alveolar bone resorption surrounding the dental implant replacing the right mandibular first molar (*arrow*). **b** Sagittal CT view. **c** Coronal CT view

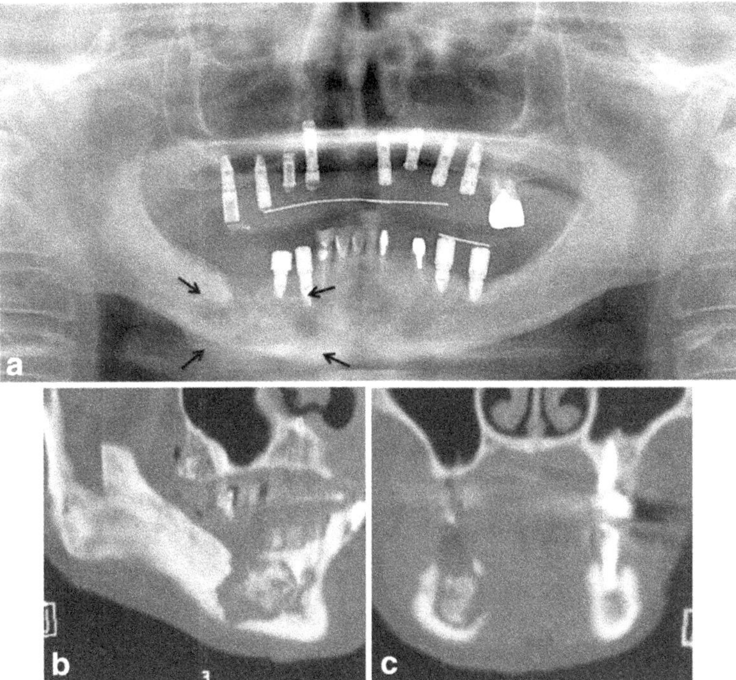

Fig. 3 a Panoramic radiograph showing the sequestrum separation after 5 months of teriparatide therapy (*arrows*). **b** Sagittal CT view. **c** Coronal CT view

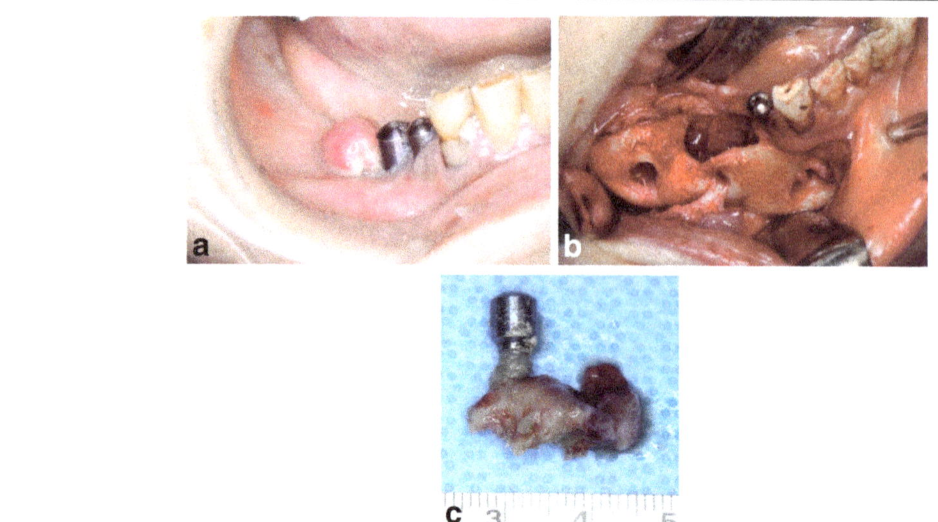

Fig. 4 a Preoperative intraoral photograph. **b** Intraoperative photograph of the sequestrectomy. **c** Removal of the dental implant with a specimen of the necrotic bone

Recently, an increasing number of peri-implant BRONJs have been described [5–9]. Peri-implant BRONJ has been classified into two types: implant surgery-triggered BRONJ, when it develops within 6 months after implant surgery, suggesting that the surgical process may be a contributing factor; and non-implant surgery-triggered BRONJ, if it develops 6 months or more after implant surgery, or when BP administration started after implant placement and osteointegration [8]. Most authors do not consider the surgical procedure of implantation as a trigger factor for MRONJ [7, 8, 14, 16–20].

It is therefore important that all patients treated with oral BPs must be given a full explanation of the potential risks of implant failure and BRONJ development in the short and long term. Because the potential role of infection in implant failure and BRONJ occurrence is still debated, great attention should be paid to the long-term oral hygiene and plaque control of implant-prosthetic restorations in patients taking oral BPs.

BPs and other antiresorptives such as denosumab increase apoptosis and inhibit osteoclast differentiation and function, all leading to decreased bone resorption and remodeling [11]. Teriparatide may counteract these mechanisms by stimulating bone remodeling. It has been shown to stimulate the activity and viability of osteoblasts from the alveolar bone of chronic bisphosphonate users [21], while indirectly increasing the metabolic activity and number of osteoclasts by affecting osteoblast function [22]. An increased number of remodeling units and increased bone formation within each unit may promote healing and the removal of damaged bone. Thus, teriparatide may offer therapeutic promise for localized bone defects of the jaw in patients with BRONJ [3, 23–25].

While it has been suggested recently that assertive surgical removal of the sequestrum appears to be effective [26–29], it can sometimes be difficult to distinguish living bone from necrotic bone. Recently, resection of BRONJ-affected tissue produced healing in patients taking oral bisphosphonates more successfully than conservative management [30]. However, bone resection

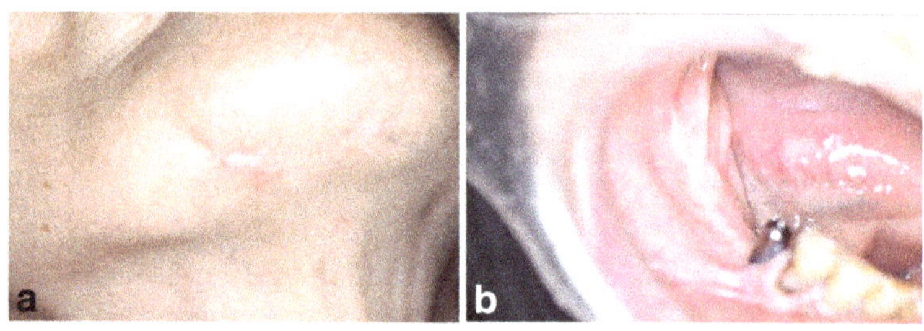

Fig. 5 a Extraoral photograph 5 months after the sequestrectomy. **b** Intraoral photograph 5 months after the sequestrectomy.

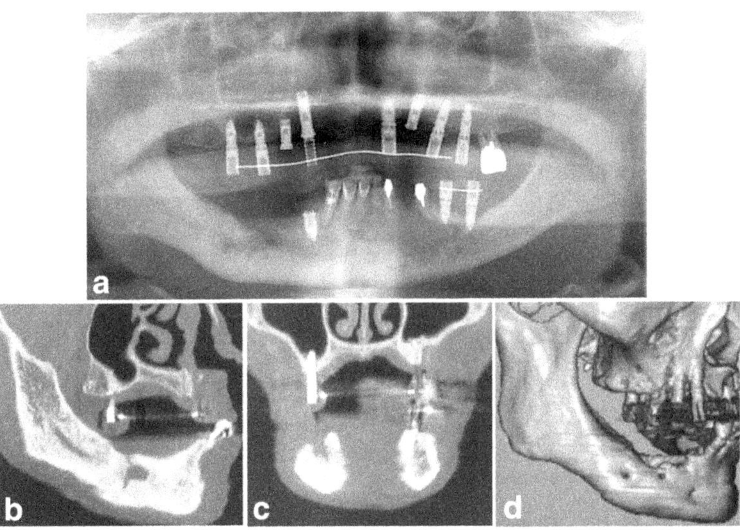

Fig. 6 **a** Panoramic radiograph 16 months after the sequestrectomy. **b** Sagittal CT view. **c** Coronal CT view. **d** 3D CT view

because of surgical treatment may lead to significant oral disability.

Activation of living bone turnover by teriparatide therapy causes progression of the separation of the sequestrum. As a result, teriparatide therapy promotes sequestrum separation followed by normal mucosal coverage of the exposed bone. After 5 months of teriparatide therapy in our patient, sequestrum separation had progressed and thus a sequestrectomy was performed under general anesthesia. After the wound in the affected area had healed, our patient did not report any problems pertaining to her ability to ingest food, despite the presence of the bone defect in the mandible. We treated the patient with teriparatide for 2 years. CT monitoring of the mandible would assist in determining whether teriparatide can allow complete recovery of the bone defect in the mandible in cases of ONJ induced by bisphosphonates.

Conclusions

We have reported a case of a severely osteoporotic elderly woman with BRONJ around her dental implants, who was treated successfully with teriparatide. Teriparatide therapy appeared to exert beneficial effects in this patient.

Funding

This report was supported by Grant-in-Aid for Researchers, Hyogo College of Medicine, 2016.

Authors' contributions

YZ and KT participated in the design of the study and drafted of the manuscript. JT and MU participated in the acquisition of data. YZ and HK participated in surgical treatment. KN and HK participated in the manuscript review. All authors read and approved the final manuscript.

Authors' information

YZ is a specialist in Oral and Maxillofacial Surgery and a research student of the Department of Oral and Maxillofacial Surgery. KT and KN are associate professors of the Department of Oral and Maxillofacial Surgery. JT is a graduate student of the Department of Oral and Maxillofacial Surgery. MU is a senior resident of the Department of Oral and Maxillofacial Surgery. HK is a professor and chief of the Department of Oral and Maxillofacial Surgery.

Competing interests

Yusuke Zushi, Kazuki Takaoka, Joji Tamaoka, Miho Ueta, Kazuma Noguchi, and Hiromitsu Kishimoto declare that they have no competing interests.

References

1. Marx RE. Pamidronate (Aredia) and zoledronate (Zometa) induced avascular necrosis of the jaws: a growing epidemic. J Oral Maxillofac Surg. 2003;61: 1115–7.
2. Marx RE, Sawatari J, Fortin M, et al. Bisphosphonate-induced exposed bone (osteonecrosis/osteopetrosis) of the jaws; risk factors, recognition, prevention, and treatment. J Oral Maxillofac Surg. 2005;63:1567.
3. Harper RP, Fung E. Resolution of bisphosphonate-associated osteonecrosis of the mandible: possible application for intermittent low-dose parathyroid hormone [rhPTH(1- 34)]. J Oral Maxillofac Surg. 2007;65:573–80.
4. Madrid C, Sanz M. What influence do anticoagulants have on oral implant therapy? A systematic review. Clin Oral Implants Res. 2009;20(Suppl4):96–106.
5. Bedogni A, Bettini G, Totola A, et al. Oral bisphosphonate-associated osteonecrosis of the jaw after implant surgery: a case report and literature review. J Oral Maxillofac Surg. 2010;68:1662–6.
6. Favia G, Piattelli A, Sportelli P, et al. Osteonecrosis of the posterior mandible after implant insertion: a clinical and histological case report. Clin Implant Dent Relat Res. 2011;13:58–63.
7. Lazarovici TS, Yahalom R, Taicher S, et al. Bisphosphonate-related osteonecrosis of the jaw associated with dental implants. J Oral Maxillofac Surg. 2010;68:790–6.
8. Kwon TG, Lee CO, Park JW, et al. Osteonecrosis associated with dental implants in patients undergoing bisphosphonate treatment. Clin Oral Implants Res. 2014;25:632–40.
9. Jacobsen C, Metzler P, Rössle M, et al. Osteopathology induced by bisphosphonates and dental implants: clinical observations. Clin Oral Invest. 2013;17:167–75.
10. Saad F, Brown JE, Van PC, et al. Incidence, risk factors, and outcomes of osteonecrosis of the jaw: integrated analysis from three blinded active-

controlled phase III trials in cancer patients with bone metastases. Ann Oncol. 2012;23:1341–7.
11. Ruggiero SL, Dodson TB, Fantasia J, et al. American Association of Oral and Maxillofacial Surgeons position paper on medication-related osteonecrosis of the jaw-2014 update. J Oral Maxillofac Surg. 2015;73:1440.
12. Koka S, Babu NMS, Norell A. Survival of dental implants in post-menopausal bisphosphonate users. J Prosthodont Res. 2010;54:108–11.
13. Bell BM, Bell RE. Oral bisphosphonates and dental implants: a retrospective study. J Oral Maxillofac Surg. 2008;66:1022–4.
14. Grant BT, Amenedo C, Freeman K, Kraut RA. Outcomes of placing dental implants in patients taking oral bisphosphonates: a review of 115 cases. J Oral Maxillofac Surg. 2008;66:223–30.
15. Goss A, Bartold M, Sambrook P, Hawker P. The nature and frequency of bisphosphonate-associated osteonecrosis of the jaws in dental implant patients: a South Australian case series. J Oral Maxillofac Surg. 2010;68: 337–43.
16. Holzinger D, Seemann R, Matoni N, et al. Effect of dental implants on bisphosphonate-related osteonecrosis of the jaws. J Oral Maxillofac Surg. 1937;2014(72):e1–8.
17. Madrid C, Sanz M. What impact do systemically administrated bisphosphonates have on oral implant therapy? A systematic review. Clin Oral Implants Res. 2009;20 Suppl 4:96–106.
18. Matsuo A, Hamada H, Takahashi H, et al. Evaluation of dental implants as a risk factor for the development of bisphosphonate-related osteonecrosis of the jaw in breast cancer patients. Odontology. 2016;104:363–71.
19. Vescovi P, Campisi G, Fusco V, et al. Surgery-triggered and non surgery-triggered bisphosphonate-related osteonecrosis of the jaws (BRONJ): a retrospective analysis of 567 cases in an Italian multicenter study. Oral Oncol. 2011;47:191–4.
20. Walter C, Al-Nawas B, Wolff T, et al. Dental implants in patients treated with antiresorptive medication e a systematic literature review. Int J Implant Dent. 2016;2:9.
21. Rao MV, Berk J, Almojaly SA, et al. Effects of platelet-derived growth factor, vitamin D and parathyroid hormone on osteoblasts derived from cancer patients on chronic bisphosphonate therapy. Int J Mol Med. 2009;23:407–13.
22. Charles JF, Aliprantis AO. Osteoclasts: more than 'bone eaters'. Trends Mol Med. 2014;20:449–59.
23. Lau AN, Adachi JD. Resolution of osteonecrosis of the jaw after teriparatide [recombinant human PTH-(1-34)] therapy. J Rheumatol. 2009;36:1835–7.
24. Cheung A, Seeman E. Teriparatide therapy for alendronate-associated osteonecrosis of the jaw. N Engl J Med. 2010;363:2473–4.
25. Bashutski JD, Eber RM, Kinney JS, et al. Teriparatide and osseous regeneration in the oral cavity. N Engl J Med. 2010;363:2396–405.
26. Abu-Id MH, Warnke PH, Gottschalk J, et al. "Bis-phossy jaws"—high and low risk factors for bisphosphonate-induced osteonecrosis of the jaw. J Craniomaxillofac Surg. 2008;36:95–103.
27. Stanton DC, Balasanian E. Outcome of surgical management of bisphosphonate-related osteonecrosis of the jaws: review of 33 surgical cases. J Oral Maxillofac Surg. 2009;67:943–50.
28. Carlson ER, Basile JD. The role of surgical resection in the management of bisphosphonate-related osteonecrosis of the jaws. J Oral Maxillofac Surg. 2009;67:85–95.
29. Wilde F, Heufelder M, Winter K, et al. The role of surgical therapy in the management of intravenous bisphosphonates-related osteonecrosis of the jaw. Oral Surg Oral Med Oral Pathol Oral Radiol Endod. 2011;111: 153–63.
30. Silva LF, Curra C, Munerato MS, et al. Surgical management of bisphosphonate-related osteonecrosis of the jaws: literature review. Oral Maxillofac Surg. 2016;20:9–17.

13

Peri-implant biomechanical responses to standard, short-wide, and double mini implants replacing missing molar supporting hybrid ceramic or full-metal crowns under axial and off-axial loading: an in vitro study

Lamiaa Said Elfadaly*, Lamiaa Sayed Khairallah and Mona Atteya Al Agroudy

Abstract

Background: The aim of this study was to evaluate the biomechanical response of the peri-implant bone to standard, short-wide, and double mini implants replacing missing molar supporting either hybrid ceramic crowns (Lava Ultimate restorative) or full-metal crowns under two different loading conditions (axial and off-axial loading) using strain gauge analysis.

Methods: Three single-molar implant designs, (1) single, 3.8-mm (regular) diameter implant, (2) single, 5.8-mm (wide) diameter implant, and (3) two 2.5-mm diameter (double) implants connected through a single-molar crown, were embedded in epoxy resin by the aid of a surveyor to ensure their parallelism. Each implant supported full-metal crowns made of Ni-Cr alloy and hybrid ceramic with standardized dimensions. Epoxy resin casts were prepared to receive 4 strain gauges around each implant design, on the buccal, lingual, mesial, and distal surfaces. Results were analyzed statistically.

Results: Results showed that implant design has statistically significant effect on peri-implant microstrains, where the standard implant showed the highest mean microstrain values followed by double mini implants, while the short-wide implant showed the lowest mean microstrain values. Concerning the superstructure material, implants supporting Lava Ultimate crowns had statistically significant higher mean microstrain values than those supporting full-metal crowns. Concerning the load direction, off-axial loading caused uneven distribution of load with statistically significant higher microstrain values on the site of off-axial loading (distal surface) than the axial loading.

Conclusions: Implant design, superstructure material, and load direction significantly affect peri-implant microstrains.

Keywords: Mini implants, Short-wide implants, Standard implants, Axial and off-axial loading, Hybrid ceramics, strain gauge analysis

* Correspondence: dr.l.fadaly@gmail.com
Fixed Prosthodontics, Cairo University, Giza, Egypt

Background

The molars are one of the first teeth to be lost over lifetime; thus, their replacement is frequently needed. Implantation is generally the preferred choice to replace a missing single tooth avoiding vital teeth preparation and bridge fabrication [1].

The mandibular bone loss occurs as knife-edge residual ridge where there is marked narrowing of the labiolingual diameter of the crest of the ridge with a compensatory internal remodeling which sometimes leads to a sharp crest of the ridge which proceeds to low, well-rounded residual ridge [2]. Because of this type of bone loss and the presence of important anatomical areas, the planning of atrophic arches' posterior sites is normally more complex [3]. The possibilities for patient's rehabilitation in such limiting situations have involved advanced surgical techniques, such as autogenous bone augmentation and inferior alveolar nerve repositioning. However, these augmentation procedures have some drawbacks such as prolonged time until tooth reconstruction, patient morbidity, and expense. Side effects of bone augmentation include profound edema, pain, and discomfort and possible risks of nerve and blood vessel injury leading to nerve disturbance and hematoma [3, 4].

The use of short implants offer, in relation to the regenerative techniques, several advantages: low cost and treatment length, simplicity, and less risk of complications. An implant is considered to be short if it has a length that is equal to or less than 10 mm [5].

In the last few years, root form implants ranging from 1.8 to slightly more than 2 mm have promoted for long-term use, a task for which the device was approved by the Food and Drug Administration [6].

In situations where there is an inadequate interdental space, reduced interocclusal space, convergent adjacent tooth roots or close proximity of adjacent tooth roots or narrow atrophic osseous contour, mini implants may be appropriate. Nevertheless, when using new available narrow-diameter implants to replace a single molar, two implants could be used even when the distance between the adjacent teeth is smaller [7]. Mini dental implants are minimally invasive since it allows conservative placement of implants in bone without bone grafting and significant trauma and expense for patient and they can be used in patients who would normally be considered high risk (e.g., patients on anticoagulant or steroid therapy). In addition the general dentist can master this technique with minimal training and surgical experience, significantly expanding his armamentarium [6].

There are several factors that affect force magnitudes in peri-implant bone. The application of functional forces induces stresses and strains within the implant prosthesis complex and affect the bone remodeling process around implants [8, 9].

While there are several methods of measuring strain, the most common is with a strain gauge, a device whose electrical resistance varies in proportion to the amount of strain in the device. The most widely used gauge, however, is the bonded metallic strain gauge [10].

Thus, this study aims to evaluate the biomechanical response of the peri-implant bone to standard, short-wide, and two mini implants replacing missing molar with full-metal and Lava ultimate crowns under two different loading conditions using strain gauges.

The hypothesis of this study is that using different implant designs with different superstructure materials would change the peri-implant microstrains.

Methods

In the present study, the following materials were used: titanium root form endosseous implants of standard diameter and length (4-mm platform, 3.8-mm diameter,12-mm length, fixture bevel 0.2 mm, Super Line System, Dentium, USA), short-wide implant (7-mm platform, 5.8-mm diameter, 7-mm length, Super Line System, Dentium, Seoul, Korea) with 1.5-mm machined surface and 5.5-mm threaded surface that were fixed and tightened to the internally hexed implants, and 2 one-piece implant with square head mini implants (2.5-mm diameter × 12 mm, Slim Line System, Dentium, Seoul Korea), in addition to titanium implant abutments (straight abutments) with 5.5-mm height and matching width for short-wide and standard implants (5.5 mm and 4.5 mm, respectively) (Fig. 1).

Two epoxy resin casts were constructed using epoxy resin material (Transparent Epoxy, Kemapoxy 150, CMB International, Egypt). A dental milling machine (bredent GmbH & Co.KG, Weissenhorner Str. 2, 89250 Senden, Germany) was used to prepare the site for the implant fixtures insertion. The holes were filled with epoxy resin; then, using a dental surveyor (Ramses, Egypt), the implant-abutment units were placed in straight line configuration into the epoxy resin cast which is mounted on surveyor table at zero tilt. The two mini implants were prepared using tapered stone with round end to create a 0.5 chamfer finish line. A total of six crowns were constructed in this study, three full-metal crowns (Kera NH, Deutschland) (Fig. 2), and three hybrid-ceramic (Lava™ Ultimate Restorative, 3M™ ESPE™, Deutschland GmbH) crowns (Fig. 3). They were constructed with standardized dimensions 7-mm height, 7-mm bucco-lingual, and 8-mm mesio-distal width.

A split silicon index was constructed. The first full-metal crown was seated over its corresponding abutment using temporary cement. A duplicating addition silicon impression material was mixed according to the manufacturer's instructions. The silicon index was split mesio-distally using sharp scalpel into two halves. The other

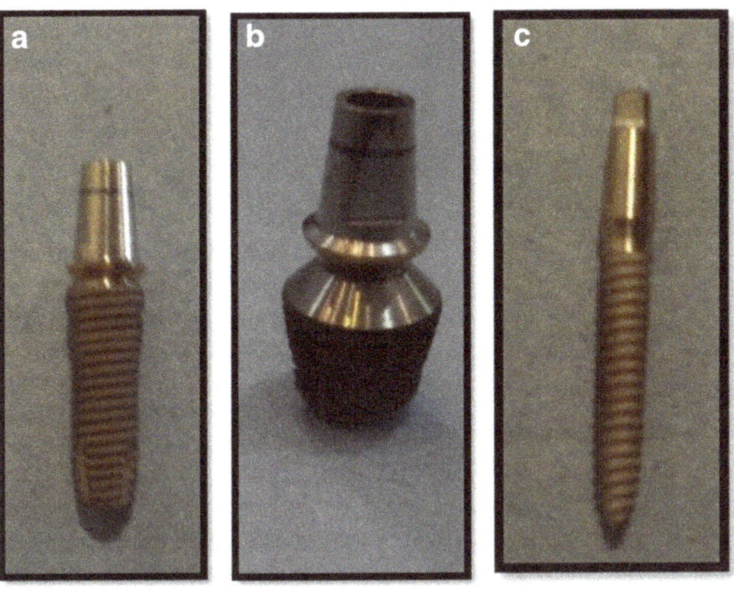

Fig. 1 **a** Standard, **b** short-wide, and **c** single-piece mini implants

wax patterns were adjusted using this index. The resin nano-ceramic crowns are milled by Computer Aided Design/Computer Aided Manufacturing (CAD/CAM) technology using CEREC inLAB MC XL (Cerec inLab, Sirona dental systems GmbH Fabrikstrasse, Bensheim, Deutschland) with inLab 3D software version 3.88. The restoration was modified to the required dimensions as the metal crowns (7 mm high, 7 mm bucco-lingual, and 8-mm mesio-distal width) by the help of the Cerec grade tool, and the occlusal table was shaped to be non-anatomical.

Each crown was cemented to its corresponding implant-abutment assembly using temporary cement (Cavex Temporary Cement, Cavex, Holland).

Each implant received 4 strain gauges (Kowa strain gages, Japan) placed on the mesial, distal, buccal, and lingual surfaces of the epoxy resin adjacent to the implants. At these selected sites, the thickness of the epoxy resin surrounding each implant was reduced to approximately 1 mm and was adjusted to be parallel to the long axis of the implant abutment units using disc and diamond stones (Fig. 4). Electric strain gauges which were 1 mm in length, 2.09 ± 1.0%, and 119.6 ± 0.4 Ω were bonded to their corresponding sites using cyanoacrylate adhesive (Amir, Egypt).They were bonded in a vertical position parallel to the implant bodies and held in place for about 5 min using adhesive tape. The lead wire from

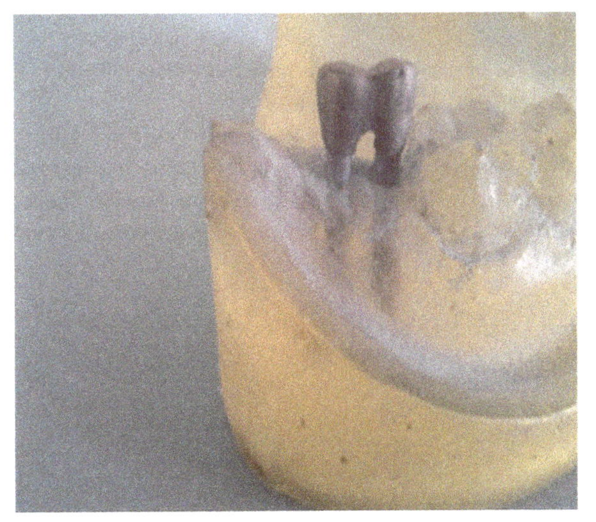

Fig. 2 Metal crown supported on two mini implants

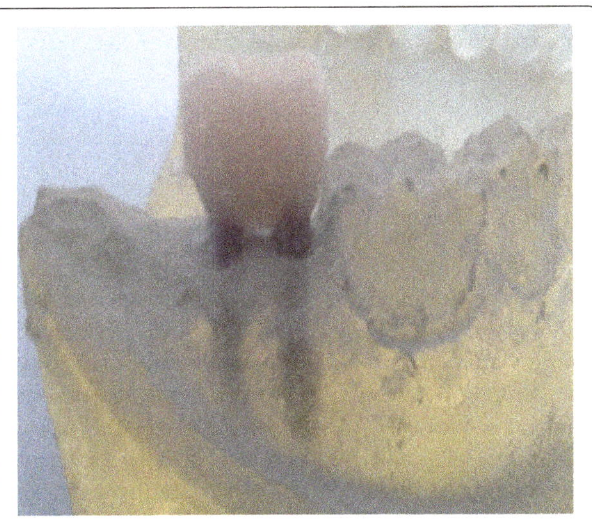

Fig. 3 Lava Ultimate Restorative crown on the two mini implants.

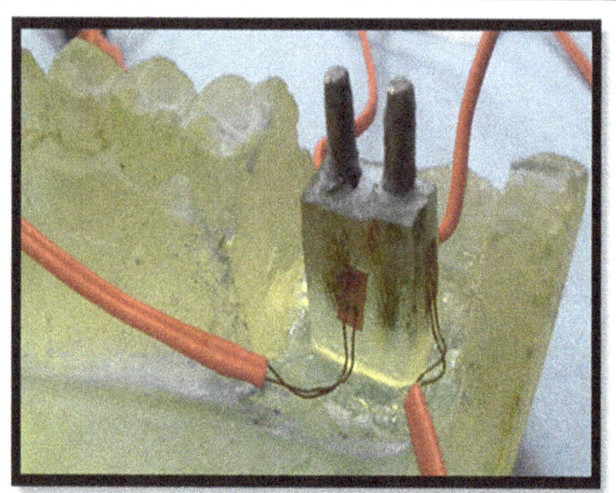

Fig. 4 Installation of strain gauges on surfaces of epoxy resin adjacent to mini implants

each active strain gauge was connected to a multichannel strain meter to register the microstrains transmitted to each strain gauge.

Functional loads of 300 N were applied to the crowns using computerized testing machine (Lloyds LR5K Plus Advance Universal Testing System, Johnson Scale CO., Inc). The machine is computer controlled by the Nexegen ver 4.3 software which permits the collection of data.

Two types of static axial loads were applied with 0.5 mm/min speed. The first load was 300 N applied axially in the position of the centric fossa of each crown Fig. 5 while the second load was 300 N applied 3 mm off-axial distally Fig. 6. The B/L and M/D strains were recorded separately for each strain gauge. Records were repeated five times, allowing the strain indicator to recover to 0 strain before reloading. A fundamental parameter of the strain gauge is its sensitivity to strain, expressed quantitatively as the gauge factor (GF). Gauge factor is defined as the ratio of fractional change in electrical resistance to the fractional change in length (strain) [10]:

$$\mathrm{GF} = \frac{\Delta \mathrm{R}/\mathrm{R}}{\Delta \mathrm{L}/\mathrm{L}} = \frac{\Delta \mathrm{R}/\mathrm{R}}{\varepsilon}$$

Data were presented as mean and standard deviation (SD) values. Data were explored for normality by checking data distribution and histograms, calculating mean and median values, and finally using Kolmogorov-Smirnov and Shapiro-Wilk tests of normality. Stress data showed non-parametric distribution, so the Kruskal-Wallis test was used to compare between the types of implants. The Mann-Whitney *U* test with Bonferroni's adjustment was used for pair-wise comparisons when the Kruskal-Wallis test is significant. The Mann-Whitney *U* test was also used to compare between the two crown types. The Wilcoxon signed-rank test was used to compare between axial and off-axial loads.

The significance level was set at $P \leq 0.05$. Statistical analysis was performed with IBM (IBM Corporation, NY, USA) SPSS (SPSS, Inc., an IBM Company) Statistics Version 20 for Windows.

Results

Effect of implant design on peri-implant microstrains

Results revealed that standard implant showed the statistically significantly highest mean microstrain values (3362.4 ± 757.4 με). Double mini implant showed statistically significantly lower mean microstrain values (801.6 ± 251.4 με), while short-wide implant showed the statistically significantly lowest mean microstrain values (697.6 ± 79.7 με), with a *P* value <0.001 (Table 1).

Effect of implant design with different crown material types under different loading directions on overall peri-implant microstrains

Under axial loading

The highest statistically significant microstrains were obtained with standard implant supporting Lava Ultimate and metal crowns (3826.5 ± 723.5 με and 2922.5 ± 218.6 με, respectively) while the lowest statistically significant microstrains were obtained with double mini implant supporting metal crown (238.2 ± 32.3 με),with a *P* value <0.001 (Table 2).

Under off-axial loading

The highest statistically significant microstrains were obtained with standard implant with Lava Ultimate and metal crowns (4286.4 ± 70.9 με and 2414.4 ± 167.6 με, respectively) while the lowest microstrain was obtained with short-wide implant with Lava Ultimate and metal crowns (382.3 ± 41.1 με and 685.8 ± 118.4 με, respectively), with a *P* value <0.001 (Table 2).

The effect of crown material type regardless of other variables

Results revealed that implants supporting Lava Ultimate crowns showed statistically significantly higher mean microstrain values (1927.3 ± 1536.6 με) than those supporting metal crowns (1313.7 ± 973.1 με),with a *P* value <0.001 (Table 3).

Table 1 Descriptive statistics and results of comparison between microstrains induced with different implant design regardless of other variables (collective microstrains)

Standard		Short-wide		Double mini		*P* value
Mean	SD	Mean	SD	Mean	SD	
3362.4[a]	757.4	697.6[c]	79.7	801.6[b]	251.4	<0.001*

Different superscripts in the same row are statistically significantly different
*Significant at $P \leq 0.05$

Table 2 Descriptive statistics and results of comparison between microstrains induced with different implant designs with each crown material (overall microstrains)

Load	Crown type	Standard		Short-wide		Double mini		*P* value
		Mean	SD	Mean	SD	Mean	SD	
Axial	Lava Ultimate	3826.5	723.5	991.5	101.4	939.8	78.3	<0.001*
	Metal	2922.5	218.6	730.8	84.9	238.2	32.3	<0.001*
Off-axial	Lava Ultimate	4286.4	70.9	382.3	41.1	1137.6	86.9	<0.001*
	Metal	2414.4	167.6	685.8	118.4	890.8	118.5	<0.001*

*Significant at $P \leq 0.05$

Effect of load direction on peri-implant microstrains

Results revealed that there was no statistically significant difference between axial loading (1608.2 ± 1339.0 με) and off-axial loading (1632.9 ± 1356.4 με) of different implant designs supporting different types of crown materials (Tables 4 and 5).

Effect of load direction on different implant designs with different crown materials on overall peri-implant microstrains

With Lava Ultimate crowns

In standard as well as double mini implants, off-axial loading showed statistically significantly higher mean microstrain values (4286.4 ± 70.9 με and 1137.6 ± 86.9 με, respectively) than axial loading (3826.5 ± 723.5 με and 939.8 ± 78.3 με, respectively). While with short-wide implant, axial loading showed statistically significantly higher mean microstrain values (991.5 ± 101.4 με) than off-axial loading (382.3 ± 41.1 με).

With metal crowns

In standard as well as short-wide implants, axial loading showed statistically significantly higher mean microstrain values (2922.5 ± 218.6 με and 730.8 ± 84.9 με, respectively) than off-axial loading (2414.4 ± 167.6 με and 685.8 ± 118.4 με), respectively. While with double mini implants, off-axial loading showed statistically significantly higher mean microstrain value (890.8 ± 118.5 με) than axial loading (238.2 ± 32.3 με).

Discussion

To replace a missing lower molar in compromised ridge, different treatment options were suggested, using either a standard size implant with surgical procedures, short-wide implant, or two mini implants. Concerning the use of mini implant, splinted multiple implants increase the surface area that interfaces with the bone to lessen the per square millimeters of force borne by the bone [11]. The implant design affects the magnitude of stresses and their impact on the bone implant interface. Screw-shaped implants were used due to the fact that threads of implants decomposes axial load into two components which are parallel and perpendicular to the plane of threads, since it was proven that distribution of the same force over a larger surface leads to lowering of the stresses [12]. The epoxy resin was used to simulate bone matrix as it has mechanical properties similar to those of trabecular bone, Young's modulus equals 3000 MPa [13].The amount of load used in this experiment, 300 N, was based on the study by Mericske-Stern et al. [14]. The rational for applying the loads on flat occlusal surfaces was to compare axial loading with absolute off-axial loading. As in the presence of cusp inclination, an additional horizontal load would be applied depending on the amount of cusp inclination, thus leading to reduction of the amount of vertical load transferred to the implants [15]. During clinical loading of an implant, the direction of loading is rarely along its central long axis, so the applied occlusal force is frequently in a direction that creates a lever arm, causing off-axial and bending moments in bone [16]. So, by measuring axial and off-axial loads, it was possible to evaluate the load transfer characteristics not only under the regular masticatory forces but also under the extreme load levels, such as those that occur during parafunction [12].

Previous studies have shown that direct correlations exist between microstrain magnitudes and bone stability/instability conditions. This has been summarized by Frost, when bone is loaded below about 2000 microstrains, bone can easily repair what little microdamage

Table 3 Descriptive statistics and results of comparison between microstrains induced by the two crown materials regardless of other variables (collective microstrains)

Lava Ultimate crowns		Metal crowns		*P* value
Mean	SD	Mean	SD	
1927.3	1536.6	1313.7	973.1	<0.001*

*Significant at $P \leq 0.05$

Table 4 Descriptive statistics and results of comparison between microstrains induced by the two load directions regardless of other variables (collective microstrains)

Axial		Off-axial		*P* value
Mean	SD	Mean	SD	
1608.2	1339.0	1632.9	1356.4	0.948

*Significant at $P \leq 0.05$

Table 5 Descriptive statistics and results of comparison between microstrains induced by the two load directions with each implant design and crown material (overall microstrains)

Crown	Implant type	Axial		Off-axial		*P*-value
		Mean	SD	Mean	SD	
Lava Ultimate	Standard	3826.5	723.5	4286.4	70.9	<0.001*
	Short	991.5	101.4	382.3	41.1	<0.001*
	Mini	939.8	78.3	1137.6	86.9	<0.001*
Metal	Standard	2922.5	218.6	2414.4	167.6	<0.001*
	Short	730.8	84.9	685.8	118.4	<0.001*
	Mini	238.2	32.3	890.8	118.5	<0.001*

*Significant at $P \leq 0.05$

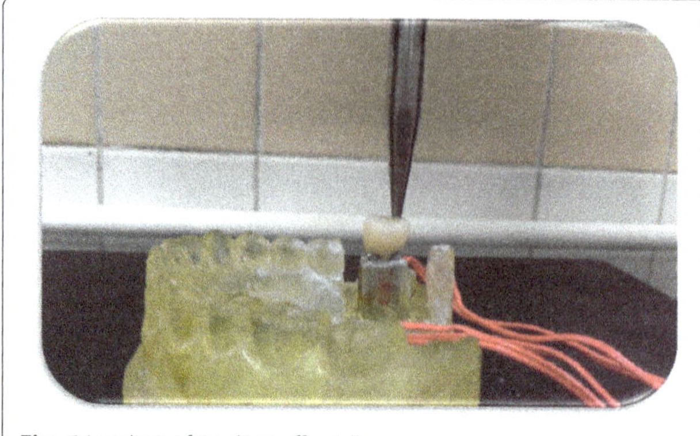
Fig. 6 Loading of implant off-axially

occurs. Yet, when pathologic overloading occurs (over 4000 microstrains), stress and strain gradients exceed the physiologic tolerance threshold of bone and cause micro-fractures at the bone-implant interface [17]. Thus, the maximum normal stress criterion, 3000 με, was used to evaluate the extent of the regions where the normal stresses were beyond the allowable tensile and compressive values in the cortical bone [12].

So the implant design that experienced the least overall amount of strain was thought to represent the best design, at least in terms of stress distribution.

Results revealed that all implant designs with different superstructure materials and under different loading conditions resulted in peri-implant microstrain values which were within the physiologic loading zone, below 3000 με, except for the standard sized implants supporting Lava Ultimate crowns under axial and off-axial loading.

Regarding the effect of implant design on peri-implant microstrains induced in the present study, standard diameter implant showed the highest microstrain values regardless of other variables (3362.4 ± 757.4 με). Microstrain value exceeded the physiologic limit in the standard implant supporting Lava Ultimate crowns. That was in approval with Balshi et al. who stated that replacing a lost molar with only one implant represents a biomechanical challenge [18]. This might be attributed to the differences in the size and morphology of natural tooth roots and the standard size implants (3.75 or 4 mm), thus providing insufficient support [19]. In the present study regardless of other variables, double mini implant showed statistically significantly lower mean microstrains (801.6 ± 251.4 με) than standard implant. Moreover, the double mini implant showed statistically significantly lowest microstrain values with metal and Lava Ultimate crowns under axial loading. Under off-axial loading, it also showed statistically significant lower microstrains value than standard implant. Moreover, the use of two implants provides more surface area for osseointegration and spreads the occlusal loading forces over a wider area while reducing the potential bending forces that would exist in a single-implant molar restoration [1, 18, 20, 21]. The one-piece design of small-diameter implants (1.8–3.0-mm diameter) provides strength to the implant in comparison with small diameter two-piece implants [22]. According to Misch [23], a solid implant with a 1.23-mm diameter has the same resistance to bending fracture as the annulus region of a 3.75-mm traditional design. Moreover, a solid 3-mm implant has an approximately 340% increase in moment of inertia over the 3.75-mm traditional two-piece root form at the annulus position. Generally, short-wide implant resulted in the lowest microstrain values in comparison with the other two implant designs. The reduced strains associated with wider implants may be due to the increased structural capacity and the enlarged resin-implant contact area offered by these implants, resulting in lower torque effect in conjunction with off-axial loading [20]. Accordingly, Balshi et al. [18] indicated that a molar crown supported by a standard or narrow size implant can easily introduce large bending moments to bone because the dimensions of crown are usually greater than the diameter of the implants. Thus, the wide implant is suggested for placement at the molar region to reduce the possibility of overload. The area that transfers the compressive and tensile loads to bone, that is, functional surface area, was proved to

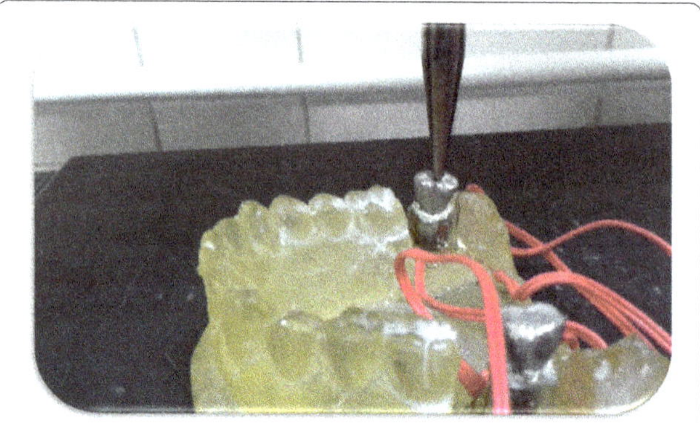
Fig. 5 Loading of implant axially

be confined to the crestal 5–7 mm [24–27]. Thus, short implant with a wider diameter provides both improved primary stability and increased functional surface area as it allows engagement of a maximal amount of bone and better distribution of stress in the surrounding bone compared with increases in implant length [28–32]. An increase in diameter by 1 mm will increase the surface area by 30–200% depending on the implant design [33]. Moreover, according to Misch [34], the large-diameter implants which have a larger prosthetic platform exhibit less force transmission.

Regarding the effect of direction of loading on induced microstrains, it was shown that changing the position of occlusal loading had a considerable effect on the amount of distribution of stresses where axial loading generated even distribution of load around the implant in comparison to off-axial loading where stresses were more pronounced in the area of load application. This might be due to the increase of the horizontal component of the applied load which was stated to generate an increase in the moment and eventually an increase in the compressive load on the side of applied force, to a level higher than the compressive load generated by only the vertical component of the force generated by axial loading [12]. Yet, regardless of other variables, there was no statistically significant difference between axial and off-axial loads. Regarding the off-axial in comparison to axial loading, a particularly high risk of traumatic overload occurred with the standard single-unit implant restoration because the restoration itself is usually wider than the implant, creating the potential for a cantilever effect with high bending moments, in off-axial loading [35]. So the loaded side implants bear more stresses on its distal part due to bending moments of the cantilever on the restorations which in turn transfer more stresses to the peri-implant bone at this side [36]. Flanagan [37] stated that mini implant smaller surface area and volume places more force per square millimeter against the encasing bone than larger diameter implants. So, mini implants may be best used in multiples to resist off-axial forces to prevent metal fatigue and fracture. According to Kheiralla and Younis [12], off-axial loading of single mini implant (3-mm diameter) supporting single molar crown induced mean microstrains value higher than the physiologic limit while in this study, the mean microstrain value of double mini implant supporting metal and Lava Ultimate crowns under off-axial loading were within the physiologic limit (890.8 με and 1137.6 με, respectively).This is in accordance with Balshi et al. [38] who stated that two implants can basically eliminate MD bending and that this situation can enable double implants to induce even less load magnification than a wide diameter implant. In this study, although short-wide implants showed mean peri-implant microstrains under axial loading higher than off-axial loading, axial loading of short-wide implant resulted in compression microstrains in all surfaces in case of metal and lava ultimate crowns, indicating that microstrains were distributed almost equally on all surfaces under both axial and off-axial loading. In this study, it was noticed that short-wide implant showed lowest off-axial loading in comparison with standard and double mini implants. Javris [39] emphasized the biomechanical advantage of wide-diameter implants, particularly in reducing the magnitude of stress delivered to the various parts of the implant. The diameter of the implant is related to the bending fracture resistance or moment of interia, and the increase in diameter decreases the risk of fracture to the power of four, provided all other geometric features remain the same. As a result, wider diameter implants may be used when offset loads (cantilevers) or greater stress conditions (i.e., parafunction, molar regions) exist. Moreover, this feature allows better distribution of occlusal forces [33, 40–42]. Rangert [43] considers that wide, single implants are the best choice to resist lateral forces. An increased width of an implant may decrease offset loads, thus increasing the amount of the implant-bone interface placed under compressive loads [34].

Regarding the effect of superstructure material on induced microstrains, generally, different implant designs supporting Lava Ultimate crowns showed higher mean microstrain values(1927.3 ± 1536.6 με), in comparison with those supporting metal crowns (1313.7 ± 973.1 με).Theoretical considerations [44, 45] and in vitro experiments [46–49] suggest that an occlusal material with a low modulus of elasticity such as acrylic resin might dampen the occlusal impact forces, thereby decreasing its effect on the bone-implant interface. Various methods have been proposed to address the issue of reducing implant loads. Yet, all these studies were in contradiction with the results of our study. In accordance with our study, in vitro studies suggested a better load distribution from high elastic modulus material [44]. It has been suggested that stiffer prosthesis materials might distribute the stress more evenly to the abutments and implants [50]. Duyck et al. [51], in an in vivo study, demonstrated a better distribution of bending moments (in contrast to acrylic) when metal was used as prosthesis material in cantilevered or longer span prostheses. Stegaroiu et al. [52, 53] demonstrated that stresses on the bone-implant interface using resin prostheses were similar to or higher than models using gold or porcelain. Desai et al. [54] concluded by 3D FEA that PFM crown reduced stresses around the implant as compared to acrylic crown. Single crowns in the present study were loaded with vertical loads that increased with time. Most in vitro studies on the influence of superstructure materials on the strain transmitted through the implant have been conducted under impact forces. However, it was proven that the mandible is decelerated prior to tooth contact, in contrast to impact forces. Since it has been suggested that impact forces occur only accidently during mastication, the shock-absorbing effect of resilient materials that has been reported under this loading in vitro might not be relevant during most actual mastication. Consequently, the use of resilient material as a superstructure material, though previously recommended to ensure shock protection of the implant-bone interface, does not seem to ease the strain in the bone around implants under simulated masticatory cycles and static loading [52, 53, 55, 56].

Conclusions

Within the limitations of this in vitro study, the following conclusions could be drawn:

1. Implant design, superstructure material, and load direction significantly affect peri-implant microstrains.
2. The recorded compressive and tensile microstrains for the tested designs were within the physiologic loading range, as they did not exceed the compressive or tensile strength of the bone-implant interface, which is more than 3000 microstrains except for the standard sized implant supporting Lava Ultimate crowns under both loading directions.
3. Off-axial loading leads to uneven distribution of loads, in standard diameter implant, due to the cantilever effect, which caused microstrain values exceeding the physiologic limit, thus causing clinical failure over time.
4. Use of splinted double mini implants and short-wide implant to restore missing mandibular molar reduces cantilever effect which leads to lowering of peri-implant microstrains under off-axial loading.
5. Usage of full-metal crown implant superstructure reduces the peri-implant microstrain values compared to using Lava Ultimate crowns.

Authors' contributions

LSE have made substantial contributions to conception and design, acquisition of data, and analysis and interpretation of data, drafted and revised the manuscript, and have given final approval of the version to be published. LSK and MAA participated in the study design and coordination. All authors read and approved the final manuscript.

Competing interests

The authors L.S.Elfadaly, L.S.Kheirallah, and M.A.Alagroudy state that they have no competing interests.

References

1. Mazor Z, Lorean A, Mijiritsky E, Levin L. Replacement of a molar with 2 narrow diameter dental implants. Implant Dent. 2012;21(1):36–8.
2. Atwood D. Postextraction changes in the adult mandible as illustrated by micrographs of midsagittal sections and serial cephalometric roentgenograms. J Prosthet Dent. 1963;13:810–24.
3. Felice P, Pellegrino G, Checchi L, Pistilli R, Esposito M. Vertical augmentation with interpositional blocks of anorganic bovine bone vs. 7-mm-long implants in posterior mandibles: 1-year results of a randomized clinical trial. Clin Oral Implants Res. 2010;21(12):1394–403.
4. Shatkin T, Petrotto C. Mini dental implants: a retrospective analysis of 5640 implants placed over a 12-year period. Compend Contin Educ Dent. 2012; 33 Spec 3(Spec 3):2–9.
5. Monje A, Chan HL, Fu JH, Suarez F, Galindo-Moreno P, Wang HL. Are short dental implants (<10 mm) effective? A meta-analysis on prospective clinical trials. J Periodontol. 2013;84(7):895–904.
6. Christensen G. The 'mini'-implant has arrived. J Am Dent Assoc. 2006;13:387–90.
7. Flanagan D, Mascolo A. The mini dental implant in fixed and removable prosthetics: a review. J Oral Implantol. 2011;37 Spec No(Special Issue):123–32.
8. Bidez M, Misch C. Force transfer in implant dentistry: basic concepts and principles. J Oral Implantol. 1992;18(3):264–74.
9. Branemark P, Zarb G, Albrektsson T. Tissue-integrated prosthesis. Osseointegration in clinical dentistry. 1987. p. 129.
10. Strain gauge measurement—a tutorial. 1998
11. Flanagan D. Fixed partial dentures and crowns supported by very small diameter dental implants in compromised sites. Implant Dent. 2008;17(2):182–91.
12. Kheiralla L, Younis J. Peri-implant biomechanical responses to standard, short-wide and mini implants supporting single crowns under axial and off-axial loading (An In-Vitro study). J Oral Implantol. 2014;40(1):42-52.
13. Renouard F, Rangert B. Risk factors in implant dentistry, Quintessence. Second editionth ed. 1999.
14. Mericske-Stern R, Assal P, Merickse E, Ing W. Occlusal force and oral tactile sensibility measured in partially edentulous patients with ITI implants. Int J Oral Maxillofac Implants. 1995;10:345–54.
15. Bozkaya D, Muftu S, Muftu A. Evaluation of load transfer characteristics of five different implants in compact bone at different load levels by finite elements analysis. J Prosthet Dent. 2004;92(6):523–30.
16. Barbier L, Vander SJ, Krzesinski G, Schepers E, Van der Perre G. Finite element analysis of non-axial versus axial loading of oral implants in the mandible of the dog. J Oral Rehabil. 1998;25(11):847–58.
17. Saime S, Murat C, Emine Y. The influence of functional forces on the biomechanics of implant-supported prostheses—a review. J Dent. 2002;30:271–82.
18. Balshi T, Hernandez R, Pryszlak M, Rangert B. A comparative study of one implant versus two replacing a single molar. Int J Oral Maxillofac Implants. 1996;11(3):372–8.
19. Sullivan D, Siddiqui A. Wide diameter implants: overcoming problems. Dent Today. 1994;13:50–7.
20. Bahat O, Handelsman M. Use of wide implants and double implants in the posterior jaw: a clinical report. Int J Oral Maxillofac Implants. 1996;11(3):379–86.
21. Petropoulos V, Wolfinger G, Balshi T. Complications of mandibular molar replacement with a single implant: a case report. J Can Dent Assoc. 2004; 70(4):238–42.
22. Jackson BJ. Small diameter implants: specific indications and considerations for the posterior mandible: a case report. J Oral Implantol. 2011;37 Spec No: 156–64.
23. Misch C. Contemporary implant dentistry. 3rd ed. St. Louis: Elsevier; 2008. p. 264–6.
24. Von Recum A. Handbook of biomaterials evaluation: scientific, technical and clinical testing of implant materials. 1986.
25. Shigley J, Mischke C. Mechanical engineering design. 5th ed. New York: McGraw-Hill; 1989. p. 325–70.
26. Bidez M, Misch C. Issues in bone mechanics related to oral implants. Implant Dent. 1992;1:289–94.
27. Sevimay M, Turhan F, Kiliçarslan M, Eskitascioglu G. Three-dimensional finite element analysis of the effect of different bone quality on stress distribution in an implant-supported crown. J Prosthet Dent. 2005;93:227–34.

28. Bidez M, Misch C. Clinical biomechanics in implant dentistry. 2005. p. 310–2. Dental implant prosthetics.
29. Misch C, Suzuki I, Misch-Dietch D. A positive correlation between occlusion between occlusal trauma and peri-implant bone loss -literature support. implant dent. 2005;14:108–16.
30. Misch C. Implant design considerations for the posterior regions of the mouth. Implant Dent. 1999;8:376–86.
31. Himmlova L, Dostalova T, Kacovsky A, Konvickova S. Influence of implant length and diameter on stress distribution: a finite element analysis. J Prosthet Dent. 2004;91(1):20–5.
32. Shetty S, Puthukkat N, Bhat S, Shenoy K. Short implants: a new dimension in rehabilitation of atrophic maxilla and mandible. Journal of Interdisciplinary Dentistry. 2014;4(2):66.
33. Misch C, Bidez M. Contemporary implant dentistry. 2nd ed. St. Louis: Mosby; 1999.
34. Misch C. Implant body size: a biomechanical and esthetic rationale, Contemporary Implant Dentistry. 2008. p. 160–77.
35. O'Mahony A, Bowles Q, Woolsey G, Robinson S, Spencer P. Stress distribution in the single-unit osseointegrated dental implant: finite element analyses of axial and off-axial loading. Implant Dent. 2000;9(3):207–18.
36. Fawzi S. The effect of dental implant design on bone induced stress distribution and implant displacement. Int J Comput Appl. 2013;74(17):15–20.
37. Flanagan D. Avoiding osseous grafting in the atrophic posterior mandible for implant-supported fixed partial dentures: a report of 2 cases. J Oral Implantol. 2011;37(6):705–11.
38. Seong W, Korioth T, Hodges J. Experimentally induced abutment strains in three types of single-molar implant restorations. J Prosthet Dent. 2000;84:318–26.
39. Jarvis W. Biomechanical advantage of wide-diameter implants. Compend Contin Educ Dent. 1997;18:687–94.
40. Rangert B, Jemt T, Jörnéus L. Forces and moments on Brånemark implants. Int J Oral Maxillofac Implants. 1989;4:241–7.
41. Misch CE. A scientific rationale for dental implant design, DENTAL IMPLANT PROSTHETICS. 2005. p. 331.
42. Misch C. Occlusal considerations for implant-supported prostheses, Contemporary Implant Dentistry. 1993.
43. Rangert B. Biomechanical considerations when choosing a platform. Nobel Biocare Global Forum. 1996;10(4):4.
44. Linish V, Peteris A. Restorative factors that affect the biomechanics of the dental implant. Stomatologija, Baltic Dental and Maxillofacial Journal. 2003;5:123–8.
45. Skalak R. Aspects of biomechanical considerations. In: Branemark PI, Zarb GA, Albrektsson, eds. Tissue integrated prostheses. 1985: p. 117–28.
46. Davis D, Rimrott R, Zarb G. Studies on frameworks for osseointegrated prostheses: part 2. The effect of adding acrylic resin or porcelain to form the occlusal superstructure. Int J Oral Maxillofac Implants. 1988;3(4):275–80.
47. Gracis S, Nicholls J, Chalupnik J, Yuodelis R. Shock-absorbing behavior of five restorative materials used on implants. Int J Prosthodont. 1990;4:282–91.
48. Skalak R. Biomechanical considerations in osseointegrated prostheses. J Prosthet Dent. 1983;49:843–8.
49. Misch C. Clinical biomechanics in implant dentistry, Contemporary Implant Dentistry. 3rd ed. 2008. p. 543–56. mosby,inc.
50. Lundgren D, Laurell L. Biomechanical aspects of fixed bridgework supported by natural teeth and endosseous implants. Periodontol 2000. 1994;4:23–40.
51. Duyck J, Van Oosterwyck H, Vander SJ, De Cooman M, Puers R, Naert I. Influence of prosthesis material on the loading of implants that support a fixed partial prosthesis: in vivo study. Clin Implant Dent Relat Res. 2000;2(2):100–9.
52. Stegaroiu R, Kusakari H, Nishiyama S, Miyakawa O. Influence of prosthesis material on stress distribution in bone and implant: a 3-dimensional finite element analysis. Int J Oral Maxillofac Implants. 1998;13(6):781–90.
53. Stegaroiu R, Khraisat A, Nomura S, Miyakawa O. Influence of superstructure materials on strain around an implant under 2 loading conditions: a technical investigation. Int J Oral Maxillofac Implants. 2004;19(5):735–42.
54. Desai S, Singh R, Karthikeyan I, Reetika J. Three-dimensional finite element analysis of effect of prosthetic materials and short implant biomechanics on D4 bone under immediate loading. J Dent Implant. 2012;2:2–8.
55. Sertgoz A. Finite element analysis study of the effect of superstructure material on stress distribution in an implant-supported fixed prosthesis. Int J Prosthodont. 1997;10(1):19–27.
56. Wang T, Leu L, Wang J, Lin L. Effects of prosthesis materials and prosthesis splinting on peri-implant bone stress around implants in poor-quality bone: a numeric analysis. Int J Oral Maxillofac Implants. 2002;17(2):231–7.

14

Novel expandable short dental implants in situations with reduced vertical bone height—technical note and first results

Waldemar Reich[1*], Ramona Schweyen[2], Christian Heinzelmann[1], Jeremias Hey[2], Bilal Al-Nawas[1] and Alexander Walter Eckert[1]

Abstract

Purpose: Short implants often have the disadvantage of reduced primary stability. The present study was conducted to evaluate the feasibility and safety of a new expandable short dental implant system intended to increase primary stability.

Methods: As a "proof of concept", a prospective clinical cohort study was designed to investigate intraoperative handling, primary and secondary implant stability (resonance frequency analysis), crestal bone changes, implant survival and implant success, of an innovative short expandable screw implant. From 2014 until 2015, 9 patients (7–9-mm vertical bone height) with 30 implants (length 5–7 mm, diameter 3.75–4.1 mm) were recruited consecutively.

Results: All 30 implants in the 9 patients (age 44 to 80 years) could be inserted and expanded without intraoperative problems. Over the 3-year follow-up period, the implant success rate was 28/30 (93.3%). The mean implant stability quotients (ISQ) were as follows: primary stability, 69.7 ± 10.3 ISQ units, and secondary stability, 69.8 ± 10.2 ISQ units ($p = 0.780$), both without significant differences between the maxilla and mandible ($p \geq 0.780$). The mean crestal bone changes after loading were (each measured from the baseline) as follows: in the first year, 1.0 ± 0.9 mm in the maxilla and 0.7 ± 0.4 mm in the mandible, and in the second year, 1.3 ± 0.8 mm and 1.0 ± 0.7 mm, respectively.

Conclusions: Compared to other prospective studies, in this indication, the success rate is acceptable. Implant stability shows high initial and secondary stability values. The system might present an extension of functional rehabilitation to the group of elderly patients with limited vertical bone height. Further long-term investigations should directly compare this compressive implant with standard short implants.

Keywords: Bone atrophy, Expandable, Macrodesign, Short implant, Implant stability

Introduction

Endosseous implants have been established over several decades. The evaluation of treatment results under biomechanical, physiological, psychological, social and economic aspects has been well documented [1]. Furthermore, patient-based outcomes reveal a predictable gain in oral health-related quality of life [2].

Especially in patients with limited vertical bone height, process of treatment is extensive. Prior to implantation, augmentation procedures are required [3]. Depending on gender, vascularisation and bone mineralisation up to 25% of the primary volume are resorbed due to remodeling of augmented alveolar ridges [4]. Recently, short dental implants have evolved into a promising and reliable treatment option in the orofacial rehabilitation of atrophic mandibles and maxillae, namely as an alternative to vertical ridge augmentation [5–8]. The prognosis of short implants and patient satisfaction is high [9–12].

The definition of short implants in the literature is not uniform. In this present study, we considered short implants with 5–8-mm length [5, 7, 13]. Other authors set the cut-off at 6 mm [8, 9, 11, 14, 15]. According to the recent consensus paper of the 11th European Consensus Conference (EuCC), dental implants are referred to as

* Correspondence: waldemar.reich@medizin.uni-halle.de
[1]Department of Oral and Plastic Maxillofacial Surgery, Martin Luther University Halle-Wittenberg, Ernst-Grube Str. 40, 06120 Halle (Saale), Germany
Full list of author information is available at the end of the article

"short" if their intrabony length measures ≤ 8 mm and considered as "ultra-short" with lengths < 6 mm [16].

Biomechanical studies show that the crestal bone is strained under axial and extra-axial loading [17]. While bone quality, implant design and position, prosthetic devices and material characteristics contribute to the character of stress distribution, the role of implant length seems to be of underpart [17, 18]. Nevertheless, implant length is crucial in D4 bone quality [19], and the crown-to-implant length itself influences stress distribution under *extra-axial* loading in the crestal bone [20] and in the abutment screw [21]. According to Petrie and Williams [22], the influence of increased implant diameter on stress reduction in the crestal bone is more efficient than increased implant length. Möhlhenrich and co-authors [23] confirmed these findings that the diameter of an implant has greater influence on primary stability than implant length. Based on in vitro analysis, they concluded additionally that especially in patients with poor bone quality, a variation of implant dimensions is expected to lead to a significant increase of primary stability. Furthermore, stress distribution on short implants is affected by the bone-to-implant contact ratio [24]. Consequently, several options to increase the implant surface of short implants are elaborated, which consecutively enhance the implant stability: thread number, thread shape, thread depth, implant diameter, implant design and surface topography [25–27].

It is known that achievement of primary stability is one precondition for osseointegration and treatment success. There are few reports of immediate [14] and early (6 weeks) functional loading of short implants [28]. This is related to good bone quality, implant design or implant site preparation (e.g. under-drilling). However, under-drilling of the crestal aspect may lead to decreased bone-to-implant contact [29]. It is desirable to reduce the periimplant stress on the crestal bone while providing sufficient primary stability for all bone densities.

Therefore, optimisation of the macro- and microdesign of short dental implants to improve the success rate and long-term stability is preferable. In fact, elderly patients with general comorbidity should benefit from the overall short treatment time [28, 30]. As previously shown, the oral health-related quality of life is compromised during the healing period after implant insertion [31], especially when augmentation procedures are required [11]. For several reasons, the overall treatment time should be reduced in patients with atrophic alveolar ridges.

The purpose of the present study was to clinically analyse the feasibility and safety of a new short dental implant system with an expandable compressive design in the apical region. We hypothesised that the innovative expandable macrodesign of this implant provides a reliable implant success rate and ensures high implant stability in vivo.

Material and methods

Study population and measures

The study was designed as a prospective monocentric longitudinal cohort study according to the STROBE criteria. The participants of this study were recruited at the university hospital of Martin Luther University Halle-Wittenberg, Department of Oral and Plastic Maxillofacial Surgery, implantological consultation from 2014 (June) until 2015 (June). Inclusion and exclusion criteria of adult patients interested in implantological treatment are summarised in Table 1. Written informed consent was obtained from all individual participants included in this study.

As a "proof of concept", the pilot study was designed to investigate the intraoperative handling and to evaluate the feasibility and safety of a new short implant system. Therefore, sample size calculation was not performed. The primary outcome variable was implant success rate, which was calculated considering known success criteria (implant in function, no sign of infection or pain, no mobility, no radiolucent area around the implant) [32, 33]. The implant survival was calculated according to the Kaplan-Meyer method. Secondary measures were implant stability (initial and secondary) and periimplant crestal bone changes. Implant stability was measured by resonance frequency analysis (RFA; Osstell AB, Göteborg, Sweden).

Primary stability was measured immediately after implant insertion and completed expansion (see below), and secondary stability after the submerged healing period (3 months in the mandible, 6 months in the maxilla; Table 2) during the re-entry operation just before the healing abutments were inserted. Implant stability quotient (ISQ) values were obtained using the Smartpegs (type 17 and 35). According to each measurement, implant stability was classified as low with ISQ values < 60,

Table 1 Patient recruitment

Inclusion criteria	Exclusion criteria
1. Adult patients, male and female	1. Comorbidity ASA category ≥ III
2. Partially/totally edentulous patients	2. Pregnancy, bruxism
3. Alveolar process atrophy Cawood et Howell category ≥ IV	3. Smoking ≥ 10 cigarettes/day
4. Minimum vertical bone height of 7–9 mm for placement of short implants (5–7-mm length)	4. Radiotherapy ≥ 50 Gy [72] or 5. Intravenous bisphosphonate therapy [73] with a significant risk of developing osteo(radio)necrosis of the jaw
5. Patients without willingness to accept vertical bone augmentation	6. Psychiatric comorbidity that could influence course of treatment
	7. Untreated or poorly controlled diabetes mellitus
	8. Highly atrophic jaws that require vertical augmentation

Table 2 Surgical treatment protocol

Surgical protocol	Bone quality			
	D1	D2	D3	D4
1. Drilling sequence (splint)	Last drill	Last drill	Second to last drill	Second to last drill
2. Condensing preparation	–	–	(Analogue to last drill)	Analogue to last drill
3. Implant insertion (maximum torque ≤ 40 N cm)				
4. Expansion (maximum torque ≤ 40 N cm)				
5. Evaluation of primary stability by resonance frequency analysis, primary wound closure				
6. Postoperative digital radiogram				
7. Re-entry after a conventional period of submerged healing (mandible 3 months, maxilla 6 months), evaluation of secondary stability by resonance frequency analysis and insertion of healing abutments				
8. Postoperative digital radiogram				

medium with ISQ values 60–70, and high with ISQ values > 70 [34].

Digital radiograms (orthopantomogram, standard periapical radiograms) were taken prior to surgery, after implant insertion and re-entry, and at yearly follow-up examinations for crestal and periapical bone evaluation (see below).

Implants

In this study, a short expandable titanium screw implant (PYRAMIDION dental implant, DenTack Implants Ltd., Kfar-Saba, Israel) was used, which leads to dynamic condensing of the apical bone. The implants had the following dimensions and special characteristics: 5, 6 and 7 mm in length, 3.75 and 4.1 mm in diameter and an internal (7-mm length) or external (5- and 6-mm length) hexagon platform. The apical expansion is performed after implant insertion using a special expansion tool and a ratchet torque, resulting in a pyramid shape (Fig. 1a–f). The implant expansion process using the expansion tool is visualised in the movie clip (Additional file 1).

Surgical and prosthetic protocol

Planning of the implantological treatment followed usual clinical and radiological examination and, concerning

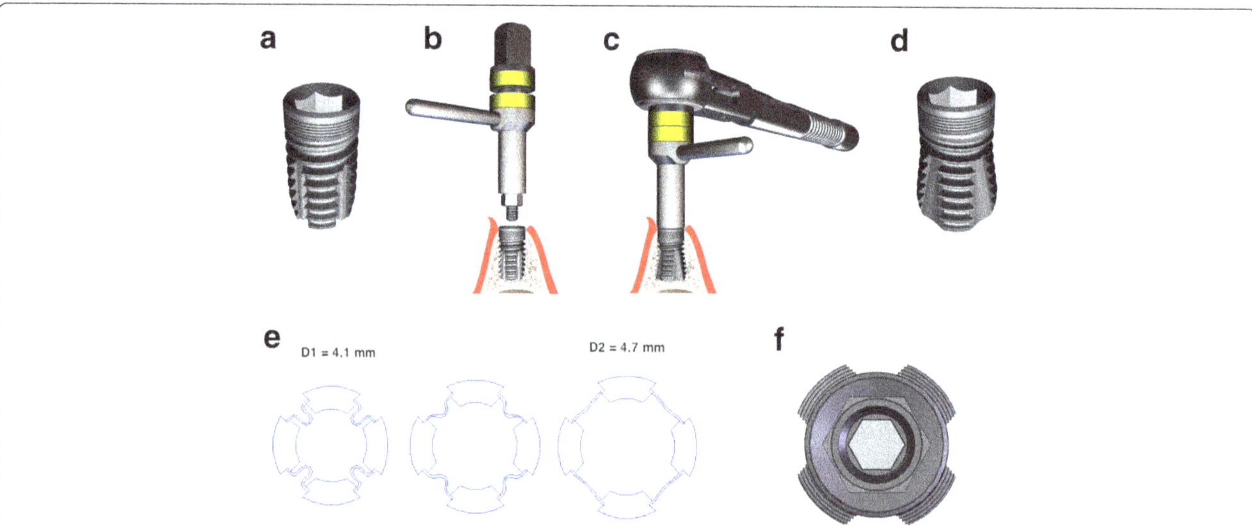

Fig. 1 a Closed short expandable dental implant (4.1 × 7 mm). The implant-abutment connection is characterised by an internal hexagon for rotation stability, combining the advantages of conical and parallel surfaces to reduce microgaps and micromovement [68]. The microthread concept and platform switching concept are implemented in the implant shoulder to reduce periimplant bone strain [53]. **b** Manual fixation of the expansion tool. Take note of the distance between both *yellow rings*. **c** Completion of the expansion process using the ratchet. Take note of the contact between both *yellow rings*. **d** Opened short expandable dental implant (4.1 × 7 mm). The expanded implant provides an increased bone-to-implant interface (*pyramid shape*) in the apical portion [54]. **e** Cross-section view of the implant apex. The apical expansion process is characterised by the unfolding of four wings, which are connected by four foils. D1: diameter of the closed implant. D2: diameter of the opened implant. **f** *Top view* of the expanded implant. The expanded implant (4.1-mm diameter) displays an apical diameter of 4.7 mm and length of the edge (base) of 4.4 mm

the position and number of implants, the recommended categories from the German consensus conference [35]. The drilling sequence, condensing preparation (where necessary) and manual implant insertion as well as expansion are described in detail in Table 2. Participants were instructed not to wear their denture 1 week after surgery. Afterwards, the conventional dentures were relined with soft material (Visco-gel, Dentsply, Salzburg, Austria). In this study, conventional periods of submerged healing were chosen: 3 months in the mandible and 6 months in the maxilla. During the re-entry surgery, a minimum of 2-mm keratinised periimplant soft tissue mucosa was considered.

All prosthetic treatments were provided at the University School of Dental Medicine, Department of Prosthetic Dentistry. At the earliest, 2 weeks after surgical re-entry, prosthetic treatment was started. All treatment steps were performed as described in detail in Table 3. The abutment screws were fixed with a torque of 15 N cm. Wherever possible, adjacent implants were primarily splinted (crowns, bar) and *extra-axial* loading during dynamic occlusion was avoided. In other cases, eccentric group guidance was achieved. To reduce overloading in the periimplant bone and implant-abutment connection, the occlusal surface was designed smaller [20, 21, 30, 36]. Patients were instructed about optimal oral hygiene, and the use of a dental water jet was recommended.

All treatments were provided by two experienced maxillofacial surgeons (WR, CH) and two experienced prosthodontists (RS, JH) to minimise bias.

Follow-up investigation

The first clinical follow-up was arranged at the latest 4 weeks after prosthetic treatment was completed. Further follow-ups were scheduled quarterly in the first year and later every 6 months. Patients were screened clinically and radiologically (yearly) for biological and technical complications. The authors applied the abovementioned success criteria according to Buser et al. [32]. Crestal bone changes were evaluated on digital radiograms (SIDEXIS imaging software, Sirona, Bensheim, Germany). The distance between the implant shoulder and first bone-implant contact at the mesial and distal aspect of each implant was measured (implant length as reference) by the first author

Table 3 Prosthetic treatment protocol

Type of prosthetic treatment		Session	Procedure
Fixed denture (bridge)		1	Open impression
		2	Abutment check, set-up • Titanium abutments • Non-precious metal framework, completely lined • Neighbouring crowns interlocked
		3	Check and insertion of the suprastructure • Cementation (ImProv™, Dentegris, Duisburg, Germany)
Combined fixed-removable denture	Telescope	1	Open impression (implants and stumps)
		2	Jaw relation (wax splint)
		3	Aesthetic check
		4	Check of the primary telescope, fixation impression
		5	Complete check
		6	Insertion of the definitive denture • Cementation of the primary telescope (Ketac™ Cem, 3M ESPE, Neuss, Germany)
Removable denture	Jaw bar	1	Open impression
		2	Abutment check
		3	Jaw relation (wax splint)
		4	Aesthetic check
		5	Jaw bar check
		6	Complete check
		7	Finishing
	Ball attachment	1	Impression of the edentulous alveolar ridge
		2	Jaw relation (wax splint)
		3	Aesthetic check
		4	Chairside insertion of the matrices

(WR), and the mean values per implant were calculated [37] 1 and 2 years after loading.

Data gathering and statistics

All patients were pseudonymised, parameters were attached to a databank and analysed statistically (Additional file 2). Statistical analyses were performed using statistics software (IBM SPSS statistics, version 20, Chicago, IL, USA). The descriptive statistics presented the frequency and distribution of several occurrences as well as combinations of certain features. Analytical statistics were performed depending on the scale: paired and independent *t* tests for differences of mean values. The implant survival was calculated according to the Kaplan-Meyer method. The level of significance was set at 5%.

Results

The first results of this longitudinal study include data from 9 patients with an average age of 57 years (range from 44 to 80) in whom 30 implants were inserted (maxilla $n = 15$, mandible $n = 15$). All 30 implants in the 9 patients could be inserted without intraoperative problems. Based on intraoperative and radiological findings, the bone quality was assessed as follows: D1 in $n = 2$, D2 in $n = 3$, D3 in $n = 2$ and D4 in $n = 2$ cases. The employed implant dimensions were as follows: 4.1 × 5 mm ($n = 2$), 4.1 × 6 mm ($n = 1$), 4.1 × 7 mm ($n = 10$) and 3.75 × 7 mm ($n = 17$). The expansion process could successfully be performed in every case. The healing period was uneventful. Patients were rehabilitated with fixed dentures in 5 cases and with removable dentures in 4 cases. Basic clinical characteristics are summarised in detail in Table 4.

Over the 3-year follow-up period, the overall cumulative implant success rate in these patients was 28/30 (93.3%). Two implants were lost in the posterior maxilla. The two affected patients had highly atrophic posterior maxillae (Cawood et Howell IV–V) [38] and a bone quality of D3–D4 (Table 4). The male patient was a smoker and suffered from a squamous cell carcinoma of mouth floor. In both cases, the manufactured removable denture was successfully relined and no technical complications were observed to date.

The Kaplan-Meyer analysis of implant survival for both jaws is visualised in Fig. 2 (log rank test, $p = 0.173$): 1-year survival 96.7% and 2-year survival 93.3%. The 3-year follow-up has not yet been completed by all patients (Table 4).

Measurements of implant stability by resonance frequency analysis (RFA) displayed the following ISQ values: primary stability 69.7 ± 10.3 95% CI (65.9; 73.6) ISQ units and secondary stability 69.8 ± 10.2 95% CI (65.8; 73.5) ISQ units (Fig. 3a, b). The differences were not statistically significant ($p = 0.780$; paired *t* test). In detail, the ISQ values for primary stability displayed in the maxilla 66.9 ± 8.9 95% CI (61.9; 71.8), and in the mandible 72.5 ± 11.1 95% CI (66.4; 78.7). The differences were not statistically significant ($p = 0.134$; independent *t* test). According to the measurement of secondary implant stability, we observed comparable ISQ values in the maxilla 66.4 ± 10.0 95% CI (60.9; 71.9) and higher ISQ values in the mandible 73.0 ± 9.7 95% CI (67.6; 78.4). The differences were as well not statistically significant ($p = 0.780$; independent *t* test).

Over the follow-up period, the mean crestal bone changes after loading were as follows (each compared to the baseline): in the first year, 1.0 ± 0.9 mm 95% CI (0.5; 1.5) in the maxilla and 0.7 ± 0.4 mm 95% CI (0.5; 1.0) in the mandible ($p = 0.011$; independent *t* test), and in the second year, 1.3 ± 0.8 mm 95% CI (0.8; 1.7) in the maxilla and 1.0 ± 0.7 mm 95% CI (0.6; 1.4) in the mandible ($p = 0.644$; independent *t* test). Clinical and radiological

Table 4 Clinical characteristics of the study cohort

Patient	Sex	Age (years)	Implant position (*FDI*)	Indication category[a]	Bone quality	Prosthetic treatment	Follow-up (months)	Implant failure
1. T. I.	F	80	Maxilla 15, 13, 11, 21, 25 (Σ = 5)	IIa	D4	Telescope	37	$n = 1$[c]
2. G. S.	F	65	Mandible 34, 32, 42, 44 (Σ = 4)	IIIb	D1	Ball attachment	34	None
3. S. Sa.	F	64	Maxilla 14, 12, 22, 24 (Σ = 4)	IIIa[b]	D4	Jaw bar	34	None
4. Th. F.	M	76	Mandible 35, 36, 37 (Σ = 3)	IIb	D1	Bridge	33	None
5. A. M.	F	44	Maxilla 16, 15, 14 (Σ = 3)	IIa	D3	Bridge	32	None
6. S. M.	M	53	Maxilla 16, 14, 12 (Σ = 3)	IIa	D3	Ball attachment	32	$n = 1$[d]
7. K. S.	F	52	Mandible 35, 36, 37 (Σ = 3)	IIb	D2	Bridge	29	None
8. R. C.	F	59	Mandible 35, 36 (Σ = 2)	IIb	D2	Bridge	24	None
9. W. K.	F	72	Mandible 47, 45, 43 (Σ = 3)	IIb	D2	Bridge	23	None

FDI implant position according to the World Dental Federation
[a]Indication categories (IIa, IIb, IIIa, IIIb) with regard to the amount of implants [35]
[b]Modified due to local conditions
[c]Implant loss before loading
[d]Implant loss after loading

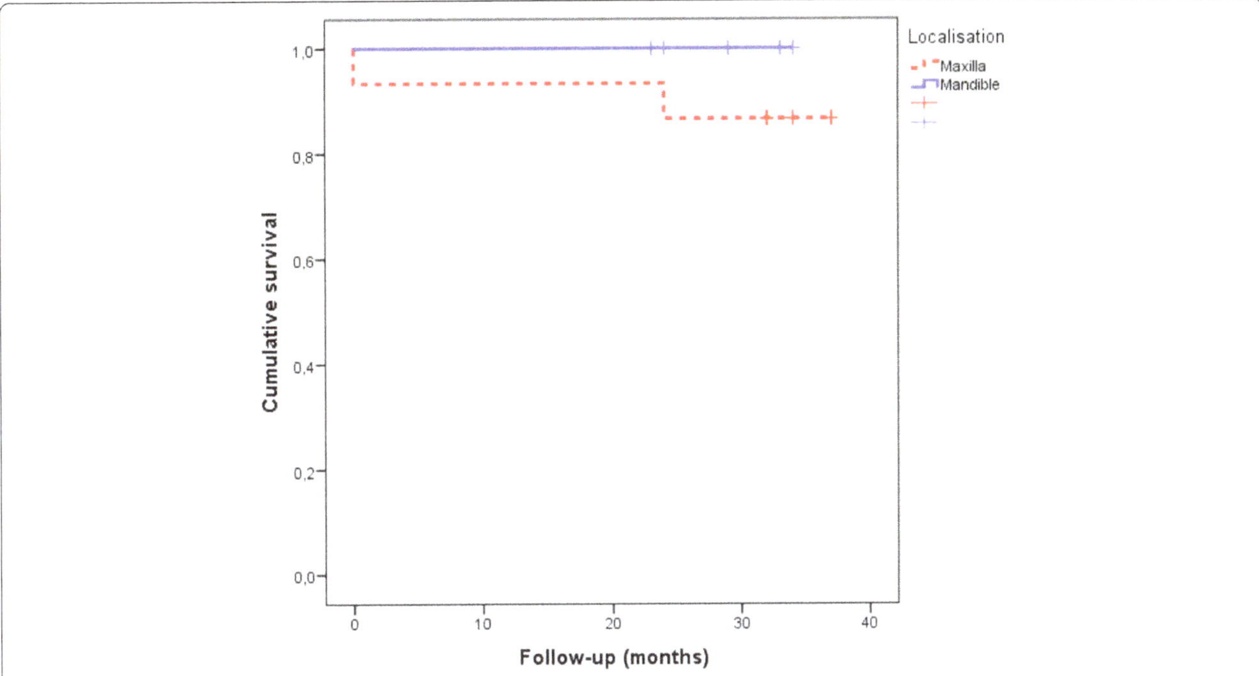

Fig. 2 Cumulative implant survival over the follow-up period. The Kaplan-Meyer diagram visualises the analysis of implant survival in the maxilla and in the mandible (log rank test, $p = 0.173$) over the follow-up period up to 37 months (Table 4)

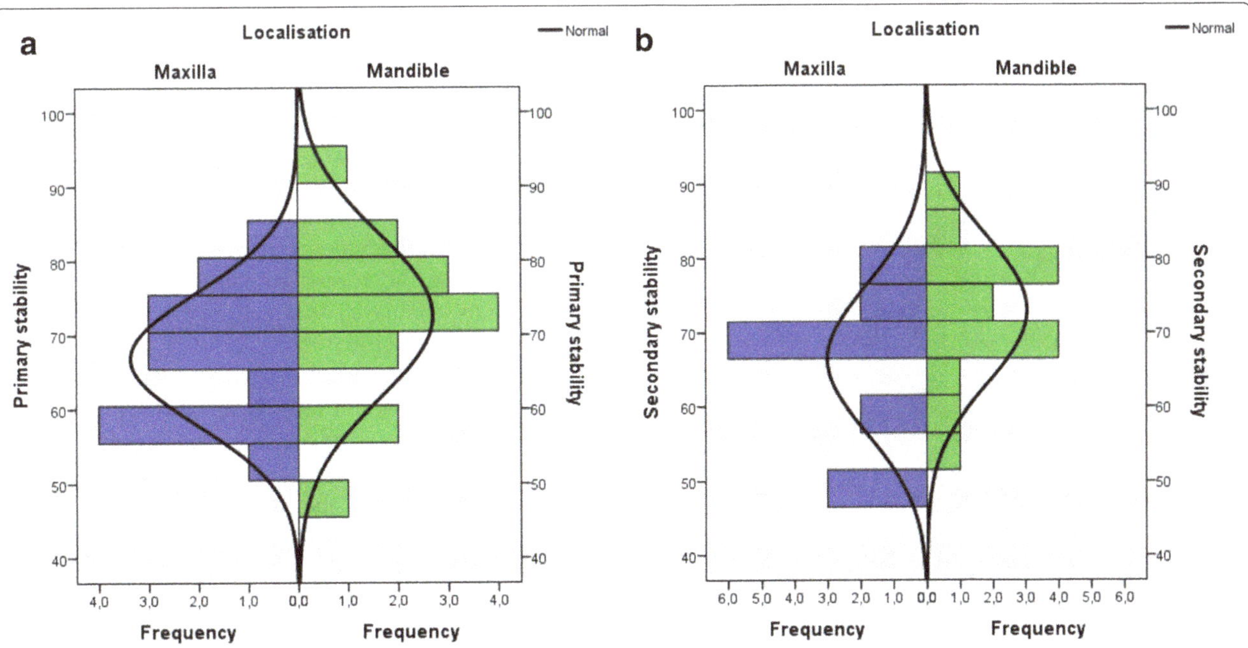

Fig. 3 a Primary implant stability. The histogram visualises the distribution of the implant stability quotients (ISQ) for both jaws measured by resonance frequency analysis (Osstell AB, Göteborg, Sweden). **b** Secondary implant stability. The histogram shows the distribution of the implant stability quotients (ISQ) of osseointegrated implants. According to the measurement implant stability was classified as *low* with ISQ values < 60, *medium* with ISQ values 60–70, and *high* with values ISQ > 70 [34]

investigations did not reveal any inflammatory signs or radiolucency in the periapical region for all inserted implants.

A representative case of a rehabilitated female patient is visualised in Fig. 4a–h and Fig. 5a–d (radiograms).

Discussion

Recent literature has shown that short implants have achieved growing acceptance in the field of oral implantology [9, 10, 39, 40]. Since the last years, concern has decreased about the length of endosseous implants; it should be noted that all extraoral screw implants are short implants [41, 42]. Nevertheless, there are local physiological and biomechanical differences regarding long-term stability.

The survival rate of short dental implants was found to increase from 80 to > 90% over time [39]. This is also confirmed in recent studies. For short dental implants supporting single crowns and fixed bridges especially in the mandible, a 2-year success rate of 97% [43] and a 5-year outcome of 92.2% [10] are reported. Otherwise, the success rate of 100% in the maxilla (3-year outcome) [15] must be critically questioned in view of our findings.

Only a few reports in the literature have addressed *expandable dental implants* [44–47]. In 2001, Jo and co-authors reported about a 40-month prospective survival of an expandable standard-length implant (10–16 mm) for immediate loading. They found a 3-year survival rate of 96.1% in the maxilla and of 94.8% in the mandible [46]. Huré and co-authors [47] performed a biomechanical and histologic canine study on early loaded expandable implants of 10- and 11.5-mm lengths. Six years later (2010), in orthopaedic surgery, an expandable implant was introduced [48]. Similar with the present study, these authors addressed implants under difficult regional bony conditions.

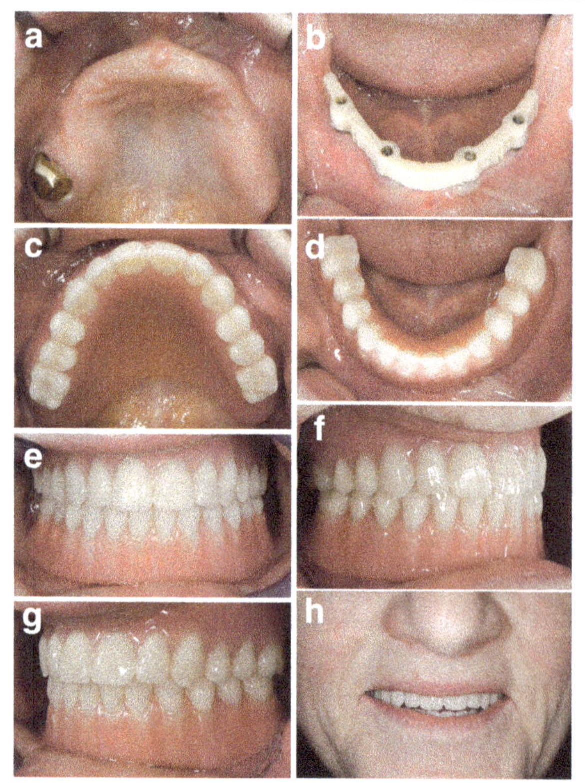

Fig. 4 a–h Prosthetic restauration—follow-up examination. Intraoral and perioral views of a rehabilitated female patient. (She asked explicitly only for implantological treatment in the mandible.)

The purpose of our study was to evaluate the intraoperative handling, safety and feasibility of a new *expandable dental implant* system in a heterogeneous study cohort. We found in the present pilot study an overall 3-year implant success rate of 93.3%, which is comparable with recent literature [39]. To the best of our knowledge (PubMed), the present clinical study is the first published investigation about the usage of an *expandable short dental implant system*. Therefore, directly comparable data from other clinical studies are missing.

Several investigators analysed the preferred indications of short dental implants in the posterior mandible or maxilla and outlined the cost efficiency compared to additional vertical augmentations. In the present trial, we used a new short implant in both jaws and nearly all possible indication categories were represented, which proves the broad versatility (Table 4).

In our study, two implant failures occurred early in the prosthetic period and under loading. In a former systematic review, 11 studies reported more short implant failures *before* loading, while 7 studies reported more implant failures *after* loading [39]. Regarding the implant success rate in the present study, it must be considered that the lost implants were associated with difficult surgical conditions. Besides biological failures, in this study cohort, no technical complications were observed. In accordance with earlier comparative studies, it is evident that when using short implants, there is a lower risk of complications compared to augmentation [4, 7, 8] and nerve lateralisation [40].

Why design modifications? This is a matter of reduction of the healing period [46], the gain of stability under difficult conditions and increased bone-to-implant contact [27, 49–51] and the fact that most complications of short implants occur in the *preprosthetic period* [39]. It is also a question of long-term crestal bone stability. Earlier biomechanical finite-element studies confirmed that apical expansion results in favourable stress reduction in the *crestal bone* of nearly 10% [52]. It is assumable that additionally to the microthread and platform-switching concept [53], the periimplant bone strain could be reduced by apical expansion. This issue requires separate consideration in further studies. The

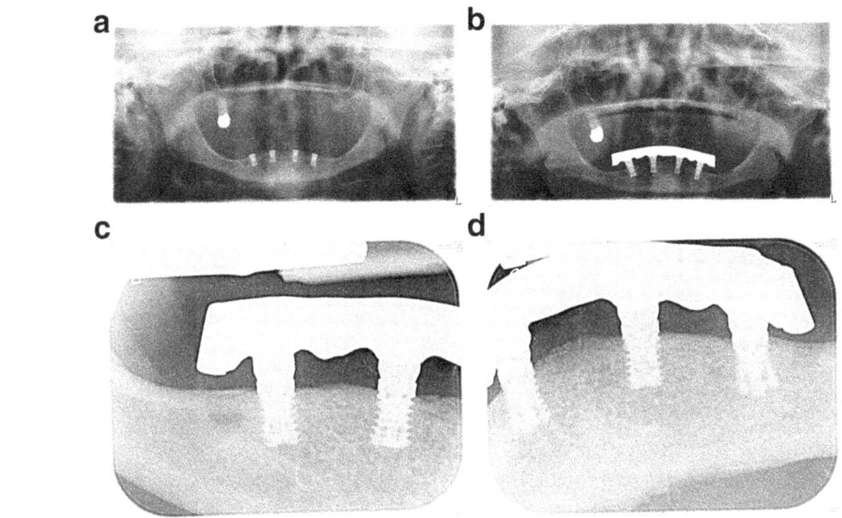

Fig. 5 **a** Postoperative orthopantomogram. **b** Follow-up orthopantomogram. **c** Follow-up standard periapical radiogram (implants i42 and i44). **d** Follow-up standard periapical radiogram (implants i32 and i34)

employed implant design (especially its 7-mm length) combines several favourable biomechanical features, which were considered in this study (Fig. 1a, d).

According to Gehrke and co-authors, and in relation to the present study, the *apical implant design* influences the implant stability and bone-to-implant contact [54]. The expansion procedure presents an additional bicortical anchorage [17] in the oro-vestibular direction. In hard bone, this might be a disadvantage and lead to asymmetrical expansion. Manufacturers' recommendations for hard bone should be strongly considered.

Regarding resonance frequency analysis, the values are related to bone quality and quantity as well as the exposed implant height above the alveolar crest, which depends on the type of implant and insertion technique [55–57]. Our results (primary stability in the maxilla 66.9 ± 8.9 ISQ units and in the mandible 72.5 ± 11.1 ISQ units; secondary stability in the maxilla 66.4 ± 10.0 ISQ units and in the mandible 73.0 ± 9.7 ISQ units) are comparable with the results from Becker and co-authors (standard-length implants): primary stability 72.1 ISQ units and secondary stability 72.6 ISQ units [58]. These values are marginally lower than those of short implants inserted only in the *posterior mandible* (79.0 ISQ units) [12]. Other authors measured in the *posterior maxilla* 68.2 ISQ units (6-mm implants) [15]. Altogether, our mean results (Fig. 2a, b) represent high stability values [34]. Huré and co-authors [47] measured in their animal study the following stability values (expandable implant of ≥ 10-mm length): for primary stability, 53.6 ± 3.0 ISQ units, and for secondary stability (3 months after insertion), 59 ± 4.5 ISQ units. The evaluation of stability values during the osseointegration period was not possible in our trial due to submerged healing. The question, whether the level of implant stability achieved at insertion can be maintained during the early healing period, remains. This should be analysed separately for all bone types in front of the known lowest stability values at 3–4 weeks after placement for all bone types [59–61] and the recent attempts of immediate [14] or early (6 weeks) functional loading of other short implant systems [28]. In relation to the results by McCullough and Klokkevold [62], who found that the macrothread design appears to play a positive role in implant stability in the early healing period, this can also be assumed for the employed implant system. Additionally, with regard to the results by Marković and co-authors [61], a critical stability drop down due to bone remodeling after bone condensing (implant site preparation and/or using expandable implants) should not be suspected; the opposite can be expected. The authors analysed the implant stability (4.1 × 10-mm screw implant) in the posterior maxilla in vivo depending on the implant site preparation (bone condensing vs. bone drilling) and confirmed that, after bone condensing, significantly higher implant stability results were achieved, immediately after implant insertion as well as during the whole observation period of 6 weeks. Especially in the third week in both groups, the following results were measured: 66.7 ± 1.64 vs. 57.1 ± 1.45 ($p < 0.001$). [61]. In the present study, we measured in the posterior maxilla 66.3 ± 10.4 ISQ units for primary stability and 66.9 ± 12.0 ISQ units for secondary stability, respectively.

Contrary to conventional hollow-screw implants (only marginal gap), a problem of the expandable implant is the presence of gaps down to the apical region. Former microbial assessment of different implant-abutment interfaces displayed that none of the marginal connections had the capacity to prevent microbial leakage [63–65].

Therefore, an apical microleakage (comparable to distractable implants and endodontically treated teeth) might be a disadvantage of the evolved implant system [66, 67]. However, according to the manufacturer's information, a microbiological study revealed no microbial leakage through the expanded implants. Over the follow-up period, we equally did not observe any inflammatory signs in the apical region, neither clinically nor radiologically (Figs. 4b and 5c–d). Nevertheless, this aspect should be analysed under mechanical loading in vitro. Based on an earlier animal histologic study [47], as well as a clinical up-to-40-month study [46], which referred to comparable apically expandable implants, authors did not report any periapical inflammatory complications. To eliminate the potential risk of deep intrabony microleakage, it is questionable whether equal biomechanical stability values can be achieved only by the macrothread design avoiding any deep microgaps.

In the present study, the crestal bone changes under loading in the first year exceeded that of the second year. Moreover, the differences between the maxilla and mandible in each year were not statistically significant, which only partially agrees with previous findings in the literature [7, 58]. Besides microbiological conditions, there are several biomechanical aspects which influence maintenance of periimplant crestal bone. Conical and parallel surfaces of the implant-abutment connection (internal hexagon) provide rotational stability and reduce microgaps and micromovement [68]. Another important factor is the thickness of the implant shoulder [69], which might be a weak point in the design of a short implant due to elastic deformity under *extra-axial* loading. This fact might be the reason for non-inflammatory periimplant crestal bone loss. We addressed this aspect by splitting adjacent implants wherever possible [50, 51]. According to Brenner and co-authors [30] as well as Pommer and co-authors [50], the following *prosthodontic factors* are to be considered to avoid screw loosening, component fracture, loss of marginal bone or even loss of osseointegration: crown-to-implant ratio (extra-axial loading), cantilever length, status of opposing dentition, splinting of adjacent implants, occlusal surface relief and dimensions.

Comparable studies displayed at 24 months a crestal bone loss of 0.5–0.6 mm [15]. Other authors reported at 2, 3 and 5 years a mean loss of 0.57, 0.55 and 0.53 mm, respectively, in the mandible (without significant change after 1 year) [10]. On the other hand, randomised controlled trials demonstrated 1 year after loading periimplant marginal bone loss of 0.7 mm [70] and 1.1 mm [7] in the mandible which is the same value measured in the present study.

Within the limitations of a pilot study design, low number of implants, single-arm study and short-term follow-up, the results show a basic improvement of functional rehabilitation especially for elderly patients with compromised general and local conditions for implantation. Controversial questions [5, 71] remain on whether (a) short implants are suitable for irradiated patients and (b) there is a need for expandable short implants in the D1 bone. Furthermore, potential bias should be eliminated in future studies by a randomised controlled trial.

Conclusion

Initial results of the ongoing study confirm the feasibility and safety of the employed system. The implant type seems to be useful for all bone qualities and shows high initial and secondary biomechanical stability in the maxilla and mandible. Long-term follow-up will be needed in validating these initial results in a larger 3-year clinical trial. Crestal bone changes should be evaluated in a larger study cohort. The novel system might extend the spectrum in functional rehabilitation.

Abbreviations

D1, D2, D3, D4: Bone quality (density); FDI: World Dental Federation; ISQ: Implant stability quotient; RFA: Resonance frequency analysis

Acknowledgements

The authors are grateful to the DenTack Company for providing some of the implants and components used in this study. The courtesy of Oz Vachtenberg is acknowledged for providing Fig. 1a–f and the movie clip. There are no financial supports or conflicts of interest associated with this publication that could have influenced its outcome. We thank the Osstell Company, which supplied the RFA device and Smartpegs used in this study. We acknowledge American Journal Experts (AJE) for providing English language editing (certificate verification key: 06DA-C0B2-2672-4103-A251). In addition, the authors thank the dental technicians from the dental laboratory Rübeling and Klar, Berlin, Germany, for their kind support in manufacturing all dental prostheses. Furthermore, we thank all involved members of the surgical and prosthodontic teams.

Funding

No funding received.

Authors' contributions

WR was responsible for the preparation of the study protocol, surgical treatment, data acquisition, statistics and preparation of the manuscript. RS was responsible for prosthetic treatment. CH was responsible for surgical treatment, radiological analysis and statistics. JH was responsible for preparation of the study protocol, prosthetic treatment and interpretation of the data. BA was responsible for interpretation of the data and approval of the final manuscript version to be submitted. AWE was responsible for the approval of the study protocol and interpretation of the data. All authors read and approved the final manuscript.

Authors' information

WR is a senior physician at the University Hospital Halle, Martin Luther University Halle-Wittenberg, Department of Oral and Plastic Maxillofacial Surgery, Halle/Saale, Germany.
RS is a clinical research associate at the University School of Dental Medicine, Department of Prosthetic Dentistry, Martin Luther University Halle-Wittenberg, Halle/Saale, Germany.
CH is a consultant at the University Hospital Halle, Martin Luther University Halle-Wittenberg, Department of Oral and Plastic Maxillofacial Surgery, Halle/Saale, Germany.
JH is an assistant professor at the University School of Dental Medicine, Department of Prosthetic Dentistry, Martin Luther University Halle-Wittenberg, Halle/Saale, Germany.
BA is professor and the head of the department at the University Hospital Halle, Martin Luther University Halle-Wittenberg, Department of Oral and Plastic Maxillofacial Surgery, Halle/Saale, Germany.
AWE is a senior assistant professor at the University Hospital Halle, Martin Luther University Halle-Wittenberg, Department of Oral and Plastic Maxillofacial Surgery, Halle/Saale, Germany.

Competing interests

Waldemar Reich, Ramona Schweyen, Christian Heinzelmann, Jeremias Hey and Alexander Walter Eckert declare no competing interest.
Bilal Al-Nawas is giving lectures for Straumann, Camlog, Dentsply, Nobel biocare, Geistlich.

Author details

[1]Department of Oral and Plastic Maxillofacial Surgery, Martin Luther University Halle-Wittenberg, Ernst-Grube Str. 40, 06120 Halle (Saale), Germany. [2]University School of Dental Medicine, Department of Prosthetic Dentistry, Martin Luther University Halle-Wittenberg, Magdeburger Straße 16, 06112 Halle (Saale), Germany.

References

1. Schwarz F, Terheyden H. Significance of dental implants for health care. Bundesgesundheitsblatt Gesundheitsforschung Gesundheitsschutz. 2011;54(9):1097–101. (German)
2. Gates WD, Cooper LF, Sanders AE, Reside GJ, De Kok IJ. The effect of implant-supported removable partial dentures on oral health quality of life. Clin Oral Impl Res. 2014;25:207–13.
3. Fretwurst T, Nack C, Al-Ghrairi M, Raguse JD, Stricker A, Schmelzeisen R, Nelson K, Nahles S. Long-term retrospective evaluation of the peri-implant bone level in onlay grafted patients with iliac bone from the anterior superior iliac crest. J Craniomaxillofac Surg. 2015;43(6):956–60.
4. Verhoeven JW, Rujiter J, Cune MS, Terlou M, Zoon M. Onlay grafts in combination with endosseous implants in severe mandibular atrophy: one year results of a prospective, quantitative radiological study. Clin Oral Implants Res. 2000;11(6):583–94.
5. Nkenke E. Short implants. Do they replace reconstruction of the alveolar crest? MKG-Chirurg. 2013;6:221–7. (German)
6. Al-Hashedi AA, Ali TB, Yunus N. Short dental implants: an emerging concept in implant treatment. Quintessence Int. 2014;45(6):499–514.
7. Esposito M, Barausse C, Pistilli R, Sammartino G, Grandi G, Felice P. Short implants versus bone augmentation for placing long implants in atrophic maxillae: one-year post-loading results of a pilot randomised controlled trial. Eur J Oral Implantol. 2015;8(3):257–68.
8. Schincaglia GP, Thoma DS, Haas R, Tutak M, Garcia A, Taylor TD, Hämmerle CH. Randomised controlled multicenter study comparing short dental implants (6 mm) versus longer dental implants (11-15 mm) in combination with sinus floor elevation procedures. Part 2: clinical and radiographic outcomes at 1 year of loading. J Clin Periodontol. 2015;42(1):1042–51.
9. Srinivasan M, Vazquez L, Rieder P, Moraguez O, Bernard JP, Belser UC. Survival rates of short (6 mm) micro-rough surface implants: a review of literature and meta-analysis. Clin Oral Implants Res. 2014;25(5):539–45.
10. Slotte C, Grønningsaeter A, Halmøy AM, Ohrnell LO, Mordenfeld A, Isaksson S, Johansson LA. Four-milimeter-long posterior-mandible implants: 5-year outcomes of a prospective multicenter study. Clin Implant Dent Relat Res. 2015;17(Suppl 2):e385–95.
11. Thoma DS, Haas R, Tutak M, Garcia A, Schincaglia GP, Hämmerle CH. Randomised controlled multicenter study comparing short dental implants (6 mm) versus longer dental implants (11-15 mm) in combination with sinus floor elevation procedures. Part 1: demographic and patient-reported outcomes at 1 year of loading. J Clin Periodontol. 2015;42(1):72–80.
12. Hentschel A, Herrmann J, Glauche I, Vollmer A, Schlegel KA, Lutz R. Survival and patient satisfaction of short implants during the first 2 years of function: a retrospective cohort study with 694 implants in 416 patients. Clin Oral Impl Res. 2016;27:591–6.
13. Fan T, Li Y, Deng WW, Wu T, Zhang W. Short implants (5-8 mm) versus longer implants (>8 mm) with sinus lifting in atrophic posterior maxilla: a meta-analysis of RCTs. Clin Implant Dent Relat Res. 2017;19(1):207–15.
14. Anitua E, Flores J, Flores C, Alkhraisat MH. Long-term outcomes of immediate loading of short implants: a controlled retrospective cohort study. Int J Oral Maxillofac Implants. 2016;31(6):1360–6.
15. Bechara S, Kubilius R, Veronesi G, Pires JT, Shibli JA, Mangano FG. Short (6-mm) dental implants versus sinus floor elevation and placement of longer (≥10 mm) dental implants: a randomized controlled trial with a 3-year follow-up. Clin Oral Implants Res. 2016. doi:10.1111/cir.12923.
16. Zöller J, Neugebauer J. Update on short, angulated and diameter-reduced implants. Consensus paper of the 11th European Consensus Conference (EuCC) 2016 in Cologne. https://www.bdizedi.org/. Accessed 01 Oct 2017 (German).
17. Pierrisnard L, Renouard F, Renault P, Barquins M. Influence of implant length and bicortical anchorage on implant stress distribution. Clin Implant Dent Relat Res. 2003;5(4):254–62.
18. Geng JP, Tan KB, Liu GR. Application of finite element analysis in implant dentistry: a review of the literature. J Prosthet Dent. 2001;85(6):585–98.
19. Baggi L, Capelloni I, Di Girolamo M, Maceri F, Vairo G. The influence of implant diameter and length on stress distribution of osseointegrated implants related to crestal bone geometry: a three-dimensional finite element analysis. J Prosthet Dent. 2008;100(6):422–31.
20. De Moraes SL, Verri FR, Santiago JF Jr, Almeida DA, de Mello CC, Pellizzer EP. A 3-D finite element study of the influence of crown-implant ratio on stress distribution. Braz Dent J. 2013;24(6):635–41.
21. Moraes SL, Pellizzer EP, Verri FR, Santiago JF Jr, Silva JV. Three-dimensional finite element analysis on stress distribution in retention screws of different crown-implant ratios. Comput Methods Biomech Biomed Engin. 2015;18(7):689–96.
22. Petrie CS, Williams JL. Comparative evaluation of implant designs: influence of diameter, length, and taper on strains in the alveolar crest. A three-dimensional finite-element analysis. Clin Oral Implants Res. 2005;16(4):486–94.
23. Möhlhenrich SC, Heussen N, Elvers D, Steiner T, Hölzle F, Modabber A. Compensating for poor primary implant stability in different bone densities by varying implant geometry: a laboratory study. Int J Oral Maxillofac Surg. 2015;44:1514–20.
24. Yazicioglu D, Bayram B, Oguz Y, Cinar D, Uckan S. Stress distribution on short implants at maxillary posterior alveolar bone model with different bone-to-implant contact ratio: finite elemnt analysis. J Oral IMplantol. 2016;42(1):26–33.
25. Sivan-Gildor A, Machtei EE, Gabay E, Frankenthal S, Levin L, Suzuki M, Coelho PG, Zigdon-Giladi H. Novel implant design improves implant survival in multirooted extraction sites: a preclinical pilot study. J Periodontol. 2014;85:1458–63.
26. Jain N, Gulati NJM, Garg M, Pathak C. Short implants: new horizon in implant dentistry. J Clin Diagn Res. 2016;10(9):ZE14–7.
27. Quaranta A, D'Isidoro O, Bambini F, Putignano A. Potential bone to implant contact area of short versus standard implants: an in vitro micro-computed tomography analysis. Implant Dent. 2016;25(1):97–102.
28. Makowiecki A, Botzenhart U, Seeliger J, Heinemann F, Biocev P, Dominiak M. A comparative study of the effectiveness of early and delayed loading of short tissue-level dental implants with hydrophilic surfaces placed in the posterior section of the mandible—a preliminary study. Ann Anat. 2017;212:61–8.
29. Cohen O, Ormianer Z, Tal H, Rothamel D, Weinreb M, Moses O. Differences in crestal bone-to-implant contact following an under-drilling compared to an over-drilling protocol. A study in the rabbit tibia. Clin Oral Investig. 2016;20(9):2475–80.
30. Brenner M, Brandt J, Lauer HC. Prothetische Versorgung auf kurzen Implantaten. Zahnmedizin up2date. 2014;2:123–42. (German)

31. Eitner S, Wichmann M, Schlegel KA, Kollmannberger JE, Nickenig HJ. Oral health-related quality of life and implant therapy: an evaluation of preoperative, intermediate, and post-treatment assessments of patients and physicians. J Craniomaxillofac Surg. 2012;40(1):20–3.
32. Buser D, Weber HP, Lang NP. Tissue integration of non-submerged implants. 1-year results of a prospective study with 100 ITI hollow-cylinder and hollow-screw implants. Clin Oral Impl Res. 1990;1:33–40.
33. Karoussis IK, Brägger U, Salvi GE, Bürgin W, Lang NP. Effect of implant design on survival and success rates of titanium oral implants: a 10-year prospective cohort study of the ITI dental implant system. Clin Oral Implants Res. 2004;15(1):8–17.
34. Sennerby L. 20 years of experience with resonance frequency analysis. Implantologie. 2013;21(1):21–33. (German)
35. Terheyden H. Indikationsklassen für Implantatversorgung zur Regelversorgung. Consensus conference implantology. 2014. https://www.konsensuskonferenz-implantologie.eu/. Accessed 05 May 2014 (German).
36. Gross MD. Occlusion in implant dentistry. A review of the literature of prosthetic determinants and current consepts. Aust Dent J. 2008;53(Suppl1):S60–8.
37. Gomez-Roman G, Schulte W, d'Hoedt B, Axman-Krcmar D. The Frialit-2 implant system: five-year clinical experience in single-tooth and immediately postextraction applications. Int J Oral Maxillofac Implants. 1997;12(3):299–309.
38. Cowood JI, Howell RA. A classification of the edentulous jaws. Int J Oral Maxillofac Surg. 1988;17:232.
39. Karthikeyan I, Desai SR, Singh R. Short implants: a systematic review. J Indian Soc Periodontol. 2012;16(3):302–12.
40. Dursun E, Keceli HG, Uysal S, Güngör H, Muhtarogullari M, Tözüm TF. Management of limited vertical bone height in the posterior mandible: short dental implants versus nerve lateralization with standard length implants. J Craniofac Surg. 2016;27(3):578–85.
41. Tjellström A, Lindström J, Nylén O, Albrektsson T, Brånemark PI, Birgersson B, Nero H, Sylvén C. The bone-anchored auricular episthesis. Laryngoscope. 1981;91(5):811–5.
42. Choi KJ, Sajisevi MB, McClennen J, Kaylie DM. Image-guided placement of osseointegrated implants for challenging auricular, orbital, and rhinectomy defects. Ann Otol Rhinol Laryngol. 2016;125(10):801–7.
43. Malmstrom H, Gupta B, Ghanem A, Cacciato R, Ren Y, Romanos GE. Success rate of short dental implants supporting single crowns and fixed bridges. Clin Oral Implants Res. 2016;27(9):1093–8.
44. Garfield RE. An expandable implant fixture. Dent Implantol Updat. 1998;9(5):37–40.
45. Nowzari H, Chee W, Tuan A, Abou-Rass M, Landesman HM. Clinical and microbiological aspects of the Sargon immediate load implant. Compend Contin Edu Dent. 1998;19(7):686–9.
46. Jo HY, Hobo PK, Hobo S. Freestanding and multiunit immediate loading of the expandable implant: an up-to-40-month prospective survival study. J Prosthet Dent. 2001;85(2):148–55.
47. Huré G, Aguado E, Grizon F, Baslé MF, Chappard D. Some biomechanical and histologic characteristics of early-loaded locking pin and expandable implants: a pilot histologic canine study. Clin Implant Dent Relat Res. 2004;6(1):33–9.
48. Folman Y, Ron N, Shabat S, Romano G, Galasso O. The fixation expandable stem hemiarthoroplasty for displaced femoral neck fracture: technical features and pilot study. Arch Orthop Trauma Surg. 2010;130(4):527–31.
49. Xiao JR, Li DH, Chen YX, Chen SJ, Guan SM, Kong L. Evaluation of fixation of expandable implants in the mandibles of ovarectomized sheep. J Oral Maxillofac Surg. 2013;71:682–8.
50. Pommer B, Hingsammer L, Haas R, Mailath-Pokorny G, Busenlechner D, Watzek G, Fürhauser R. Denture-related biomechanical factors for fixed partial dentures retained on short dental implants. Int J Prosthodont. 2015;28(4):412–4.
51. Kim Y, Oh TJ, Misch CE, Wang HL. Occlusal considerations in implant therapy: clinical guidelines with biomechanical rationale. Clin Oral Implants Res. 2005;16(1):26–35.
52. Xiao JR, Li YF, Guan SM, Song L, Xu LX, Kong L. The biomechanical analysis of simulation implants in function under osteoporotic jawbone by comparing cylindrical, apical tapered, neck tapered, and expandable type implants: a 3-dimensional finite element analysis. J Oral Maxillofac Surg. 2011;69:e273–81.
53. Yun HJ, Park JC, Yun JH, Jung UW, Kim CS, Choi SH, Cho KS. A short-term clinical study of marginal bone level change around microthreded and platform-switched implants. J Periodontal Implant Sci. 2011;41(5):211–7.
54. Gehrke SA, Pérez-Albacete Martinez C, Piattelli A, Shibli JA, Markovic A, Calvo Guirado JL. The influence of three different apical implant designs at stability and osseointegration process: experimental study in rabbits. Clin Oral Implants Res. 2017;28(3):355–61.
55. Herrero-Climent M, Santos-Garcia R, Jaramillo-Santos R, Romero-Ruiz MM, Fernandez-Palacin Lazaro-Calvo P, Bullon P, Rios-Santos JV. Assesment of Osstell ISQ's reliability for implant stability measurement: a cross-sectional clinical study. Medicina Oral Pathologia Oral y Cirugia buccal. 2013;18:e877–82.
56. Gupta RK, Padmanabhan TV. Resonance frequence analysis. Indian J Dent Res. 2011;22(4):567–73.
57. Kang IH, Kim CW, Lim YJ, Kim MJ. A comparative study on the initial stability of different implants placed above the bone level using resonance frequence analysis. J Adv Prosthodont. 2011;3(4):190–9.
58. Becker W, Becker BE, Hujoel P, Abu Raz Z, Goldstein M, Smidt A. Prospective clinical trial evaluating a new implant system for implant survival, implant stability and radiographic bone changes. Clin Implant Dent Relat Res. 2013;15(1):15–21.
59. Barewal RM, Oates TW, Meredith N, Cochrane DL. Resonance frequency measurement of implant stability in vivo on implants with a sandblasted and acid-etched surface. Int J Oral Maxillofac Implants. 2003;18(5):641–51.
60. Huwiler MA, Pjetursson BE, Bosshardt DD, Salvi GE, Lang NP. Resonance frequency analysis in relation to jawbone characteristics and during early healing of implant instillation. Clin Oral Implants Res. 2007;18(3):275–80.
61. Marković A, Calasan D, Colić S, Stojčev-Stajčć L, Janjić B, Mišić T. Implant stability in posterior maxilla: bone-condensing versus bone-drilling: a clinical study. Oral Surg Oral Med Oral Pathol Oral Radiol Endod. 2011;112(5):557–63.
62. McCullough JJ, Klokkevold PR. The effect of implant macro-thread design on implant stability in the early post-operative period: a randomized, controlled pilot study. Clin Oral Implants Res. 2016. doi:10.1111/cir.12945.
63. Teixeira W, Ribeiro RF, Sato S, Pedrazzi V. Microleakage into and from two-stage implants: an in vitro comparative study. Int J Oral Maxillofac Implants. 2011;6(1):56–62.
64. Canullo L, Penarrocha-Oltra D, Soldini C, Mazzocco F, Penarrocha M, Covani U. Microbial assessment of the implant-abutment interface in different connectioins: cross-sectional study after 5 years of functional loading. Clin Oral Implants Res. 2015;26(4):426–34.
65. Mishra SK, Chowdhary R, Kumari S. Microleakage at different implant abutment interface: a systematic review. J Clin Diagn Res. 2017;11(6):ZE10–5.
66. Feichtinger M, Gaggl A, SChultes G, Kärcher H. Evaluation of distraction implants for prosthetic treatment after vertical alveolar ridge distraction: a clinical investigation. Int J Prosthodont. 2003;16(1):19–24.
67. Pradeep PR, Kasti KJ, Ananthakrishna S, Raghu TN, Vikram R. Evaluation of different dentin adhesive systems and its effect on apical microleakage: an in vitro study. J Int Oral Health. 2015;7(5):44–8.
68. Streckbein P, Streckbein RG, Wilbrand JF, Malik CY, Schaaf H, Howaldt HP, Flach M. Non-linear 3D evaluation of different oral implant-abutment connections. J Dent Res. 2012;91(12):1184–9.
69. Pellizzer EP, de Mello CC, Santiago Junior JF, de Souza Batista VE, de Faria Almeida DA, Verri FR. Analysis of the biomechanical behavior of short implants: the photo-elasticity method. Mater Sci Eng C Mater Biol Appl. 2015;55:187–92.
70. Felice P, Pistilli R, Barausse C, Bruno V, Trullenque-Eriksson A, Esposito M. Short implants as an alternative to crestal sinus lift: a 1-year multicentre randomised controlled trial. Eur J Oral Implantol. 2015;8(4):375–84.
71. Schwartz SR. Short implants: are they a viable option in implant dentistry? Dent Clin N Am. 2015;59(2):317–28.
72. Granström G. Osseointegration in irradiated cancer patients. An analysis with respect to implant failures. J Oral Maxillofac Surg. 2005;63:579–85.
73. Grötz KA, Schmidt BLJ, Walther C, Al-Nawas B. In which bisphosphonate patients am I allowed to place implants? A systematic review. Z Zahnärztl Impl. 2010;26(2):153–61. (German)

15

Maxillary segmental osteoperiosteal flap with simultaneous placement of dental implants

Tibebu Tsegga[1,2] and Thomas Wright[1,2*]

Abstract

Dental restorative space from the opposing dentition requires adequate distance for restorative material for an acceptable restoration. Typically, long-standing edentulous alveolar ridges will have vertical and or horizontal defects that require alveolar ridge augmentation for ideal dental implant restorations. Along with these defects, one will see the opposing dentition supra erupt which can obliterate the restorative space. Multiple surgical techniques have been described to address these dilemmas. The use of osteoperiosteal flaps has been described to address vertical height deficiencies. The purpose of this paper is to document and introduce a maxillary segmental osteoperiosteal flap intrusion to increase the restorative space with simultaneous dental implant placement. As with most dilemmas in treatment planning dental implants, multiple acceptable treatment options are available to the practitioner. This technique is another of many that can be added to the available options. When appropriately planned in select cases, this technique will result with ideal dental implant restorations without compromising the esthetic and functional harmony of the native dentition.

Background

Obtaining proper occlusal clearance to allow for a single unit crown restoration is a fundamental prerequisite for dental implant restoration. Long-standing edentulous sites are often fraught with disuse atrophy and unopposed supra-eruption of the opposing dentition. In the posterior maxillae/mandible, there are vital structures that have to be mobilized in order to allow space for either bone transposition or onlay/inlay grafting. There are several predictable techniques described to address these preprosthetic alveolar deficiency dilemmas [1–3].

The osteoperiosteal flap technique has made a strong contribution towards management of these defects. Mobilizing a segment of alveolus attached to the overlying soft tissue can obtain uni- or bi-directional augmentation. This case report describes an amplification of a vertical osteoperiosteal flap with concomitant placement of dental implants in a partially edentulous dental arch.

* Correspondence: Thomas.L.Wright2.mil@mail.mil
[1]Department of Oral & Maxillofacial Surgery, San Antonio Military Medical Center, 3551 Roger Brooke Dr., Ft. Sam Houston 78234, TX, USA
[2]Department of Oral & Maxilofacial Surgery, Wilford Hall Ambulatory Surgical Center, 2200 Bergquist Dr, Suite 1, Lackland AFB, TX 78236, USA

Case Presentation

A 35-year-old female with a 10-year history of partial acquired edentulism at site numbers 3 and 4 presented to our clinic for dental implant evaluation. Preoperative clinical examination revealed a reproducible intercuspation, well-delineated band of keratinized tissue, and decreased inter-occlusal clearance to allow for optimal dimension of prosthetic crowns (Fig. 1). Radiographs demonstrated excessive pneumatization of the antrum in the respective area. The preoperative planning included fabrication of two surgical splints. The first splint was fabricated for transmucosal positioning of the implant osteotomy sites in the existing alveolus position. The second splint was fabricated from the predetermined augmented vertical position of the dentoalveolar segment with ideal inter-occlusal clearance. Our surgical treatment began with a horizontal incision 3 mm apical to the mucogingival junction, a full thickness mucoperiosteal flap was created exposing the anterior and posterior boundaries of the proposed segmental osteotomy (Fig. 2). Similar to alveolar distraction techniques, minimal mucosa was elevated off of the transport or movable segment to maintain adequate blood supply. A

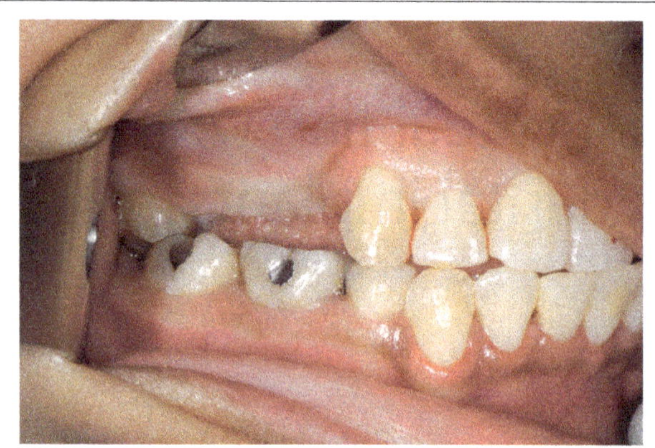

Fig. 1 Edentulous site with supra-eruption of opposing dentition

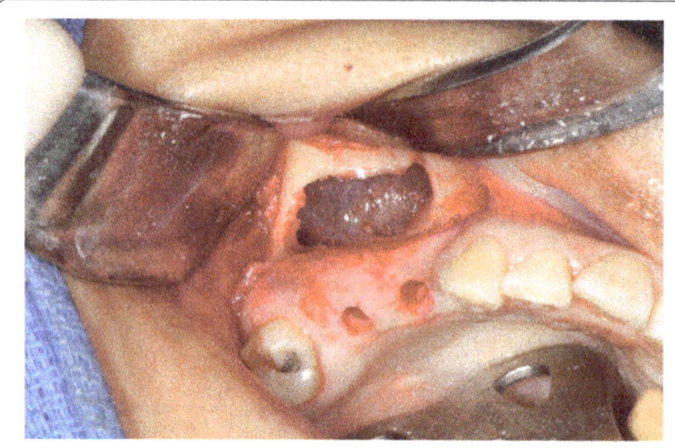

Fig. 3 Direct sinus lift with implant osteotomy preparation

lateral sinus window technique was used to access the antrum, and the associated Schneiderian membrane was elevated and completely cleared from all boundaries of the respective dentoalveolar segment (Fig. 3). A right angle piezosurgery blade (Piezosurgery Inc., Piezosurgery3 Unit, OT1 insert, OT2 insert) was used to initially create the horizontal/apical osteotomy, which was followed by crestally diverging full thickness vertical osteotomies at the mesial/anterior and distal/posterior areas of the edentulous dentoalveolar segment at site numbers 3 and 4. Before mobilization of the osteoperiosteal flap, the predetermined implant osteotomies were made using the initial surgical splint, and the respective implants (Nobel Biocare, NobelReplace Tapered Groovy) were placed into the predetermined location. Mobilization of the osteoperiosteal flap with a T-handle osteotome confirmed successful separation from the maxillae proper. With the sinus membrane lifted and protected, the vertical repositioning of the osteoperiosteal flap with the positioned implants was accomplished using the second prefabricated splint. In an effort to control torque movement of the mobile segment, we placed the implant placement driver and with the shaft coming through the pilot drill holes of the second guide. The mobile segment was then secured to the anteriorly and posteriorly intact lateral wall of the antrum using an eight-hole 0.6 mm profile curvilinear plate (KLS Martin 1.5 mm, 0.6 mm profile) (Fig. 4). The region under the lifted sinus membrane was then packed with mineralized allograft (Medtronic Sofamor Danek, 0.6–1.25 mm cortical and cancellous chips) in a routine manner. A resorbable membrane (Geistlich Bio-Gide) was then placed over the grafted sinus and fixation mini-plate. The platform of the respective transmucosal placed implants were tactically interrogated to confirm approximation with the alveolar crest. The cover screws were then placed (Fig. 5), and the patient underwent a 4-month healing period. Normal progression to healing abutments and final prosthesis was accomplished (Fig. 6). Pt was followed up 2 years after loading of the implant without any untoward sequelae and radiographic evidence of osseointegrated dental implants (Fig. 7).

Discussion

A suitable alternative surgical management of this particular case might have been to simply perform an alveoloplasty to produce the desired inter-occlusal clearance and proceed with placement of implant and simultaneous

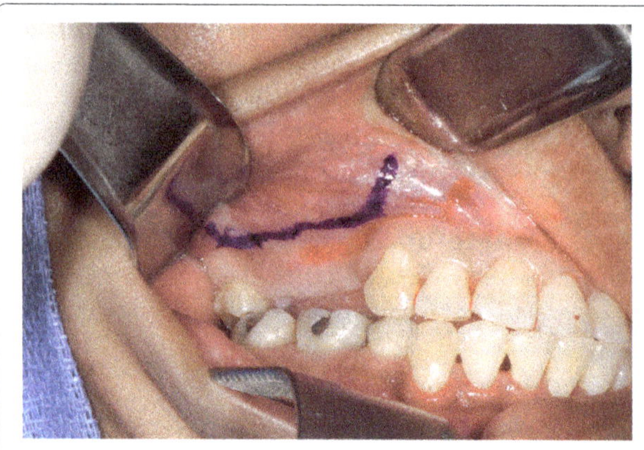

Fig. 2 Marked incision site for surgical access

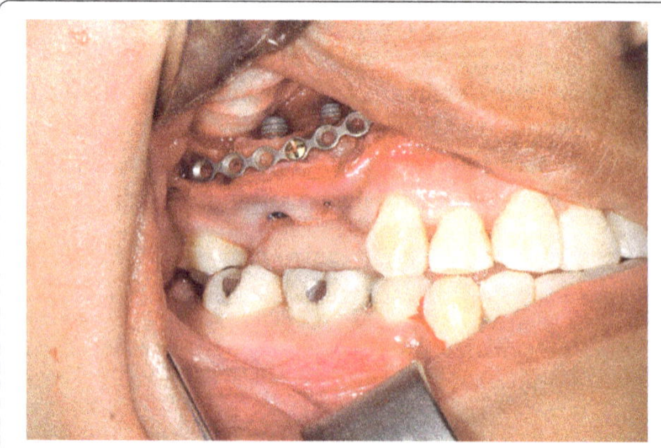

Fig. 4 Vertical repositioning of dental alveolus segment with placement of dental implants

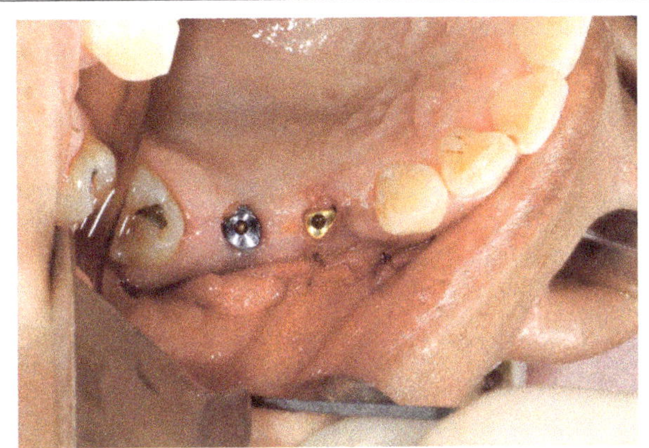

Fig. 5 Occlusal view of implants after vertical repositioning of the dental alveolus segment showing proper mesiodistal space and buccolingual spacing

direct sinus lift. That would have left more of the apical portion of the implant within the grafted sinus and possibly modified the location of keratinized band of tissue. The location of the dental alveolar segment in relation to any antral septae also needs to be appreciated, as this described technique can be fraught with complication if such anatomical obstacles are not accounted for preoperatively [4].

The osteoperiosteal flap or "bone flap" commonly used in segmental orthognathic surgery is a bone fragment moved in space without detachment of the investing periosteum [5]. The prerequisite for simultaneous implant placement in a vertical repositioning bone flap is adequate width within the transport segment. It is always a fine balance between allowing enough exposure to place the fixation device without significantly compromising periosteal vascular input into the bone segment. As it is well documented both clinically and experientially, full thickness mucoperiosteal releases will cause some degree of bone resorption at the labial plate [6].

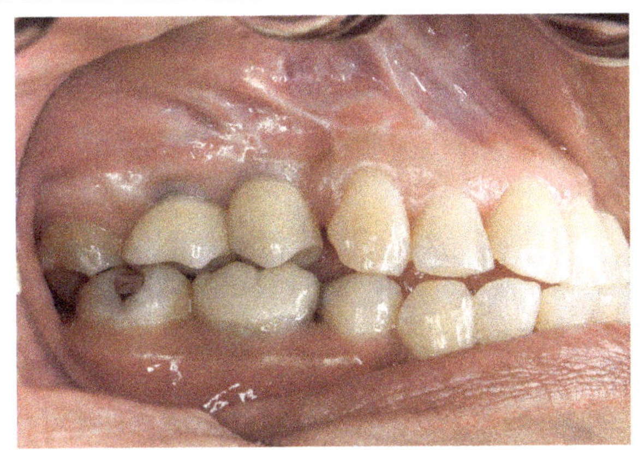

Fig. 6 Clinical picture 2 years after implant placement

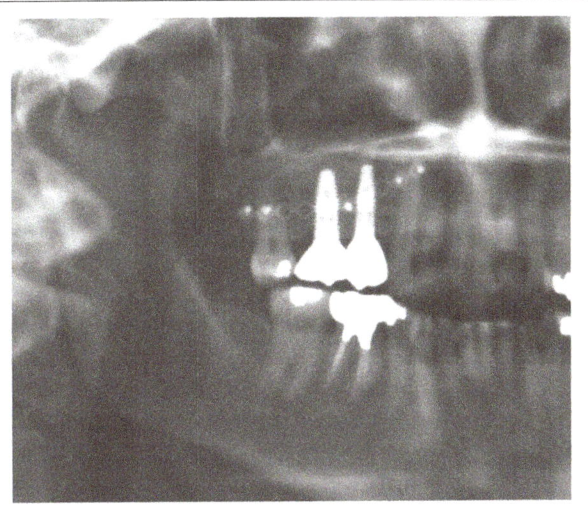

Fig. 7 Orthopantomograph 2 years after implant placement

Due to the presence of fixation plate and a sizeable sinus window, we decided to use a long-lasting resorbable membrane. In our experience and supported by the literature, placement of a membrane over the osteotomy site has been shown to increase the amount of bone formation [7]. Considering we were only able to obtain one monocortical screw fixation on the mobilized portion of the maxillae, maintaining immobility during the critical phase of bone healing was an obvious liability. Animal studies which have investigated the biology of small segment wound healing have noted that after 2 weeks, revascularization of the small dento-osseous segment was noted [8]. The cross application of such animal studies are helpful but do not completely capture the additional challenges in this case report. The studies in animals were looking at segmental dental alveolar segments which encompassed the natural teeth. In our case illustration, there were osteotomies made within the transport segment and healing of the overlying particulate allograft was contingent on biological stability of the respective segment. This is a clear illustration of how animal models can begin to provide a platform towards technical innovation, but there is always a parameter of uncharted terrain in translating to human clinical application.

A critical appraisal of the gingival architecture in the final end point of this case demonstrates some radiolucency through the soft tissue outlining the platform of the Nobel Biocare TiUnite implant. This would lead us to believe that either the transmucosal bone level placement attempt was inaccurate or excessive reflection of the labial tissue has caused some degree of resorption. This is another liability that needs to be carefully addressed if this application is recaptured within the esthetic zone. Perhaps slight subcrestal placement of the dental implant or platform switched body feature would minimize this outcome. In our application, we utilized an implant platform topography that is purported by the manufacture to allow soft tissue adhesion and minimize crestal bone loss.

Conclusions

This case highlights the evolving variations in dentoalveolar augmentation with an emphasis on concomitant implant placement. In the most traditional sense, a vertical osteoperiosteal flap technique would be bound with a stable basal bone that can be used to anchor simultaneous dental implant placement. Further refinement should consider minimizing crestal reflection and overall labial bone resorption.

Authors' contributions

TT was the staff surgeon for the case being presented and gave the final approval for submission. TW was the resident surgeon for the case being presented and was involved in drafting the manuscript and finalizing it for submission. Both authors read and approved the final manuscript.

Competing interests

Tibebu Tsegga and Thomas Wright declare that they have no competing interests.

References

1. Irinakis T. Efficacy of injectable demineralized bone matrix as graft material during sinus elevation surgery with simultaneous implant placement in the posterior maxilla: clinical evaluation of 49 sinuses. J Oral and Maxillofac Surg. 2011;69:134–41.
2. Chiapasoo M, Casentini P, Zaniboni M. Bone augmentation procedures in implant dentistry. Int J Oral Maxillofac Implants. 2009;24:237–69.
3. Jenson OT. The osteoperiosteal flap: a simplified approach to alveolar bone reconstruction. Quintessence Pub; 2010.
4. Stern A, Green J. Sinus lift procedures: an overview of current techniques. Dent Clin N Am. 2012;56:219–33.
5. Jenson OT. Dentoalveolar modification by osteoperiosteal flaps. In: Fonseca RJ, editor. Oral and maxillofacial surgery. 2nd ed. St. Louis, MO: Saunders; 2000. p. 471–8.
6. Jensen OT, Cullum DR, Baer D. Marginal bone stability using three different flap approaches for alveolar expansion for dental implants—a one year clinical study. J Oral Maxillofac Surg. 2009;67:19–21.
7. Herford AS, Nguyen K. Complex bone augmentation in alveolar ridge defects. Oral Maxillofacial Surg Clin N Am. 2015;27:227–44.
8. Jenson OT, Bell W, Cottam J. Osteoperiosteal flaps and local osteotomies for alveolar reconstruction. Oral Maxillofacil Surg Clin N Am. 2010;22:331–46.

16

Ridge preservation using an in situ hardening biphasic calcium phosphate (β-TCP/HA) bone graft substitute - a clinical, radiological, and histological study

Ashish Kakar[1*], Bappanadu H. Sripathi Rao[1], Shashikanth Hegde[1], Nikhil Deshpande[2], Annette Lindner[3], Heiner Nagursky[3], Aditya Patney[4] and Harsh Mahajan[4]

Abstract

Background: Post-Extraction ridge preservation using bone graft substitutes is a conservative technique to maintain the width of the alveolar ridge. The objective of the present study was to evaluate an in situ hardening biphasic (HA/β-TCP) bone graft substitutes for ridge preservation without primary wound closure or a dental membrane.

Methods: A total of 15 patients reported for tooth extraction were enrolled in this study. Implants were placed in average 5.2 ± 2 months after socket grafting. At this visit, Cone Beam CT (CBCT) images and core biopsies were taken. Implant stability (ISQ) was assessed at the insertion as well as at the day of final restoration.

Results: CBCT data revealed 0.79 ± 0.73 mm ridge width reduction from grafting to implant placement. Histomorphometric analysis of core biopsy samples revealed in average 21.34 ± 9.14% of new bone in the grafted sites. Primary implant stability was high (ISQ levels 70.3 ± 9.6) and further increased until final restoration.

Conclusions: The results of this study show that grafting of intact post-extraction sockets using a biphasic in situ hardening bone graft substitute results in an effective preservation of the ridge contour and sufficient new bone formation in the grafted sites, which is imperative for successful implant placement.

Background

Following tooth extraction, the alveolar ridge will decrease in volume and change its morphology [1, 2]. These changes are clinically significant [3] and can complicate the placement of a conventional bridge or an implant-supported crown. Post-extraction maintenance of the alveolar ridge following the principles of ridge preservation using bone graft substitutes minimizes ridge resorption and, thus, facilitate subsequent placement of an implant that satisfies esthetic and functional criteria, limiting the need of additional bone augmentation procedures [4–8].

Bone graft substitutes have been in use for several decades to replace autogenous bone grafts. The first experimental use of calcium phosphates as bone graft substitutes was reported in the 1920s [9]. These materials were recognized early on as promising candidates due to their chemical similarity to native bone, which is mainly composed of calcium phosphate hydroxyapatite (70% of dry weight). Synthetic calcium phosphate ceramics belong to the group of alloplastic biomaterials and are nowadays widely used. Synthetic materials are osteoconductive and free of any risk of transmitting infections or diseases in contrast to animal-derived xenografts or materials from human cadaver (allografts). Synthetic calcium phosphates comprise of resorbable ß-tricalcium phosphates, nonresorbable hydroxyapatites, and combinations of these two materials that are named biphasic calcium phosphate materials (BCP). ß-TCP materials resorb completely and are replaced by the body's own tissue whereas hydroxyapatite-containing materials do not resorb but are integrated in the host's bone [10–13].

Both ß-TCP and BCP materials have been successfully used in clinical practice, and their efficacy and safety have been demonstrated in a multitude of clinical

* Correspondence: kakar_ashish@yahoo.com
[1]Yenepoya University Dental College, University Road, Mangalore 575018, India
Full list of author information is available at the end of the article

studies [14–17]. However, it is still a matter of discussion whether resorbable ß-TCP materials can provide sufficient support to adequately maintain the ridge in contrast to nonresorbable hydroxyapatite-containing BCP materials.

The aim of this clinical, radiological, and histological study was to evaluate the potential of the use of poly(lactide-co-glycolide) acid (PLGA)-coated alloplastic BCP particles to preserve the ridge profile while supporting the formation of new bone in intact socket defect after tooth extraction. The PLGA coating of the BCP granules provide additional initial in situ hardening properties and, therefore, allow stabilization of the bone graft substitute in the empty extraction socket without the use of a barrier membrane to stabilize the graft and to cover the defect without achieving primary wound closure [18].

To our knowledge, this is the first systematic clinical, radiographic, and histological evaluation that assesses bone formation and ridge width preservation after socket grafting using an in situ hardening biphasic bone graft substitute in healthy patients.

Methods

This study was approved by the Yenepoya University Ethics committee, Mangalore, India (Approval Number YOEC83/8/3/2014). Fifteen patients who required extraction of a maxillary or mandibular tooth and subsequent single-tooth implant placement and who met the inclusion and exclusion criteria were included in this prospective single-arm clinical study. The patients (4 females and 11 males) had a mean age of 51.3± 14.8 years (range: 27 to 75 years). The site-specific areas and teeth numbers for the study are shown in Table 1.

All patients were systemically healthy at the time of consultation and study inclusion. The reasons for extraction included endodontic treatment failures and advanced caries lesions and tooth fractures. If more than one tooth was extracted (maximum of three teeth), all teeth were treated but only the most anterior tooth with intact socket wall was selected for the study. Standard exclusion criteria for bone grafting procedures were applied including allergy, systemic chronic disease, alcoholism and drug abuse, pregnancy, or nursing mothers. Smokers and patients with any oral tobacco use/habits were excluded. Patients using dentures were also excluded. Patients with acute abscesses or active infections localized in the proximity of the prospective surgical field and those with heavily scarred mucosa at the site and patients who had malignant diseases or other diseases treated with radiotherapy or chemotherapeutic agents (chemotherapy) during the past 5 years were excluded.

Surgical technique

All surgical procedures were performed by one surgeon in this study. The following procedures were planned for all sites. Tooth extraction was performed under local anesthesia without flap elevation (Fig. 1a, b). Periotomes and luxators (Directa, Sweden) were gently used for all extraction procedures. Extraction forceps were only used when the tooth was mobile in the extraction socket. All multi-rooted teeth were sectioned with a Lindemann burr (Komet Inc., Lemgo, Germany) under copious irrigation with sterile saline to minimize extraction trauma. Each root of the multi-rooted teeth was independently mobilized and carefully luxated. Attention was given not to damage the surrounding soft and hard tissues, especially in the buccal aspect. All sockets were thoroughly curetted to remove granulation tissue, followed by irrigation and rinsing with sterile saline. A ball-ended probe was then utilized to explore the buccal plate. All teeth included for this study had an intact buccal and lingual plate (four-wall post-extraction sockets). A biphasic alloplastic in situ hardening bone graft substitute (GUIDOR easy-graft CRYSTAL, Sunstar Suisse SA, Etoy, Switzerland) was used to graft the site according to the manufacturer's instructions. Attention was given not to overfill the extraction socket to avoid any displacement of the entire graft mass after mechanical irritation during the first phases of healing. A saline-wet gauze was used to further compact the granules and accelerate the hardening of the graft in situ so that after a few minutes the alloplastic bone substitute formed a stable, solid, porous scaffold for the host osseous regeneration (Fig. 1c). An interrupted tension-free nonresorbable 4-0 sutures (Black Silk, Ethicon, Johnson & Johnson, Somerville, NJ, USA) was placed over the filled socket to achieve soft tissue stability (Fig. 1d). All sites were left uncovered without obtaining primary closure in order to heal by secondary intention. The patients did not wear any prosthesis during the healing period.

Antibiotic therapy consisting of 1 g amoxicillin every 12 h for 4 days and mouth rinsing with 0.2% chlorhexidine every 8 h for 10 days were prescribed. The suture was removed 1 week postoperatively. After 3 to 8 months (average 5.2 ± 2 months), the sites (Fig. 2a) were reentered for implant placement. A site-specific full thickness mucoperiosteal flap was elevated to expose the regenerated hard tissue. A bone core biopsy was taken with a minimum depth of 7 mm from the center of the site using a trephine drill with a diameter of 2.3 mm (Komet Inc., Lemgo, Germany) (Fig. 2b). Following the harvesting of the bone sample, the preparation of the bony bed was completed at the same site and a dental implant was placed (Fig. 2b, c) according to the manufacturer's surgical protocol. Immediately after placement, the initial stability was measured by resonance frequency analysis (Osstell ISQ, Gothenburg, Sweden). For each implant, two ISQ measurements were recorded, palatally (or lingually) and bucally, according to the guidelines of the company. The measurement was repeated after

Table 1 Buccal and palatal ISQ values at implant placement and time of loading

		ISQ level at implant placement			ISQ level at loading		
Patient no.	Tooth no.	Buccal	Palatal	Average	Buccal	Palatal	Average
1	17	67	71	69	70	70	70
2	17	73	72	72.5	76	76	76
3	36	76	78	77	84	80	82
4	26	48	48	48	61	66	63.5
5	25	49	49	49	71	66	68.5
6	37	71	78	74.5	69	78	73.5
7	45	76	74	75	72	74	73
8	36	80	82	81	85	85	85
9	37	74	74	74	72	72	72
10	46	76	72	74	74	74	74
11	27	71	71	71	74	72	73
12	47	72	72	72	74	71	72.5
13	36	71	71	71	76	72	74
14	36	80	82	81	82	82	82
15	17	70	62	66	66	66	66
Mean		70.3	70.4	70.3	73.7	73.6	73.7
Standard deviation		9.5	10.2	9.7	6.5	5.8	5.9

placement of the final restoration 4 months after implant placement. Average of the ISQ measurements was then reported. The mucoperiosteal flap was closed with interrupted nonresorbable 4-0 sutures (Silk, Ethicon, Johnson & Johnson, Somerville, NJ, USA), and Fig. 3 shows the postoperative radiograph of the implants placed in the preserved ridge. Figure 4a shows the second surgery followed by impression making, and Fig. 4b shows implant crowns placed and loaded after 3 months of placement.

Assessment of ridge width changes by cone beam computer tomography

The area of interest (site of socket preservation and grafting) was identified in accordance with the site which was

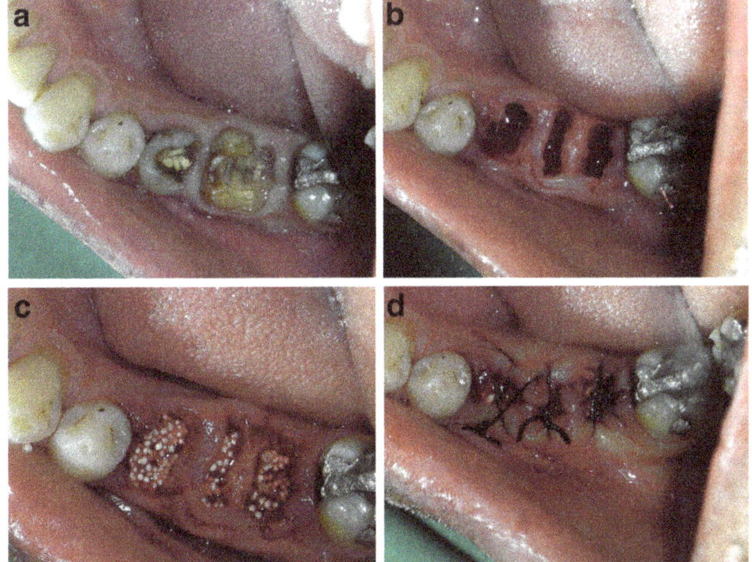

Fig. 1 **a** Clinical occlusal view with fractured 45 and 46. **b** Post-extraction view of the socket. Note minimal trauma to the soft tissue and no flap reflection on the surgical site. **c** Graft material condensed into the extraction sockets showing good initial graft stability. **d** Black silk sutures placed with tissue approximation and no releasing incision in the flaps

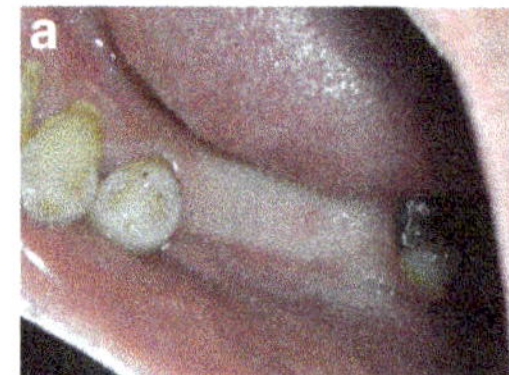

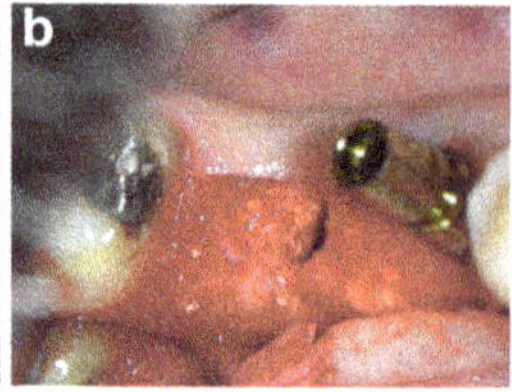

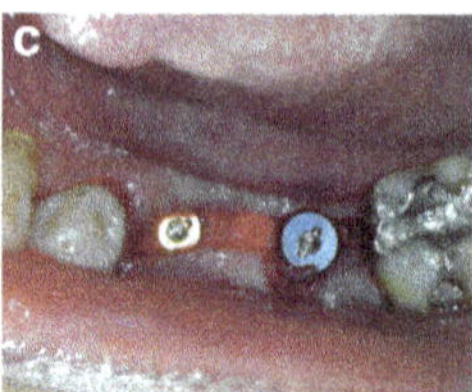

Fig. 2 **a** Clinical postoperative view after 4 months. Note that the healing was achieved only with tissue approximation. A good width of keratinized tissue is visible along with ridge preservation. Ready for implant placement in the grafted areas. **b** Implant placed in 45 area. Core biopsy sample taken from area 46. Note the integration of graft particles in the preserved alveolar ridge also inside the osteotomy site of 46. **c** Two Xive (Dentsply) implants placed in the preserved ridge. **d.** Postoperative X ray showing the implant positions in the mandible where the teeth were extracted and ridge preservation was accomplished

grafted (Fig. 5a–d). Axial correction of the view was performed in conformity with angulation of the alveolar ridge. Contours of the crestal bone were identified, considering apical recession of the alveolar crestal level, if any on buccal or lingual/palatal aspect. Buccolingual/palatal width of the alveolus was then determined 2 mm below the alveolar crestal level before tooth extraction and at the time of implant placement. Ridge width changes were calculated by subtracting preoperative measurements from postoperative ridge width measurements (Fig. 6a–c).

Histological and histomorphometric evaluation

Bone biopsies were harvested using a trephine bur at the site of implant placement. The trephine burs including the bone biopsies were fixed in 4% formalin for 5–7 days, rinsed in water, and dehydrated in serial steps of ethanol (70, 80, 90, and 100%), remaining for 1 day in each concentration. Specimens were then infiltrated, embedded, and polymerized in resin (Technovit 9100, Heraeus Kulzer, Wehrheim, Germany) according to the manufacturer's instructions. After polymerization, samples were cut in 500-μm sections using a precision cutting machine Secotom 50 (Struers, Ballerup, Denmark). The sections were mounted on acrylic slides (Maertin, Freiburg, Germany) and ground to a final thickness of approximately 60 μm on a rotating grinding plate (Struers, Ballerup, Denmark). Specimens were subsequently stained with Azur II and Pararosanilin (Merck, Darmstadt, Germany), which allowed for a differentiation between graft granules, and preexisting and newly formed bone. Imaging was performed with an Axio ImagerM1 microscope equipped with a digital AxioCamHRc (Carl Zeiss,Göttingen, Germany). Histomorphometric analysis was performed by one observer digitally using the analySIS FIVE software (Soft Imaging System, Munster, Germany). The reference area for the histomorphometric evaluation was the entire area in the biopsy excluding old bone from the defect margins. Values measured in percent of the examined area were taken for remnants of graft material, newly formed bone, and soft tissue/ bone marrow (Fig. 7a–c).

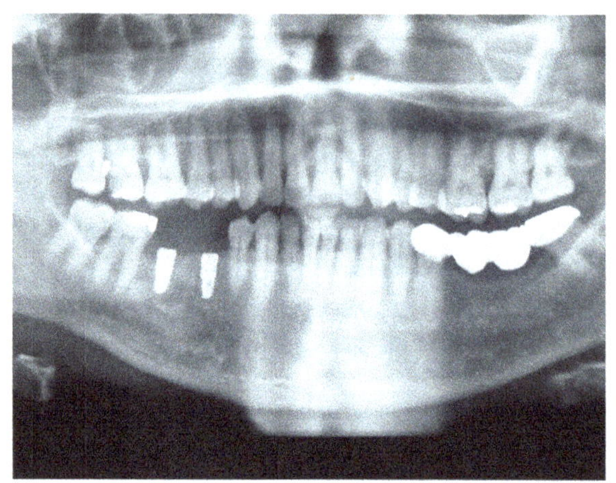

Fig. 3 Postoperative X ray showing the implant positions in the mandible where the teeth were extracted and ridge preservation was accomplished

Statistics

Data were expressed as means ± standard deviations (SD). A two-sided paired t test was used to assess significance of intra-group longitudinal changes for ridge width changes and changes of ISQ. Statistical significance was set to $p < 0.05$ for a two-sided test.

Results

Fifteen patients (4 females and 11 males) with a mean age of 51.3 ± 14.8 years (range: 27 to 75 years) participated in this randomized clinical trial. The site specific areas and teeth numbers for the study are shown in Table 1.

In all cases, the postoperative healing was uneventful. Clinically, the soft tissue healing pattern observed was very similar in all cases. The soft tissue on all sites was completely closed and healed at the 4-month recall period (Fig. 2a). There was no loss or sequestration of bone graft granules observed during the healing period although the sites were left uncovered to heal for secondary intention. Due to the specific in situ hardening biomechanical properties of the grafting material, the stable granules provided a solid immobile scaffold over

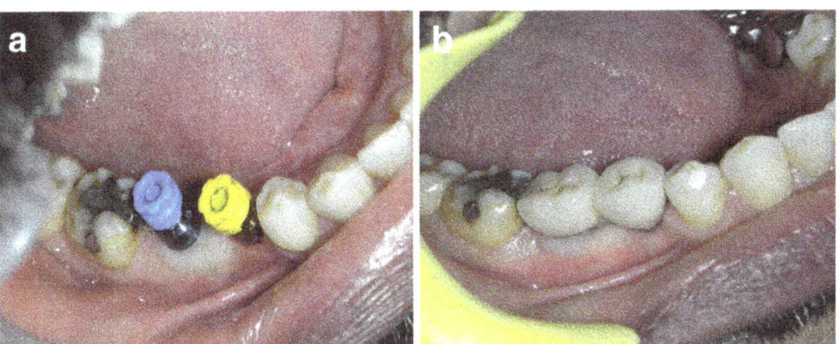

Fig. 4 **a** Second stage surgery followed by impression making. Note the excellent width of keratinized tissue which was also preserved. **b** Implant crowns placed and loaded after 3 months of placement

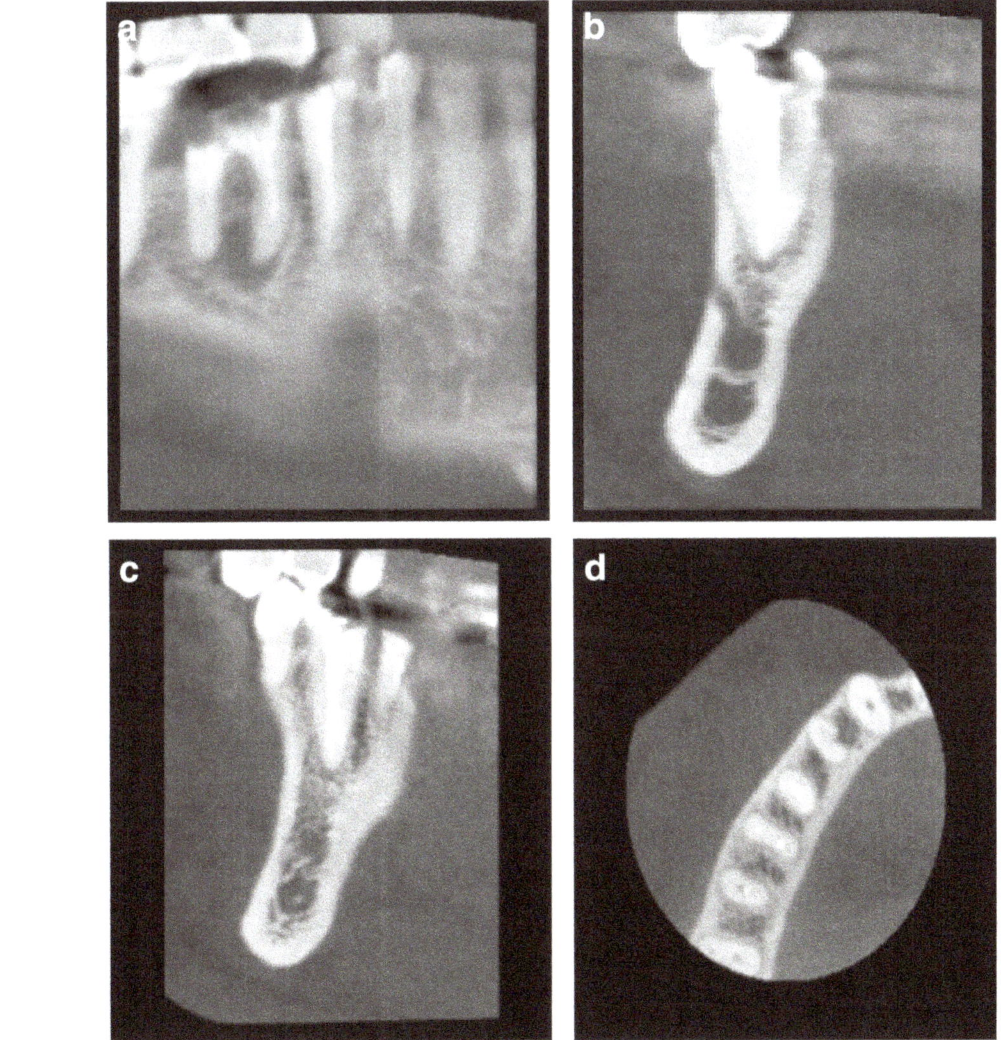

Fig. 5 CBCT images of the extraction site. **a** Preoperative CBCT showing fractured and un-restorable teeth #45 and #46 planned to be extracted. **b**–**d** Cross sectional views

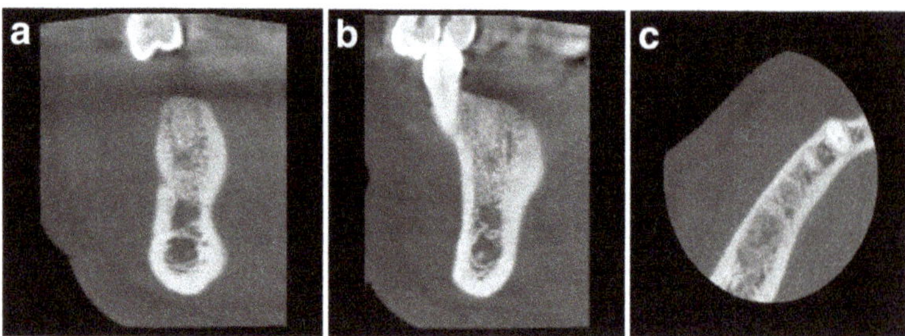

Fig. 6 a–c Four-month postoperative CBCT showing graft integration and preservation of ridge without collapse of the buccal or lingual cortical plates also showing the cross sections in the grafted area

which newly formed soft tissue migrated from the margins of the sockets, achieving secondary intention soft tissue healing. In the first stage, graft particles were embedded in fibrin matrix that was slowly replaced by a layer of connective tissue that slowly covered the occlusal aspect of the exposed graft starting from the wound edges. Subsequently, epithelial tissue proliferated from the periphery over the connective tissue layer and after 4 months all areas were completely covered with newly formed keratinized epithelium. At this time point, clinical examination showed that the volume and architecture of the ridges were adequately preserved. Reentry for implant placement was between 3.3 and 8.4 months and on average 5.2 ± 2 months after socket grafting. At this time point, the grafted areas were filled with newly formed bone with particles of the bone graft substitute (BGS) visible in the regenerated hard tissue. All implants were placed at the precise 3D position showing excellent initial stability, and the potential implant sites had a good resistance to drilling clinically. At implant placement, the mean

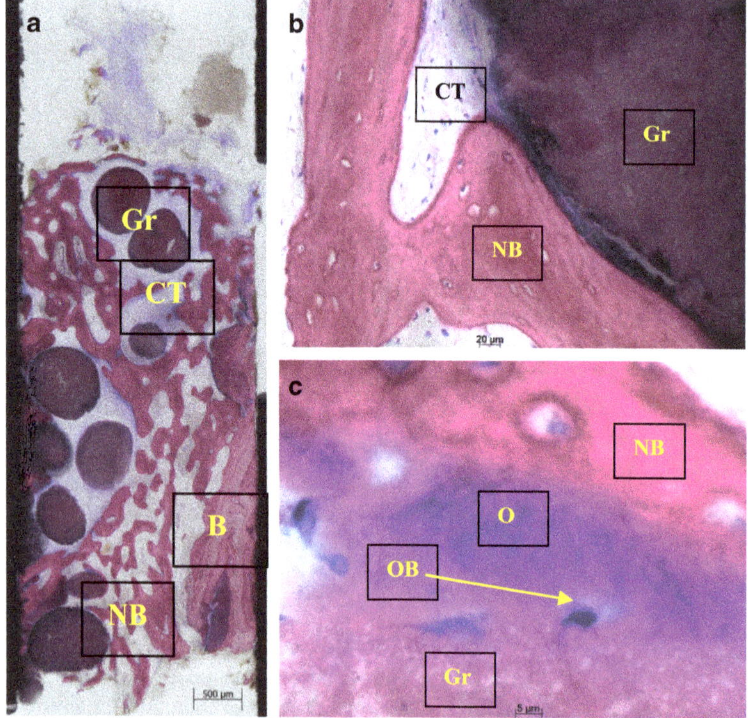

Fig. 7 a–c Histological sections of bone core biopsy taken from the site of implantation using a trephine bur. **a** Overview image of coronal-apical cut through the entire core biopsy showing formation of new bone (*NB*) next to old bone of the extraction socket (*B*). easy-graft CRYSTAL particles (*Gr*) are embedded in well perfused connective tissue (*CT*) and new bone (*NB*) (Azur II and Pararosanilin, original magnification ×50). **b** Integration of easy-graft CRYSTAL particle (*Gr*) into newly formed bone (*NB*) and connective tissue (*CT*) showing tight contact between graft particle and new bone. **c** High magnification (×200) images of the interface between graft particle (*Gr*) and new bone (*NB*) showing osteoblasts (*OB*) forming osteoid (O) and formation of new bone (*NB*) on the surface of easy-graft CRYSTAL particles (*Gr*) (Azur II and Pararosanilin, original magnification ×200)

final ISQ measurements were 70.3 ± 9.6 (Table 1) showing excellent initial stability for the majority of the cases.

Cone beam computer tomography (CBCT) was performed before tooth extraction and at the time point of implant placement. Mean ridge width reduction before tooth extraction to implant placement was calculated to effect in 0.79 ± 0.73 mm horizontal bone loss (Table 2). Primary implant stability was achieved in all 15 cases, showed in average high ISQ levels 70.3 ± 9.7 (buccal/palatal), and further increased until final restoration to an average level of 73.7 ± 6.0 (Table 3) showing commenced osseointegration of the dental implant in the grafted sites.

Histologically, all analyzed biopsies contained newly formed bone, residual graft material, and well vascularized uninflamed connective tissue (Fig. 7a–c). No necrosis or foreign body reactions were detected. The graft granules were in contact with active osteoblasts forming osteoid and new woven bone, demonstrating persistent osteogenesis. Active cellular resorption of the BCP particles was not observed. In many areas, active bone remodeling was evident with mature lamellar bone replacing the woven bone. Histomorphometric analysis revealed that the grafted site was occupied with an average of 21.34% ± 9.14% new bone, 26.19 ± 9.38% residual graft material, and 53% ± 7.51% connective tissue (Table 3). In all cases, 3–4 months after implant placement, a vertical crestal incision was made and a healing abutment was placed. After allowing 2 weeks for the maturation of the soft tissues, the final restoration was fabricated with successful functional and esthetic results.

Discussion

Ridge preservation following dental extractions is fundamental, preserving the ridge profile for subsequent implant placement and providing a sustained function and esthetics. This clinical trial reports on the successful application of an in situ hardening biphasic alloplastic bone graft substitute for ridge preservation and subsequent implant placement in 15 healthy patients. A routine but minimally invasive surgical protocol was followed in all cases. Extractions and grafting were performed without raising a flap. After grafting, the augmented sites were not covered with a barrier membrane or an advanced buccal flap for primary closure. Elevating the periosteum from the buccal bone to create a mucoperiosteal flap can compromise the blood supply of the exposed bone surface, leading to osteoclastic activity and increased bone resorption [19]. Moreover, this approach was selected in order to minimize patient morbidity, surgical time, and cost, but mostly in an attempt not to displace the mucogingival junction and to allow for the spontaneous formation of new keratinized soft tissue over the grafted site. According to the clinical findings of this report, it seems that secondary intention soft tissue healing of grafted post-extraction sites can be achieved when filling the sockets with in situ hardening bone graft substitutes without the use of barrier membranes. The findings and parameters for soft tissue healing are in alignment with observations previously reported on in situ hardening β-TCP materials [18] as well as in situ hardening biophasic calcium phosphate (BCP) materials [20]. Both authors have reported

Table 2 Width ridge changes assess by cone beam computer tomography (CBCT)

Patient no.	Tooth no.	Ridge width baseline [mm]	Ridge width implant placement [mm]	Ridge width changes [mm]
1	17	8.2	7.4	0.8
2	17	12.6	12.3	0.3
3	36	12	11.6	0.4
4	26	8.4	8.2	0.2
5	25	7.5	7.2	0.3
6	37	9.4	6.2	3.2
7	45	8.4	7.9	0.5
8	36	13.3	12.8	0.5
9	37	14.2	13.6	0.6
10	46	16.2	14.8	1.4
11	27	14.2	13.6	0.6
12	47	12.6	11.8	0.8
13	36	13.6	12.7	0.9
14	36	17.4	16.9	0.5
15	17	9.6	8.7	0.9
Mean		11.84	11.05	0.79
Standard deviation		3.10	3.22	0.73

Table 3 Histomorphometric evaluation of core biopsy sections

Patient no.	Gender	Patient's age	Tooth no.	Time post extraction [month]	% New bone	% Residual graft	% Connective tissue
1	M	48	17	8.4	17.9	31.3	50.8
2	F	68	17	8.4	23.5	17	59.4
3	M	54	36	3.9	17	25.8	57.2
4	M	39	26	4.5	22.7	26.3	51
5	F	40	25	4.5	14.3	30.7	55
6	M	50	37	4.5	21.1	26.6	52.2
7	F	32	45	4.0	39.4	16	44.6
8	M	55	36	3.8	9.6	20.2	70.2
9	M	44	37	3.3	12.8	22.9	64.3
10	F	27	46	5.1	22.5	25.7	51.8
11	M	76	27	5.7	9.6	41.6	48.8
12	M	74	47	4.6	34.3	23.8	41.9
13	M	75	36	8.0	25.6	28.6	45.8
14	M	74	36	4.4	35	9.6	47.6
15	M	47	17	5.0	14.8	46.8	54.4
Mean				5.2	21.3	26.2	53.0
Standard deviation				2.0	9.2	9.4	7.5

excellent and uneventful soft tissue healing without achieving primary closure or covering the site with a barrier membrane or soft tissue punch. The coating of calcium phosphate granules with PLGA results in a stable, solid alloplastic bone substitute, deterring the loss of exposed granules. In contrast, a flap and/or a barrier membrane may be necessary to provide the necessary stability and protection for loose particulate bone grafts without self-hardening characteristics. Furthermore, the approach using reflection of a mucosal flap brings significant disadvantages as elevation of the periosteum from the bone will compromise the vascular supply to the bone surface leading to osteoclastic activity and increased bone resorption [21, 22]. After analyzing the existing evidence, the authors concluded that achieving primary closure did not present beneficial effects on preserving the ridge width. On the other hand, patients experience more discomfort and the mucogingival junction was significantly more coronally displaced when primary flap closure was achieved compared to secondary intention healing [23–25].

As previously reported, secondary intention soft tissue healing of grafted post-extraction sites can be well achieved when using an in situ hardening and in situ stabilizing bone graft substitutes without the need of a dental membrane [18, 20]. Findings of the present report corroborate these results. The authors found that all sites healed uneventfully with coverage of soft tissue and no local complications. In the present study, all sites were fully covered with newly formed keratinized soft tissue while the buccal keratinized soft tissues were preserved. As the presence of an adequate zone of keratinized gingiva is an important parameter in achieving esthetic implant restorations [26], preventing future mucosal recessions, and improving the overall long-term implant stability, the use of flapless techniques by taking advantage of the biomechanical properties of in situ hardening alloplastic grafts seems to be a benefit for the clinicians and patients when applicable.

Following tooth extraction, the width of the alveolar ridge seems to undergo pronounced shrinkage which can render subsequent implant placement challenging [5]. In all patients, the dimensions of the ridge were adequately preserved at the time of implant placement (5.1 ± 2 months) and bone resorption was marginal. Mean ridge width reduction assessed by CBCT was 0.79 ± 0.73 mm (Table 2), which is well below the results reported for ridge preservation techniques using both bone substitute material in combination with membranes or soft tissue grafts [26, 27]. A recent meta-analysis [27] further suggested that the choice of the biomaterial did not have a significant influence on the ridge preservation after tooth extraction and that all materials sufficiently maintained the ridge dimensions.

At reentry, all sites were filled with sufficient bone, allowing for the precise placement of an implant at the optimal position. The histomorphometric analysis of the harvested samples revealed pronounced new bone formation. In order to investigate the remineralization of the grafted sites, it is of outmost importance to discriminate between the old and new bone and only assess the new bone that is found within the graft site of the biopsy. Displaying only the total amount of mineralized bone found in the biopsy, including old bone from the defect margins, will falsify the true de novo bone formation and defect fill. In this study, 21.34 ± 9.14% of the grafted area was occupied by newly formed vital bone (Table 1). Similar levels of new bone formation have been reported in rabbit calvaria defects model published by Schmidlin et al. [28] using the same material and revealing 20.16 ± 5.27% of new bone in the defect site after 4 weeks of healing. Moreover, the amount of new bone formation in the grafted site is comparable to that reported for other BCP materials and xenografts used in sinus augmentation [14, 29]. In this histomorphometric study including core biopsies from 38 sinus augmentations, a mean percentage of new bone of 21.6 ± 10.0% was reported for particulate BCP and 19.8 ± 7.9% for particulate xenograft bone substitutes.

Likewise, the reported amount of residual grafting material in the defect site was similar. In average, only 26.2 ± 9.4% of the defect was occupied with residual graft material in this study which is well in line with 26.6 ± 5.2% reported for BCP but below the 37.7 ± 8.5% reported for xenograft [14].

All 15 implants could be placed without the need for additional bone augmentation. ISQ values measured after implant placement revealed adequate primary stability of the implants. It is important to note that primary stability is not only affected by the geometry of the implant placed (i.e., length, diameter, and type) and the placement technique used (relation between drill size and implant size, tapping) but also positively related to the quality, density, and quantity of the local bone [29–31]. Considering that in the present study the same implant type and technique were utilized, the reported high primary stability values might suggest good quality of the regenerated bone at 4 months postoperatively.

Conclusions

The results of this clinical study support the use of a biphasic in situ hardening alloplastic bone graft substitute for ridge preservation in intact post-extraction sites without the use of a dental membrane. Therefore, grafting of sockets without primary wound closure or using dental membranes or a soft tissue punch can be an effective minimally invasive method of preserving the contour and architecture of the alveolar ridge while supporting sufficient bone formation for implant placement. The hardening characteristics of the grafting material used seem to be of great importance for the stability of the healing site, secondary wound healing, and the success of the above technique. Additional prospective studies using control groups, larger patient populations, and other time frames are needed in order to confirm and supplement the present findings.

Acknowledgements

We acknowledge Sunstar Suisse SA, Etoy, Switzerland, for partly supporting this clinical study with a study grant. The authors declare that there is no conflict of interest regarding the publication of this paper.

Competing interests

Ashish Kakar, Bappanadu H. Sripathi Rao, Shashikanth Hegde, Nikhil Deshpande, Annette Lindner, Heiner Nagursky, Aditya Patney, and Harsh Mahajan declare that they have no competing interests.

Authors' contributions

AK performed all the surgical procedures post-extraction and prosthetic procedures. BHSR performed all the extractions. ND and SH performed all the core biopsies. AL and HN performed all the histomorphometric analysis. AP and HM performed all the CBCT data calculations. All authors read and approved the final manuscript.

Author details

[1]Yenepoya University Dental College, University Road, Mangalore 575018, India. [2]Dental Foundations and Research Centre, Malad, Mumbai 400064, India. [3]Department of Oral and Maxillofacial Surgery, Center for Dental Medicine, Medical Center—University of Freiburg, Hugstetter Str. 55, 79106 Freiburg, Germany. [4]Mahajan Imaging Center, K-18 Hauz Khas Enclave, New Delhi 110016, India.

References

1. Araujo MG, Sukekava F, Wennstrom J, Lindhe J. Ridge alterations following implant placement in fresh extraction sockets: an experimental study in the dog. J Clin Periodontol. 2005;32:645–52.
2. Van der Weijden F, Dell'Acqua F, Slot DE DE. Alveolar bone dimensional changes of post-extraction sockets in humans: a systematic review. J Clin Periodontol. 2009;36(12):1048–58.
3. Schropp L, Wenzel A, Kostopaulos L, Karring T. Bone healing changes and soft tissue contour changes following single-tooth: a clinical and radiographic 12-month prospective study. Int J Periodontol Restor Dent. 2003;23:313–23.
4. Fickl S, Zuhr O, Wachtel H, Stappert CF, Stein JM, Hürzeler MB. Dimensional changes of the alveolar ridge contour after different socket preservation techniques. J Clini Periodontol. 2008;35(10):906–13.
5. Barone A, Orlando B, Cingano L, Marconcini S, Derchi G, Covani U. A randomized clinical trial to evaluate and compare implants placed in augmented versus non-augmented extraction sockets: 3-year results. J Periodontol. 2012;83(7):836–46.
6. Wang RE, Lang NP. Ridge preservation after tooth extraction. Clinical Oral Implants Res. 2012;23 Suppl 6:147–56.
7. Vignoletti F, Nuñez J, de Sanctis F, Lopez M, Caffesse R, Sanzet M, et al. Healing of a xenogeneic collagen matrix for keratinized tissue augmentation. Clin Oral Implants Res. 2015;26(5):545–52.
8. Araujo MG, da Silva JCC, de Mendonc AF, Lindhe J. Ridge alterations following grafting of fresh extraction socketsin man. A randomized clinical trial. Clin Oral Implants Res. 2015;26(4):407–12.
9. LeGeros RZ. Properties of osteoconductive biomaterials: calcium phosphates. Clin Orthopedic Related Research. 2002;395:81–98.
10. Artz Z, Weinreb M, Givol N, Rohrer MD, Nemcovsky CE, Prasad HS, Tal H. Biomaterial resorption rate and healing site morphology of inorganic bovine bone and beta-tricalcium phosphate in the canine: a 24-month longitudinal histologic study and morphometric analysis. Int J Oral Maxillofac Implants. 2004;19(3):357–68.

11. Jensen SS, Broggini N, Hjørting-Hansen E, Schenk R, Buser D. Bone healing and graft resorption of autograft, anorganicbovine bone and beta-tricalcium phosphate. A histologic and histomorphometric study in the mandibles of minipigs. Clin Oral Implants Res. 2006;17(3):237–43.
12. Nair PNR, Luder H-U, Maspero FA, Fischer JH, Schug J. Biocompatibility of beta-tricalcium phosphateroot replicas in porcine tooth extraction sockets—a correlativehistological, ultrastructural, and x-ray microanalytical pilotstudy. J Biomater Appl. 2006;20(4):307–24.
13. Jensen SS, Terheyden H. Bone augmentation procedures in localized defects in the alveolar ridge: clinical results with different bone grafts and bone-substitute materials. Int J Oral Maxillofac Implants. 2009;24(Suppl):218–36.
14. Cordaro L, Bosshardt DD, Palattella P, Rao W, Serino G, Chiapasco M. Maxillary sinus grafting with Bio-Oss or Straumann Bone Ceramic: histomorphometric results from arandomized controlled multicenter clinical trial. Clin Oral Implants Res. 2008;19(8):796–803.
15. Handschel J, Simonowska M, Naujoks C, Depprich RA, Ommerborn MA, Meyer U, Kübler NR. A histomorphometric meta-analysis of sinus elevation with various grafting materials. Head Face Med. 2009;11(5):12.
16. Zijderveld SA, Schulten EA, Aartman IH, ten Bruggenkate CM. Long-term changes in graft height after maxillary sinus floor elevation with different graftingmaterials: radiographic evaluation with a minimum follow-up of 4.5 years. Clin Orallmplants Res. 2009;20(7):691–700.
17. Troedhan A, Schlichting I, Kurrek A, Wainwright M. Primary implant stability in augmented sinuslift-sites after completed bone regeneration: a randomized controlled clinical study comparing four subantrally inserted biomaterials. Sci Rep. 2014;4:5877.
18. Leventis MD, Fairbairn P, Kakar A, Leventis AD, Margaritis V, Lückerath W, Horowitz RA, Rao BH, Lindner A, Nagursky H. Minimally invasive alveolar ridge preservation utilizing an in situ hardening β-tricalcium phosphate bone substitute: a multicenter case series. Int J Dent. 2016;2016:5406736.
19. Wang HL, Tsao YP. Istologic evaluation of socket augmentation with mineralized human allograft. Int J Periodontics Restorative Dent. 2008;28:231–7.
20. Jurisic M, Manojlovic-Stojanoski M, Andric M, Kokovic V, Danilovic V, Jurisic T, Brkovic BB. Histological and morphometric aspects of Ridge preservation with a moldable, in situ hardening bone graft substitute. Arch Biol Sci. 2013;65(2):429–37.
21. Brkovic BM, Prasad HS, Konandreas G, Milan R, Antunovic D, Sándor GK, Rohrer MD. Simple preservation of a maxillary extraction socket using beta-tricalcium phosphate with type I collagen: preliminary clinical and histomorphometric observations. J Can Dent Association. 2008;74(6):523–8.
22. Lang NP, Pun L, Lau KY, Li KY, Wong MC. A systematic review on survival and success rates of implants placed immediately into fresh extraction sockets after at least 1 year. Clin Oral Implants Res. 2012;23 Suppl 5:39–66.
23. Smukler H, Landi L, Setayesh R. Hostomorphometric evaluation of extraction sockets and deficient alveolar ridges treated with allografts and barrier membrane. A pilot study. Int J Oral Maxillofac Implants. 1999;14:407–16.
24. Dies F, Etienne D, Bou Abboud N, Ouhayoun JP. Bone regeneration in extraction sites after immediate placement of an e-PTFE membrane with or without a biomaterial. Clin Oral Implnts Res. 1996;7:277–85.
25. Briunami F, Then P, Moroi H, Kabini S, Leone C. GBR in human extraction sockets and ridge defects prior to implant placement: clinical and histologic evidence of osteoblastic and osteoclastic activities in DFDBA". Int J Periodontics Restorative Dent. 1999;19:259–67.
26. Weng DS, Schliephake H. Are socket and ridge preservation techniques at the day of tooth extraction efficient in maintaining the tissues of the alveolar ridge? Systemic review, consensus statements and recommendations of the 1st DGI Consensus Conference in September 2010, Aerzen, Germany. Eur J Implantol. 2011;4:59–66.
27. Vignoletti F, Matesanz P, Rodrigo D, Figuero E, Martin C, Sanz M. Surgical protocolsfor ridge preservationafter tooth extraction. A systemic review. Clin Oral ImplantsRes. 2012;23(Suppl):22–38.
28. Schmidlin PR, Nicholls F, Kruse A, Zwahlen RA, Weber FE. Evaluation of moldable, in situ hardening calcium phosphate bone graft substitutes. Clin Oral Implants Res. 2013;24(2):49–57.
29. Darby I, Chen ST, Buser STD. Ridge preservation techniques for implant therapy. Int J Oral Maxillofac Implants. 2009;24(Suppl):260–71.
30. Fuster-Torres MA, Pe˜narrocha-Diago M, Pe˜narrocha-Oltra D, Pe˜narrocha-Diago M. Relationships between bone density values from cone beam computed tomography, maximum insertion torque, and resonance frequency analysis at implant placement: a pilot study. Int J Oral Maxillofac Implants. 2011;26(5):1051–6.
31. Da Cunha HA, Francischone CE, Nary Filho H, Gomes De Oliveira RC. A comparison between cutting torque and resonance frequency in the assessment of primary stability and final torque capacity of standard and Ti Unite single-tooth implants under immediate loading. Int J Oral Maxillofac Implants. 2004;19(4):578–85.

17

In vitro surface characteristics and impurity analysis of five different commercially available dental zirconia implants

B. Beger[1*], H. Goetz[2], M. Morlock[1], E. Schiegnitz[1] and B. Al-Nawas[1]

Abstract

Background: The aim of this study was to assess surface characteristics, element composition, and surface roughness of five different commercially available dental zirconia implants.
Five zirconia implants (Bredent whiteSKY™ (I1), Straumann® PURE Ceramic (I2), ceramic.implant vitaclinical (I3), Zeramex® (I4), Ceralog Monobloc M10 (I5)) were evaluated.

Methods: The evaluation was performed by means of scanning electron microscopy (SEM), energy-dispersive X-ray spectroscopy (EDX), and confocal laser scanning microscopy (CLSM).

Results: The semi-quantitative element composition showed no significant impurity of any implant tested. Both the machined and the rough areas of the investigated implants were predominated by zirconium, oxygen, and carbon. Roughness values (S_a) showed highest values for I2 and I5.

Conclusions: The investigated zirconia implants showed surface characteristics and roughness values close to those of conventionally produced titanium implants, making them a promising alternative. However, zirconia implants have yet to prove themselves in clinical practice and clinical controlled trials.

Keywords: Zirconia, Dental implant, Ceramic, Implant surface, Implant material, Roughness, Titanium

Background

Dental implants have become a well-established treatment method for oral rehabilitation after tooth loss. Pure titanium is still the material of choice when it comes to dental intraosseous implants and has been used for decades. However, titanium implants have esthetic limitations, especially in the front aspect of the maxillary jaw. The recession of the gingiva can lead to visible implant necks. Furthermore, titanium may cause immunological reactions with early local infection and possible risk for implant loss [1]. Ceramic implants are proclaimed as a new alternative to titanium implants. The first tooth-colored ceramic implants were inferior to titanium-based implants due to their biomechanical characteristics such as low fracture toughness [2]. In the 1980s, the Tübinger immediate implant was introduced, fully made of aluminum oxide (AL_2O_3), but was withdrawn from the market because of high fracture rates [3]. Other investigations on different AL_2O_3 implants found less bone-implant contact compared to titanium [4] as well as reduced survival rates [2, 5]. Since the introduction of yttrium-stabilized tetragonal zirconia polycrystalline (Y-TZP)-based implants, it could be shown that these implants show high similarity in osseointegration compared to titanium implants [2].

Titanium implants with smooth or roughened surfaces have shown high success rates in various indications [2, 6, 7]. Surface characteristics of dental implants, as a new development over the last decades, are seen as an important factor that affects osseointegration, especially in compromised patients (e.g., following radiation therapy, bone augmentation, class D4 bone) [8]. By improving the implant design, implant material, and implant surface characteristics as well as surgical techniques and implant loading conditions,

* Correspondence: Benjamin.beger@unimedizin-mainz.de
[1]Department of Maxillofacial Surgery, University Medical Center of the Johannes Gutenberg-University Mainz, Augustusplatz 2, 55131 Mainz, Germany
Full list of author information is available at the end of the article

osseointegration can be affected [9]. Several new techniques are performed nowadays to speed up the osseointegration process by altering the surface of the implant chemically (incorporating inorganic phases onto the titanium oxide layer) or physically (increasing the level of roughness) [10, 11]. Advantages of surface-modified implants include (a) establishing a greater contact area followed by better primary stability, (b) providing surface-retaining blood clots, and (c) stimulating bone formation [10, 12]. In vitro tests of surface roughness showed higher proliferation, cytokine, and growth factor production of osteoblast-like cells. Those factors are known to affect proliferation, differentiation, and matrix synthesis of chondrocytes [13–16]. Many studies on surface characteristics of titanium implants were performed over the last years. Due to the renaissance and new development of zirconia implants, it is now necessary to study their behavior and surface characteristics and to compare them to titanium implants. However, data regarding the surface characteristics of these zirconia implants are very rare. Therefore, the aim of this study was to examine the surface characteristics, element composition, and surface roughness of the five different commercially available dental zirconia implants.

Methods

Investigated implants

The following five commercially available dental zirconia implants were used in this study (Table 1). Bredent whiteSKY™ implant (I1) is made from unground Brezirkon™, an yttrium oxide (Y_2O_3)-stabilized tetragonal polycrystalline zirconium oxide and is sandblasted. Zirconium oxide is endowed with 3 mol% yttrium oxide to gain a rectangle and room temperature stable structure [17]. Straumann® PURE Ceramic Implant (I2) is generally made from yttrium oxide-stabilized tetragonal polycrystalline zirconium oxide. The surface due to the manufacturer is coated with a special process called ZLA™ which shall be similar to the SLA™ process (Sandblasted, Large-grit, Acid-etched) of titanium implants. Ceramic.implant vitaclinical (I3) is made from zirconium oxide. The Zeramex® implant (I4) is made from zirconium and has a sandblasted and etched surface structure with their so-called ZERAFIL™ technology. Camlog's Ceralog Monobloc M10 ceramic implant (I5) is also made from yttrium-stabilized zirconium dioxide. Unlike the other ceramic implants, it is produced with ceramic injection molding (CIM) technique. This technique requires no sandblasting or etching. The implants' geometrical design and the surface structure are already molded via CIM before the sintering and hot isostatic pressing (HIP) process.

Scanning electron microscopy

For a more detailed illustration of the implant surface topology, the technique of scanning electron microscopy (SEM) was used. A Quanta 200 FEG (FEI Company, Netherlands) field emission SEM equipped with environmental low vacuum mode makes it possible to avoid the typical surface charging-up problems of uncoated highly insulating ceramic implants without the need for sample preparation. Therefore, high-resolution SEM images with magnifications up to 25,000 are possible to demonstrate the micro-structured appearances at different locations. Comparable areas for all implants under investigation are selected by splitting up the cylindrical shape of the implant into sections (Fig. 1). For the comparison of

Table 1 Five commercially available ceramic implants and surface characteristics

	WhiteSKY (implant 1)	Pure ceramic (implant 2)	Vitaclinical (implant 3)	Zeramex (implant 4)	Ceralog (implant 5)
	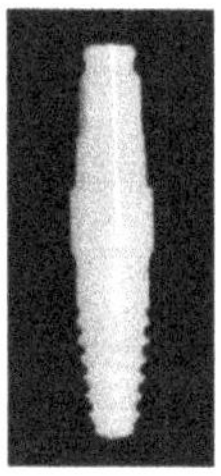	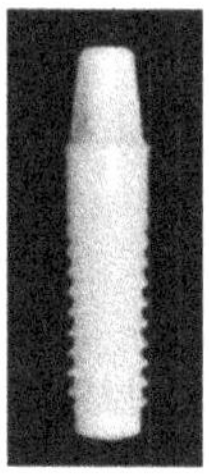	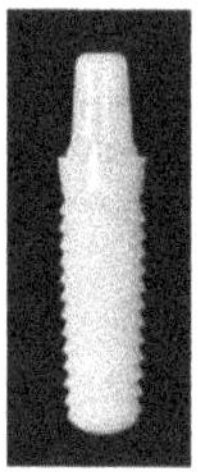	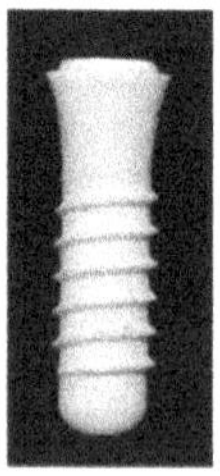	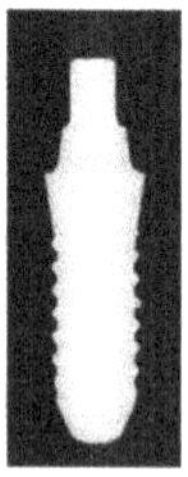
Sandblasted	Yes	Yes	N.A.	Yes	No*
Etched	N.A.	Yes	N.A.	Yes	No*
Special coating	N.A.	ZLA™	N.A.	ZERAFIL™	No*

*Due to the processes CIM and HIP, see the "Methods" section

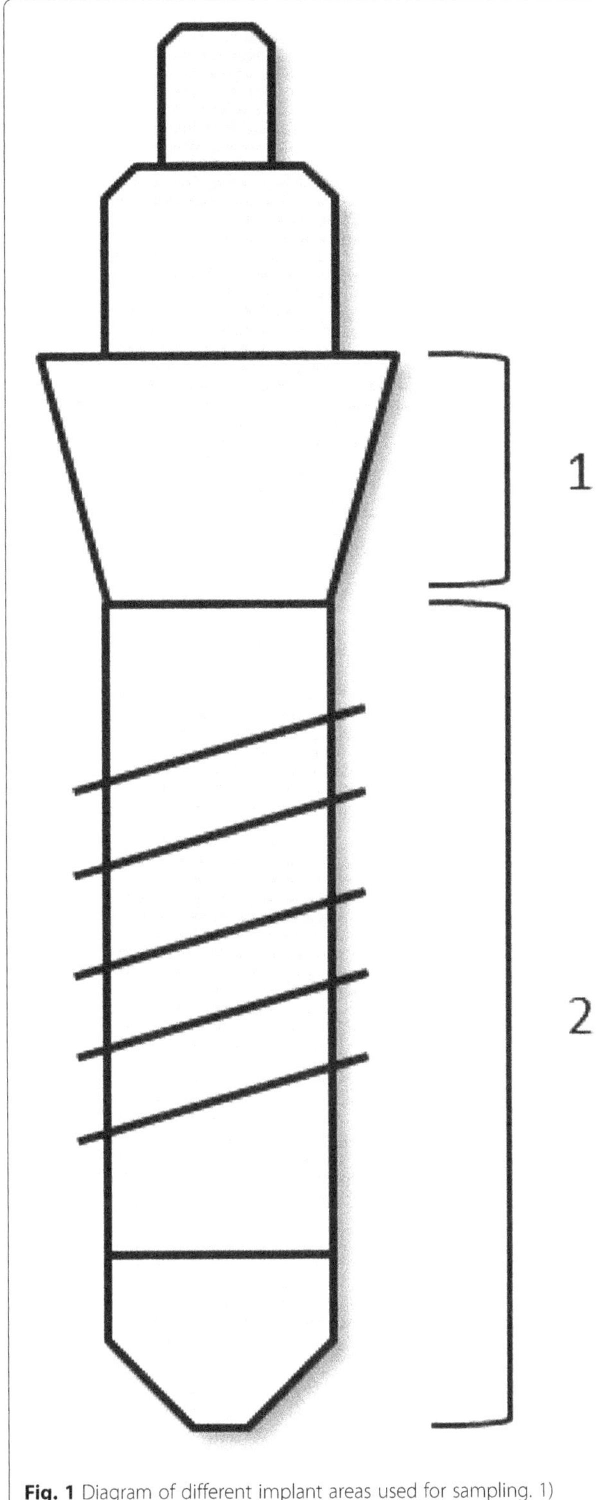

Fig. 1 Diagram of different implant areas used for sampling. 1) Machined (untreated) area. 2) rough (treated) area

surface structures between the tested implants, two regions of interest were selected: machined and rough area (compare Figs. 1 and 3). Each section was observed under different degrees of magnifications (× 2000, × 10,000, × 25,000) with the same microscope parameters (HV 20 kV, Det LFD, pressure 0.90 mbar). The low vacuum pressure in the sample chamber was reduced until charging levels on the sample surface were reduced to the level at which electron imaging of the sample surface was possible.

Energy-dispersive X-ray spectroscopy

Analysis of the element composition of the implant surfaces by means of energy-dispersive X-ray spectroscopy (EDX) was performed with an INCA Energy 350 system (Oxford Instruments, Wiesbaden, Germany) coupled with the SEM Quanta 200 FEG (Fig. 2). Similar to the micro-morphological presentation, each implant was divided into comparable sites of interest. Typical areas were selected and evaluated (Fig. 3). With the "Point &ID" mode of the INCA Energy software, both points of interest and the areas of interest are selected for the EDX analysis. Microscopic conditions (magnification × 2000) and excitation energy (HV 20 kV) are kept constant for all types of implants. For a semi-quantitative approach, the main components identified on all of the sample surfaces are evaluated as shown in Table 2. Intervals of minimum and maximum values are presented to demonstrate the high inhomogeneous situation found at most of the selected areas.

Confocal laser scanning microscopy

Evaluation of the zirconia implant surface roughness as well as their surface texture parameters is carried out by means of confocal laser scanning microscopic technique. A Leica TCS SP2 (Leica Microsystems, Wetzlar, Germany) upright microscope with a red He-laser (633 nm) and a high-performance objective (HC PL FLUOTAR × 50/0.80) was used to acquire high spatial resolution images (1024 × 1024 pixels). Image stacks are created by capturing all the light reflected from the deepest to the highest point of the selected sample surface area. The image stacks are created in defined steps and acquired for five uniformly distributed points at the circumferences of representative-treated and none-treated locations on each type of implant (compare Fig. 4). The step size was calculated for optically optimized values by the LCS Leica confocal software. Because of the cylindrically shaped surface character, a zoom factor of 2 which generates an image size of 150 × 150 μm was used to avoid artificial height values.

Maximum projections and height distribution images (depth map) are calculated by LCS software from the image stacks and viewed exemplary in Fig. 5.

Subsequently, the depth map images are imported in the SPIP™ 4.2.6 (Image Metrology) software for roughness and texture evaluation. According to the

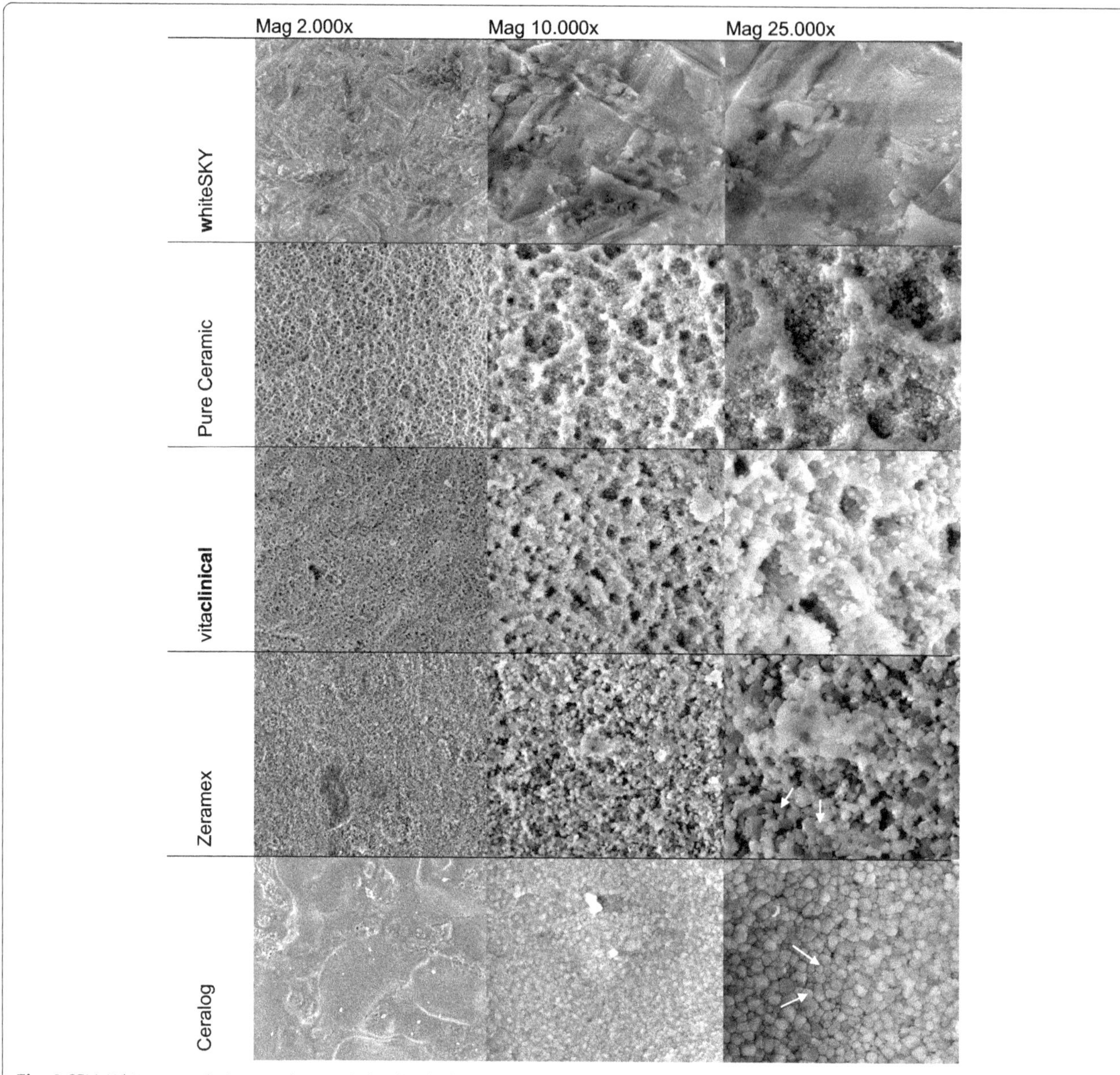

Fig. 2 SEM. White arrow (→) exemplary mark the droplet like shape of surface as described in the text

ISO 25178-2 reference, all surface roughness parameters implemented in SPIP™ are evaluated and classified as amplitude, hybrid, functional, and spatial parameters. Selected values are shown in Table 3.

Results

SEM

SEM micrographs presented in Fig. 2 demonstrate the dissimilarity of the sample surface microstructure. Implant 1 shows an overall smoother surface and a slaty-like surface without evidence of a typical etching process. The surface shows sparse roughness. Implants 2–4 show deep markings from their brand's specific etching and sandblasting processes. In × 10,000 magnification, immersions can be found that look like little craters. Implant 2 shows the biggest immersions, and implant 4 shows the smallest. In a × 25,000 magnification, implants 2–5 show droplet-like-shaped particles on the outer surface as a basic structure of the immersions under × 10,000 magnification. The finest droplets can be found on implant 2, and the biggest droplets can be found on implants 4 and 5. Implant 5 stands out from the other implants. It shows very evenly spread droplets on the surface in every magnification (Fig. 2).

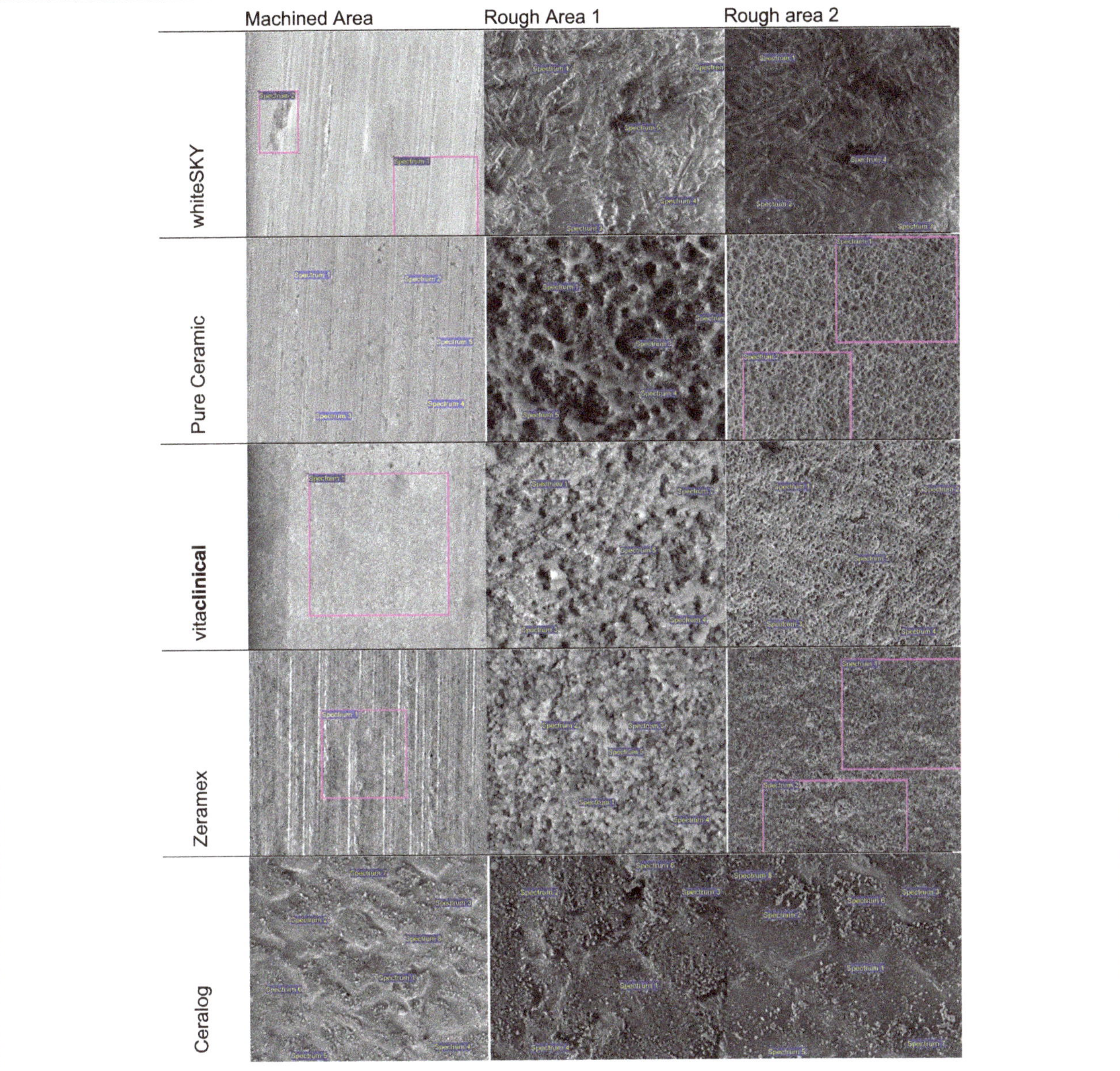

Fig. 3 SEM for localization of EDX analysis

EDX analysis

The semi-quantitative element composition showed no significant impurity of any implant tested (Table 2). Both the machined and the rough areas (Fig. 3) were predominated by zirconium, oxygen, and carbon. Yttrium could be found in implants 1–3. Implants 4 and 5 showed yttrium under the detection limit and just less than 1.7 atomic % in the apical aspect of implant 4. Minor traces of hafnium could be shown in all implants 1–5. Implants 1, 4, and 5 showed traces of aluminum on the surface. The highest amount of aluminum could be found on the surface of implant 4.

Confocal laser scanning microscopy (CLSM)

CLSM images including the topological information of all five implants are shown in Fig. 4.

Untreated areas (machined areas) of implants 1–4 showed parallel grooves of the machining process in the interface area of the neck (Fig. 4). Treated areas (rough areas) show roughened surfaces due to special treatment with acid and sandblasting. Implant 5 showed roughened surface in both areas and no sign for a machined neck part.

Roughness analysis (SPIP)

Implant 2 (S_a 1.27 μm ± 0.24) and implant 5 (S_a 1.22 μm ± 0.36) show the highest roughness values

Table 2 EDX

Element composition/semi-quantitative evaluation								
Location	Type	Zr at $\%_{min}$–at $\%_{max}$	Hf at %	Y at $\%_{min}$–at $\%_{max}$	Al at $\%_{min}$–at $\%_{max}$	O at $\%_{min}$–at $\%_{max}$	C at $\%_{min}$–at $\%_{max}$	N at $\%_{min}$–at $\%_{max}$
Machined area	WhiteSKY	16.0–19.5	< 0.25	1.47–1.67	< 0.5	55–58	17.6–24.0	< 1.0
	Straumann ZLA	19.4–22.4	< 0.35	1.6–1.8	< 0.12	48.5–52.1	20.6–22.3	5.2–7.2
	Vitaclinical	23.7	< 0.30	< 1.5	< 0.13	56	9.8	None
	ZERAMEX	17.7	< 0.23	< Det. limit	< 9.6	57.5	7.7	7.7
	Monobloc M10	4.0–11.0	< 0.09	< Det. limit	0.4–2.3	12.0–21.0	63.0–80.0	0–11.0
Rough area	WhiteSKY	15.6–19.3	< 0.23	0–2.8	1.1–3.8	49.8–80.7	0–20.7	0–6.3
	Straumann ZLA	17.4–28.9	< 0.25	1.7–3.4	< 0.13	48.8–63.7	7.4–15.4	8.2–14.7
	Vitaclinical	17.2–23.4	< 0.26	1.3–2.6	< 0.24	48.6–64.5	11.5–18.9	3.8–8.2
	ZERAMEX	6.9–18.3	< 0.23	< 1.7	7.8–18.7	67.1–71.5	3.0–6.7	6.1–7.8
	Monobloc M10	4.6–28.0	< 0.40	< Det. limit	2.9–13.9	12.0–69.0	28.0–79.0	None

(S_a) of all tested implants: Straumann's pure ceramic implant was blasted and etched and shows the overall highest S_a value in the rough area. Implant 3 (vitaclinical) shows correspondingly lower S_a around 1.05 μm (± 0.17) (Table 3). The lowest S_a value could be found in implant 4, which was only sandblasted due to manufacturer's specifications. However, the Zeramex implant despite being sandblasted and etched shows the lowest roughness value around 0.73 μm (± 0.95). Nevertheless, Zeramex shows a fine distribution of small pores all over the surface in the SEM sample images. Camlog's Ceralog shows the highest roughness in the untreated area with 0.61 μm (± 0.03). Figure 6 shows the box plot of the roughness analysis with implant 5 having the widest distribution of measured values.

Discussion

Implant surface characteristics are of ongoing scientific interest. Implants made from titanium are still the most common to be used. Titanium implants are made from alpha-beta alloy which consists of 6% aluminum and 4% vanadium (Ti-6Al-4V). These materials have low density, high strength, and resistance to fatigue and corrosion, and their modulus of elasticity is closer to the bone than any other implant material [18]. However, titanium implants are discussed to trigger hypersensitivity reactions due to surface corrosion [1, 19]. Titanium implant surfaces are machined, etched, sandblasted, and sometimes coated with special (company-specific) coatings. For titanium implants, roughness values (Ra) around 1.5 μm are known to provide successful osseointegration [20].

Ceramic implants experienced a renaissance since their reentry into the market. New ceramic implants with yttria (Y_2O_3)-stabilized tetragonal zirconium polycrystalline (Y-TZP) material have superior corrosion and wear resistance in comparison to titanium implants as well as high flexural strength (800 to 1000 MPa) [18]. However, due to manufacturing imperfections or flaws created during zirconia implant fabrication and because of special surface treatments, their strength can be compromised [18, 21]. Due to their brittle nature, ceramic implants tend to fracture. Especially sharp, deep, and thin threads can easily lead to implant failures [18, 21]. The surface treatment on ceramic is developed due to a process of sandblasting, etching, and heat treatment [22]. Sandblasting is usually done with alumina particles that lead to sharp edges and scratches on the surface. The treatment with hydrofluoric acid as the following procedure may smoothen the surface again [22–24]. However, in zirconia implants, due to stress caused by sandblasting, a tetragonal to monoclinic phase transition may be caused [22, 25]. This monoclinic volume fraction can be seen in 10–15% of the cases [26] and initially leads to a surface compression of the zirconia material [22]. According to Fischer et al., the long-term effects and the implant stability after this procedure are not yet proven [22]. However, it can be reversed by a thermal treatment that is higher than the transition temperature [22, 27].

The surface shape (droplet-like surface), which was observed in the SEM samples, can be caused due to the sintering process in which ceramic powder was melted and then formed. Different particle,

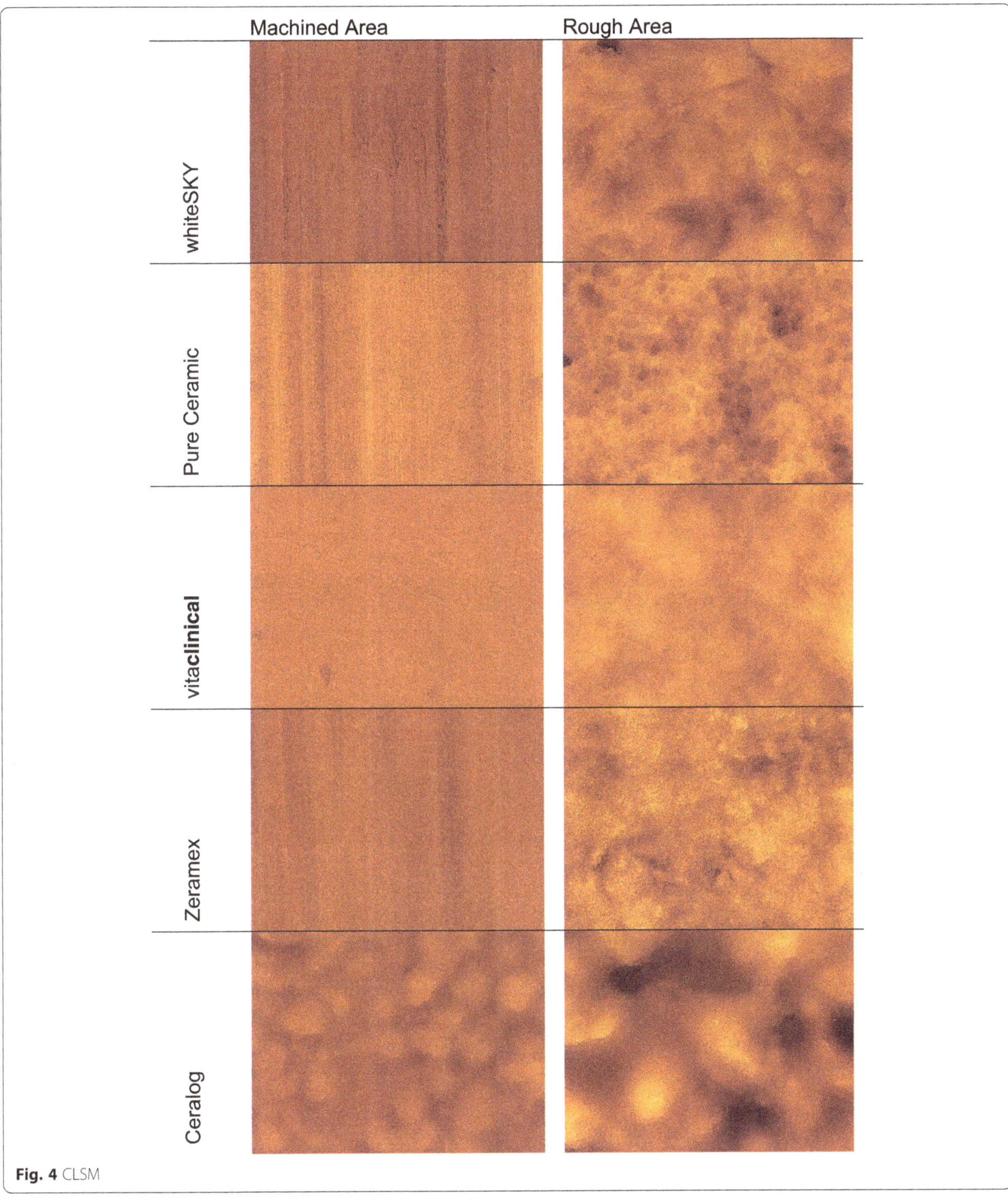

Fig. 4 CLSM

immersion, and droplet sizes can also change due to possible reasons like usage of various types and dosages of acid for the etching process and change of exposure time to acid effect. A longer exposure time to etching process could also be responsible for lowering aluminum corundum from sandblasting processes. However, despite a very fine surface microstructure, implant 4 shows the highest amount of aluminum on the outer surface. This could be explained by sandblasting with aluminum-containing corundum particles followed by a shorter etching process. The higher amount of aluminum in implants

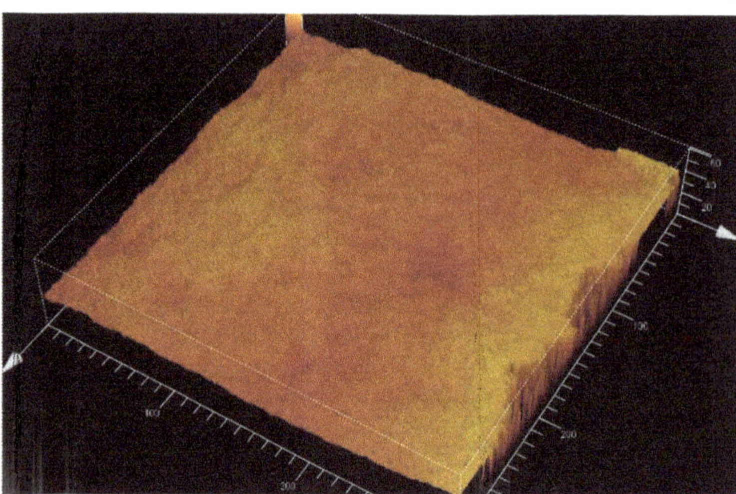

Fig. 5 3D profile

1, 4, and 5 might be due to the individual material composition while sintering the material mixture or to corundum particles of the machining and sandblasting process. Implants with aluminum under the detection limit could be caused by a final etching process. Implants 1 and 5 are not advertised with a special etching process. However, implant 4 is supposed to be etched. The etching could have happened before sandblasting, or the acid used was not strong enough to eliminate all aluminum particles.

All implants excluding the Ceralog Monobloc (implant 5) show typical parallel grooves of the machining process in the confocal laser scan and rougher surfaces in the treated areas. Ceralog is the only implant with a rough surface that can also be found in the machined area. Zirconia implants which are treated with a process of sandblasting, etching, and heat treatment are showing a micro-structured surface resulting in a surface roughness in the range of 1.2 μm [22]. In this study, implants 2 and 5 showed roughness values in the range of 1.2 μm. The other implants showed different roughness values. The surface porosity of titanium implants after sandblasting and etching processes is much more rigorous than that of the ceramic implants that were investigated. In this study, implants 2 and 5 can approximately be compared to titanium surface characteristics in the SEM samples. However, implant 5 was not sandblasted and etched because of a special "injection molding technique" and shows a wide distribution of roughness values. A similarity to the surface structure of titanium implants cannot be proven yet.

Table 3 Roughness analysis

Group	Name	Amplitude parameters S_a (μm)
Machined area	WhiteSKY	0.24 ± 0.04
	Straumann ZLA	0.36 ± 0.03
	Vitaclinical	0.20 ± 0.06
	ZERAMEX	0.30 ± 0.05
	Monobloc M10	0.61 ± 0.03
Rough area	WhiteSKY (Impl1)	0.91 ± 0.13
	Straumann ZLA (Impl2)	1.27 ± 0.24
	Vitaclinical (Impl3)	1.05 ± 0.17
	Zeramex (Impl4)	0.73 ± 0.95
	Monobloc M10 (impl5)	1.22 ± 0.36

The semi-quantitative energy-dispersive X-ray spectroscopy (EDX) can be used to further analyze the components of the implant surface. None of the implants showed any impurity or unexpected results. Implants 4 and 5 showed yttrium under the detection limit in the EDX analysis. This could be caused by the lower dosage of yttrium endowment in the stabilization processing in comparison to other implants [17].

This investigation shows results on a sample basis with one implant tested and shall not be used for generalization.

Conclusions

New ceramic implants are showing a variety of surface characteristics due to different manufacturing

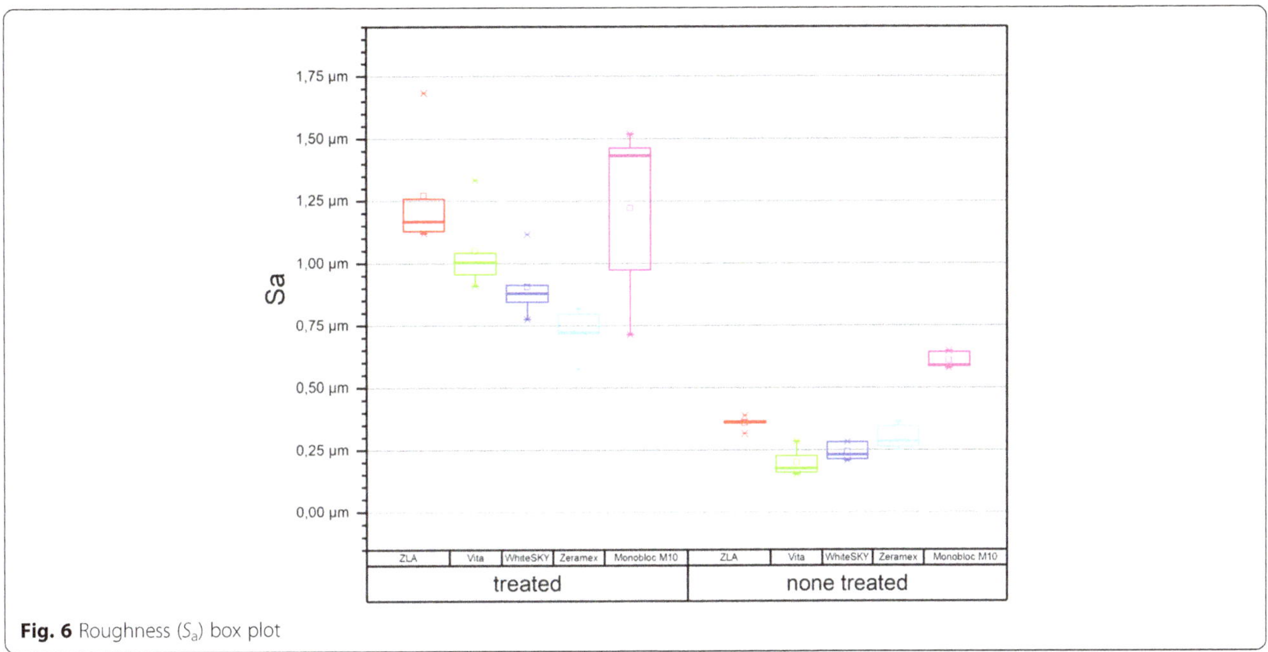

Fig. 6 Roughness (S_a) box plot

processes as shown by other groups [2, 28]. The surface structures of the investigated implants are close to titanium implants. If the surface characteristics really have a high influence on osseointegration, ceramic implants cannot yet compare to the long experience with titanium. However, there are several indications for using ceramic implants. In the future, ceramic implants have to prove themselves in clinical practice and clinical controlled trials.

Abbreviations

AL_2O_3: Aluminum oxide; CIM: Ceramic injection molding; CLSM: Confocal laser scanning microscopy; EDX: Energy-dispersive X-ray spectroscopy; HIP: Hot isostatic pressing; I: Implant; kV: Kilovolt; mbar: Millibar; MPa: Megapascal; nm: Nanometer; S_a: Area roughness parameter; SEM: Scanning electron microscopy; SLA™: Sandblasted, Large-grit, Acid-etched; Y-TZP: Yttrium-stabilized tetragonal zirconium polycrystalline; µm: Micrometer

Authors' contributions

BB carried out the concept, the design, and the analysis and interpretation of the data. BB drafted the manuscript. GH carried out the SEM, CLSM, and EDX analysis and revised the manuscript. All authors read and approved the final manuscript.

Competing interests

Beger B, Goetz H, Morlock M, Schiegnitz E, and Al-Nawas B declare that they have no competing interests.

Author details

[1]Department of Maxillofacial Surgery, University Medical Center of the Johannes Gutenberg-University Mainz, Augustusplatz 2, 55131 Mainz, Germany. [2]Biomaterials in Medicine (BioAPP), University Medical Center of the Johannes Gutenberg-University Mainz, Mainz, Germany.

References

1. Jacobi-Gresser E, Huesker K, Schutt S. Genetic and immunological markers predict titanium implant failure: a retrospective study. Int J Oral Maxillofac Surg. 2013;42(4):537–43.
2. Wenz HJ, Bartsch J, Wolfart S, Kern M. Osseointegration and clinical success of zirconia dental implants: a systematic review. Int J Prosthodont. 2008; 21(1):27–36.
3. Shulte W. The intra-osseous Al2O3 (Frialit) Tuebingen implant. Developmental status after eight years (I). Quintessence Int. 1984;15(1):9.
4. Steflik DE, Lake FT, Sisk AL, Parr GR, Hanes PJ, Davis HC, et al. A comparative investigation in dogs: 2-year morphometric results of the dental implant—bone interface. Int J Oral Maxillofac Implants. 1996;11(1):15–25.
5. Berge TI, Gronningsaeter AG. Survival of single crystal sapphire implants supporting mandibular overdentures. Clin Oral Implants Res. 2000;11(2):154–62.
6. Branemark PI, Adell R, Breine U, Hansson BO, Lindstrom J, Ohlsson A. Intra-osseous anchorage of dental prostheses. I. Experimental studies. Scand J Plast Reconstr Surg. 1969;3(2):81–100.
7. Adell R, Eriksson B, Lekholm U, Branemark PI, Jemt T. Long-term follow-up study of osseointegrated implants in the treatment of totally edentulous jaws. Int J Oral Maxillofac Implants. 1990;5(4):347–59.
8. Grötz KA, Wahlmann UW, Krummenauer F, Wegener J, Al-Nawas B, Kuffner H-D, et al. Prognosis and factors affecting prognosis for enossal implants in the irradiated jaw. Mund Kiefer Gesichtschir. 1999;3(1):S117–S24.
9. Albrektsson T, Branemark PI, Hansson HA, Lindstrom J. Osseointegrated titanium implants. Requirements for ensuring a long-lasting, direct bone-to-implant anchorage in man. Acta Orthop Scand. 1981;52(2):155–70.
10. Karamian E, Khandan A, Motamedi MR, Mirmohammadi H. Surface characteristics and bioactivity of a novel natural HA/zircon nanocomposite coated on dental implants. Biomed Res Int. 2014;2014:410627.
11. Dohan Ehrenfest DM, Coelho PG, Kang BS, Sul YT, Albrektsson T. Classification of osseointegrated implant surfaces: materials, chemistry and topography. Trends Biotechnol. 2010;28(4):198–206.
12. Wennerberg A, Albrektsson T. Effects of titanium surface topography on bone integration: a systematic review. Clin Oral Implants Res. 2009;20(Suppl 4):172–84.
13. Kieswetter K, Schwartz Z, Dean DD, Boyan BD. The role of implant surface characteristics in the healing of bone. Crit Rev Oral Biol Med. 1996;7(4):329–45.
14. Ong JL, Carnes DL, Cardenas HL, Cavin R. Surface roughness of titanium on bone morphogenetic protein-2 treated osteoblast cells in vitro. Implant Dent. 1997;6(1):19–24.
15. Schwartz Z, Kieswetter K, Dean DD, Boyan BD. Underlying mechanisms at the bone-surface interface during regeneration. J Periodontal Res. 1997;32(1 Pt 2):166–71.

16. Al-Nawas B, Gotz H. Three-dimensional topographic and metrologic evaluation of dental implants by confocal laser scanning microscopy. Clin Implant Dent Relat Res. 2003;5(3):176–83.
17. Schweiger M. Zirkoniumdioxid–hochfeste und bruchzähe Strukturkeramik. Ästhetische Zahnmedizin. 2004;5:248–57.
18. Osman R, Swain M. A critical review of dental implant materials with an emphasis on titanium versus zirconia. Materials. 2015;8(3):932.
19. Javed F, Al-Hezaimi K, Almas K, Romanos GE. Is titanium sensitivity associated with allergic reactions in patients with dental implants? A systematic review. Clin Implant Dent Relat Res. 2013;15(1):47–52.
20. Wennerberg A, Hallgren C, Johansson C, Danelli S. A histomorphometric evaluation of screw-shaped implants each prepared with two surface roughnesses. Clin Oral Implants Res. 1998;9(1):11–9.
21. Osman RB, Ma S, Duncan W, De Silva RK, Siddiqi A, Swain MV. Fractured zirconia implants and related implant designs: scanning electron microscopy analysis. Clin Oral Implants Res. 2013;24(5):592–7.
22. Fischer J, Schott A, Martin S. Surface micro-structuring of zirconia dental implants. Clin Oral Implants Res. 2016;27(2):162–6.
23. Bachle M, Butz F, Hubner U, Bakalinis E, Kohal RJ. Behavior of CAL72 osteoblast-like cells cultured on zirconia ceramics with different surface topographies. Clin Oral Implants Res. 2007;18(1):53–9.
24. Gahlert M, Rohling S, Wieland M, Eichhorn S, Kuchenhoff H, Kniha H. A comparison study of the osseointegration of zirconia and titanium dental implants. A biomechanical evaluation in the maxilla of pigs. Clin Implant Dent Relat Res. 2010;12(4):297–305.
25. Chevalier J, Grandjean S, Kuntz M, Pezzotti G. On the kinetics and impact of tetragonal to monoclinic transformation in an alumina/zirconia composite for arthroplasty applications. Biomaterials. 2009;30(29):5279–82.
26. Guazzato M, Quach L, Albakry M, Swain MV. Influence of surface and heat treatments on the flexural strength of Y-TZP dental ceramic. J Dent. 2005; 33(1):9–18.
27. Papanagiotou HP, Morgano SM, Giordano RA, Pober R. In vitro evaluation of low-temperature aging effects and finishing procedures on the flexural strength and structural stability of Y-TZP dental ceramics. J Prosthet Dent. 2006;96(3):154–64.
28. Ewais OH, Al Abbassy F, Ghoneim MM, Aboushelib MN. Novel zirconia surface treatments for enhanced osseointegration: laboratory characterization. Int J Dent. 2014;2014:203940.

18

Evaluation of effectiveness of concentrated growth factor on osseointegration

Cagasan Pirpir, Onur Yilmaz*, Celal Candirli and Emre Balaban

Abstract

Background: Growth factor-containing products have been reported to increase implant stability and accelerate osseointegration. Concentrated growth factor (CGF) can be used for this purpose with the growth factors it contains. The aim of this study is to assess the effect of CGF on implant stability and osseointegration.

Methods: Twelve patients with maxillary anterior toothless were included in the study. Implant cavities prepared in the study group were covered with CGF membrane before implant placement, but conventional implant placement was performed in the control group. Resonance frequency measurements were performed with the Osstell device intra-operatively, post-operatively, at the 1st week, and at the 4th week.

Results: The mean ISQ values were found to be 79.40 ± 2.604 for the study group and 73.50 ± 5.226 for the control group at 1st week, 78.60 ± 3.136 for the study group and 73.45 ± 5.680 for the control group at 4th week. The differences between the groups were statistically significant ($p < 0.05$).

Conclusions: It was observed that the concentrated growth factor had positive effects on implant stabilization. The ISQ measurements at week 1 and week 4 were notably higher in the study group. Application of this material seems to accelerate osseointegration.

Keywords: Dental implants, Growth factors, Osseointegration, Osteogenesis, Wound healing

Background

Osseointegration of dental implants is important for long-term success and stability. There is no standardization in terms of the time of osseointegration and the timing of prosthetic loading. This process varies between 0–6 months [1]. Various strategies are being explored to shorten this period. Changes in implant surface properties and design have increased primer stability and helped the peri-implant tissue remain healthy. These changes have aimed to increase bone-implant surface connectivity and accelerate healing. Another method of accelerating osseointegration is the modulation of healing after the placement of the implant [2]. This modulation, in turn, can be achieved by bioactive molecules that increase osteoblastic differentiation and accelerate bone healing around the implant [2].

Growth factors are bioactive proteins that control the wound healing process. The platelet-containing preparations derived from human blood contain many growth factors such as bone morphogenetic protein (BMP), platelet-derived growth factor (PDGF), insulin-like growth factor (IGF), vascular endothelial growth factor (VEGF), transforming growth factor-β1 (TGF-β1), and transforming growth factor-β2 (TGF-β2), which also play a key role in bone healing [3–5]. These growth factors attract the undifferentiated mesenchymal cells to the wound site, thus facilitating angiogenesis, chemotaxis, and cell proliferation [2].

Various platelet concentrates such as platelet-rich plasma (PRP), platelet-rich fibrin (PRF), and concentrated growth factor (CGF) are used to reconstruct bone defects [6]. PRF has been shown to have very successful results in tissue engineering in many studies [7–9]. Furthermore, a study by Sohn et al. has shown the higher regeneration capacity and multipurpose use of CGF in 2009 [10].

This preparation's potential is because it contains growth factor-containing fibrin network; it contains fibroblast, platelet, leukocyte, and endothelial cell for angiogenesis and tissue remodeling; and it provides matrix for cell migration [11]. Platelets, in particular, contain biologically

* Correspondence: onuryilmaz590@hotmail.com
Faculty of Dentistry, Department of Oral and Maxillofacial Surgery, Karadeniz Technical University, Trabzon, Turkey

active proteins at high concentrations and support healing, growth, and cell morphogenesis [12–14].

That the implant has sufficient stability after placement is important for providing the necessary bone formation around the implant and for the optimal distribution of functional forces at the implant-bone interface during healing [15–17].

It can be said that resonance frequency analysis (RFA) is a very important tool for tracking the osseointegration process [18, 19]. RFA is a technique that allows tracking the changes in stability not only during implant placement but also during healing and later periods [20].

Growth factor-containing products have been shown to accelerate bone healing and osseointegration [2, 4]. In this study, it is aimed to evaluate the effect of CGF on implant stability. Based on the results obtained in the study, it will be possible to reduce the amount of time required for osseointegration.

Methods

This study was conducted in compliance with the principles of the Declaration of Helsinki, and approval of the ethics committee required for the study was obtained from the Ethics Committee of the Karadeniz Technical University (2015/21). The procedures to be performed were explained in detail and patients signed the consent forms. The study was carried out on individuals who applied to Karadeniz Technical University, Faculty of Dentistry, Department of Oral and Maxillofacial Surgery to get dental implants for upper jaw tooth deficiencies. In terms of standardization, only patients with implants applied to maxillary anterior and premolar region were included in the study. Cylindrical implants were used in each patient. The diameter of the implant was 3.5 or 4.0 mm, and the length was 10 mm. In patients who underwent tooth extraction, implants were placed 6 months after extraction. Patients rehabilitated with a fixed prosthesis, such as a single crown or bridge, were included in the study. Patients included in the study were randomly assigned to two groups: study and control groups.

Exclusion criteria were identified as:

- Presence of systemic diseases preventing implantation
- Having blood disease to prevent centrifugation
- Previous implantation or augmentation of the same region
- The need for additional bone augmentation procedures (such as maxillary sinus augmentation, distraction osteogenesis)
- Allergy to one of the materials to be used during operation
- Pregnancy
- Smoking

The implanted regions were evaluated preoperatively with panoramic radiography and computed tomography (CT) images. In the study group, the socket walls were laid with CGF membrane while the implant surfaces were washed with the thrombocyte-deprived part of the tube. No different procedure was done to the implants and socket in the control group.

CGF preparation

A standard, disposable, 10-ml non-anticoagulant tube and a matching centrifuge device (MEDIFUGE, Silfradentsrl, S. Sofia, Italy) were used. Intravenous blood samples from the patients were placed in centrifuge tubes without anticoagulants and accelerated for 30 s, centrifuged at 2700 rpm for 4 min, 2400 rpm for 4 min, 2700 rpm for 4 min, and 3000 rpm for 3 min, and decelerated for 36 s to stop. All of these acceleration and deceleration processes are adjusted automatically due to the centrifugal device's feature. Three layers were observed in the tube: red blood cell layer at the bottom, platelet-deprived plasma layer (without cell) at the top, and fibrin gel with concentrated growth factor and platelet aggregation in the middle. First, the uppermost platelet-deprived fraction was removed with a sterile syringe. The layer in the form of a membrane containing the concentrated growth membrane was held with the aid of a hemostatic clamp, separated from the red blood cell layer by cutting with a pair of scissors and then pressed to form a membrane (Fig. 1).

Surgical procedure

All surgical procedures were performed under local anesthesia by the same surgeon. A full-thickness mucoperiosteal flap was removed by incision on the alveolar

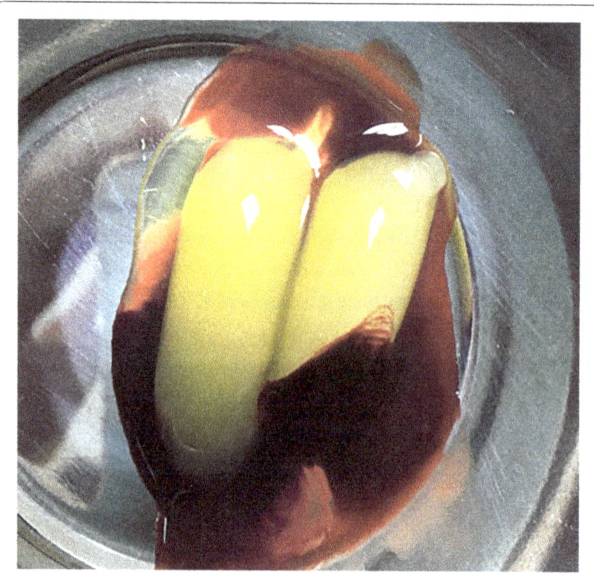

Fig. 1 CGF was obtained after centrifugation

crest. Implant cavities were prepared according to the surgical protocol of the Bego Semados implant system (BEGO Implant Systems GmbH & Co. KG, Bremen, Germany). The final osteotomy diameters were the same as the placed implants. In the study group, the implant cavity walls were laid with CGF membranes all around (Fig. 2). The implants in the study group were irrigated with CGF fluid on their surface and placed in the corresponding socket (Fig. 3). The implants representing the control group were placed in the corresponding socket without any additional procedure. The implant surgery was completed in one session by attaching gingival formers to the implants in both groups. Gingival formers were not covered with soft tissue and mucoperiosteal flaps were sutured with 3/0 silk suture material.

The patients were recommended to apply cold compresses after the surgery. Patients were prescribed antibiotic (amoxicillin + clavulanic acid combination 1000 mg 2 × 1), analgesic (arveles tablet, 25 mg 2 × 1), and antiseptic mouthwash (0.2% chlorhexidine gluconate mouthwash, 3 × 1) for 1 week. The patients were controlled at the 1st week, 4th week and 12th week.

Resonance frequency analysis measurements

The stability of implants by RFA was done using Osstell instrument (Integration Diagnostics, Goteborg, Sweden) with Smartpeg™ (Integration Diagnostics, Goteborg, Sweden), a transducer suitable for implants. The measurement result is obtained from the resonance frequency values by an arithmetic algorithm and given as the ISQ (implant stability quotient) value. At measurement time, the transducer, Smartpeg™, was placed in the region where the prosthetic part is located in the implants.

For measurements, the Osstell™ probe was approximated to the Smartpeg™ from the buccal, palatal, mesial, and distal sides. For each implant, resonance frequency values were obtained in four different directions. The ISQ values were averaged to determine the mean ISQ value for each implant. The ISQ values of the implants were measured during the operation, at the first week and at the fourth week after the operation.

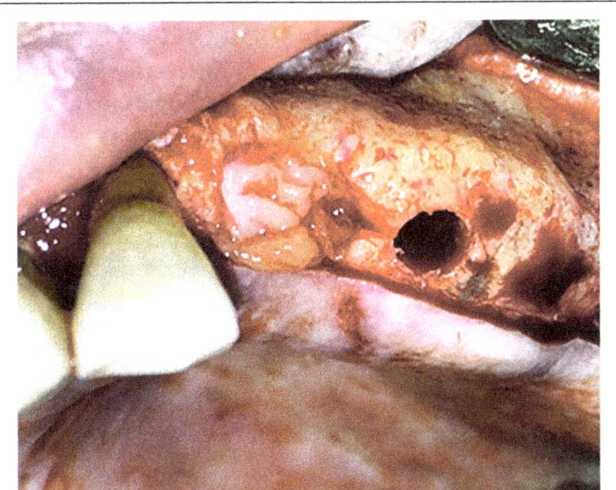

Fig. 2 CGF membrane was applied in study group implant sockets

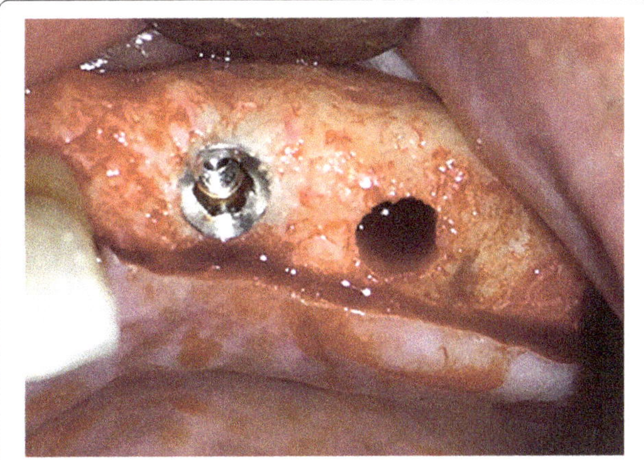

Fig. 3 Implants were placed after application of CGF membrane

Statistical analysis

Independent sample t test was applied between the two groups by taking the differences between the data obtained in these periods. Two-way ANOVA and Fisher's LSD test was used for evaluating the associations among group and insertion torque.

A value of $p < 0.05$ was considered statistically significant. All evaluations were performed with Windows SPSS (version 17.0, IBM Corp., NY, USA) software.

Results

The study includes 12 patients (5 males, 7 females). Patients participating in the study are between 20–68 years of age and the mean age is 44 years. A total of 40 implants were placed, 20 of these were included in the study group (50%), and the other 20 were included in the control group (50%). Twenty-one implants were placed in type 2 bone, 19 implants in type 3 bone (Table 1). The distribution of gender, installed implant diameter, and bone quality between the control group and the experimental group did not show any statistically significant difference. No complications occurred during the postoperative period.

At the implant placement, the average torque for study group was 31,700 ± 2,696 Ncm and for control group was 30,55 ± 2,163 Ncm; there was no significant difference between the two groups ($p = 0.098$).

The mean ISQ values measured after the placement of the implants were 75.75 ± 5.552 for the control group and 78.00 ± 2.828 for the study group. There was no statistically significant difference between control and study groups in terms of initial ISQ values ($p > 0.05$).

Table 1 Demographic data of patients

Case no.	Age	Sex	Group	Implant number
1	20	F	Study	1
2	28	M	Control	3
3	35	F	Study	4
4	32	F	Study	4
5	60	M	Control	5
6	64	F	Study	5
7	52	F	Study	5
8	34	M	Study	1
9	45	F	Control	3
10	48	F	Control	2
11	42	M	Control	3
12	68	F	Control	4

The postoperative ISQ values were found to be 79.40 ± 2.604 for the study group and 73.50 ± 5.226 for the control group at 1st week, 78.60 ± 3.136 for the study group and 73.45 ± 5.680 for the control group at 4th week (Table 2). It was determined that the differences between the groups were statistically significant ($p < 0.05$) and the ISQ measurements at week 1 and week 4 were notably higher in the study group (Fig. 4).

The increase and decrease rates of ISQ values between periods were evaluated by paired t test. Immediate postoperative measurements and 1st week measurements were compared. An increase of 1.40 ± 1.847 was observed in the study group while there was a decrease of 2.25 ± 1.713 in the control group; this difference was statistically significant ($p < 0.001$). When the difference between the immediate postoperative measures and the 4th week measurements were evaluated, an increase of 0.60 ± 2.798 was observed in the study group while a decrease of 2.30 ± 2.774 was observed in the control group; this difference was statistically significant ($p = 0.002$). When the difference between the measurements of the control group and the study group at 1st week and 4th week was evaluated, a decrease of 0.05 ± 1.572 was observed in the control group while a decrease of 0.80 ± 2.215 was observed in the study group; this difference was not statistically significant ($p = 0.224$) (Table 3).

Discussion

Implant stability is one of the important parameters that assess the loading time and dental implant success. Investigators have recommended that implants with ISQ < 49 measured when placed should not be loaded during the 3-month healing period; implants with ISQ ≥ 54 may be loaded. It is emphasized that implants with low primer stabilization value should be waited to reach a stabilization value adequate for prosthetic loading and that they must be protected against mechanical trauma and infection during this time [21].

Table 2 Mean ISQ values in the study and control groups

	Control group	Study group
Immediate	75.75 ± 5.552	78.00 ± 2.828
1st week	73.50 ± 5.226	79.40 ± 2.604
4th week	73.45 ± 5.680	78.60 ± 3.136

In some studies, there is a meaningful reduction in ISQ values measured sometime after the placement of implants [22–24]. Huwiler et al. [24] have indicated that this reduction occurs during 2nd–4th week period while Monov et al. [23] have stated that it occurs as early as 4 days after the operation. In this study also, a decrease in the 1st week ISQ values was observed in the control group. Investigators have suggested that this decrease in stability values and subsequent increase are due to remodeling occurring during bone healing [22–24]. In the implants in the study group, an increase or stability was observed. A statistically significant difference was found between the study and control groups in each period of analysis. This suggests that CGF administration affects the implant primer stability by accelerating the osseointegration process.

Growth factors indicate that they accelerate tissue healing when they function effectively. Studies in the literature have reported that thrombocytes secrete growth factors from α-granules and that these releasing growth factors promote collagen synthesis. Increased collagen synthesis is thought to play a role in increasing soft tissue resistance and in the initiation of callus formation in bone tissue [14, 25–27].

Thrombocytes (platelets) also coexist with other thrombocytes, allowing the fibrin network to remain stable [28]. Within this stable, fibrin clot formation are chemical attractants in surrounding cells such as cell adhesion proteins, thrombocytes, and plasma growth factor; some of these mitogens are related to direct osteogenic cell function [29].

Introduced in 1998 by Marx, PRP is used in oral and maxillofacial surgeries to speed up the recovery of grafts in bone-grafted areas [14, 26–30]. Although many studies have shown that platelet-rich plasma affects bone healing positively, the results of some other studies suggest otherwise [31, 32].

In recent years, the platelet-rich fibrin (PRF) was described by Choukroun as a second-generation platelet concentrate [33]. PRF is defined as leukocyte and platelet-rich fibrin biomaterial. PRF is used to accelerate healing in maxillary sinus augmentation, socket healing after tooth extraction, filling of the cyst cavity, treatment of furcation defects in periodontology, and soft tissue injuries [34].

The positive effects of blood products on healing have also triggered the development of products in different concentrations. One of these products, the concentrated

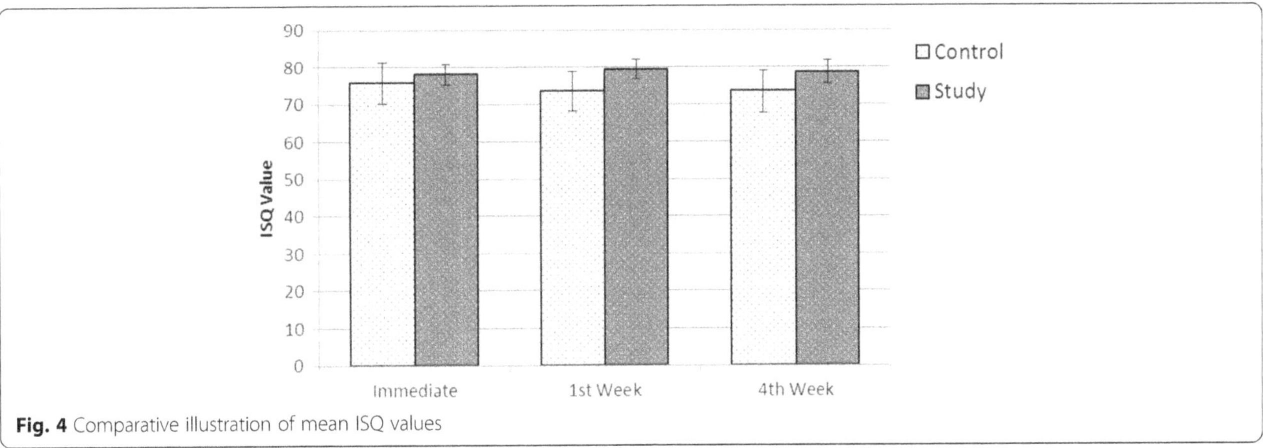

Fig. 4 Comparative illustration of mean ISQ values

growth factor (CGF), was defined by Sacco in 2006 [35]. CGF also has its own centrifugal technique in a manner similar to PRF. A longer and denser fibrin matrix with higher growth factor content was obtained by the different centrifugation technique [35].

Regional CGF administration increases FGF-β or VEGF release, which plays an active role in angiogenesis, as well as enhancing neutrophil migration by performing integrin release. It has also been shown that CGF contains such growth factors and CD34-positive cells [35]. It has been reported that CD34-positive cells in the cells also provide angiogenesis, neovascularization, and vascular continuity [36, 37].

In an animal study, CGF, PRF, and PRP were placed separately in the defects formed in the rabbit skull in the study group; the defects were left empty in the control group. Histomorphometric analysis revealed statistically significant differences between control and study groups in the growth of new bone formation at 6 and 12 weeks. In the study group, the greatest bone formation was observed in the CGF-treated group but this difference was not statistically significant [38]. In a study by Takeda et al. performed on rats, it was observed that cell proliferation and osteoblastic differentiation in the cell culture from the CGF-treated group was significantly higher than in the other groups [39].

In a study by Monov et al. using PRP around the implant, a higher stability value was obtained in the study group during the early recovery period (6 weeks) although difference between the groups was not statistically significant [23]. Kim et al. reported in a study that there was a statistically significant increase in bone-implant contact with PRP administration in the vicinity of the implant [40].

Table 3 Mean ISQ value changes between study and control groups

	Control group	Study group
Immediate–1st week	−2.25 ± 1.713	1.40 ± 1.847
Immediate–4th week	−2.30 ± 2.774	0.60 ± 2.798
1st Week–4th week	−0.05 ± 1.572	−0.80 ± 2.215

Based on all these results, it can be said that CGF and PRF accelerated the implant osseointegration process and affected the stabilization values positively. It has been reported that CGF contains more growth factors than other platelet preparations [35]. It was observed in our study that CGF has favorable effects on implant healing period. There is no publication on the effect of CGF on the stability of dental implants during healing period. For this reason, we investigated the effect of CGF on the stability of dental implants in our study.

Conclusions

Considering this data, it appears that application of CGF enhanced stability of implants and accelerated osseointegration in the early period. CGF has positive effects on the ISQ value at the first week and fourth week. Further laboratory studies are needed to demonstrate the positive effects of blood products on the osseointegration process at the histopathological level.

Abbreviations

BMP: Bone morphogenetic protein; CGF: Concentrated growth factor; CT: Computed tomography; IGF: Insulin-like growth factor; PDGF: Platelet-derived growth factor; PRF: Platelet-rich fibrin; PRP: Platelet-rich plasma; RFA: Resonance frequency analysis; TGF-β1: Transforming growth factor-β1; TGF-β2: Transforming growth factor-β2; VEGF: Vascular endothelial growth factor

Funding

The authors declare no funds for the research.

Authors' contributions

CP, OY, CC, and EB designed the study, performed the experiments, and wrote the manuscript. CP, OY, and CC collected the data in this study. EB analyzed the date statistically. All authors read and approved the final version of the manuscript

Competing interests

Cagasan Pirpir, Onur Yilmaz, Celal Candarli and Emre Balaban declare that they have no competing interests.

References

1. Raghavendra S, Wood MC, Taylor TD. Early wound healing around endosseous implants: a review of the literature. Int J Oral Maxillofac Implants. 2005;20(3):425–31.
2. Oncu E, Bayram B, Kantarci A, Gulsever S, Alaaddinoglu EE. Positive effect of platelet rich fibrin on osseointegration. Med Oral Patol Oral Cir Bucal. 2016; 21(5):e601–7.
3. Anitua E. Plasma rich in growth factors: preliminary results of use in the preparation of future sites for implants. Int J Oral Maxillofac Implants. 1999; 14(4):529–35.
4. Anitua E, Andia I, Ardanza B, Nurden P, Nurden AT. Autologous platelets as a source of proteins for healing and tissue regeneration. Thromb Haemost. 2004;91(1):4–15.
5. Anitua E, Orive G, Pla R, Roman P, Serrano V, Andia I. The effects of PRGF on bone regeneration and on titanium implant osseointegration in goats: a histologic and histomorphometric study. J Biomed Mater Res A. 2009;91(1): 158–65.
6. Bhanot S, Alex JC. Current applications of platelet gels in facial plastic surgery. Facial Plast Surg. 2002;18(1):27–33.
7. Coetzee JC, Pomeroy GC, Watts JD, Barrow C. The use of autologous concentrated growth factors to promote syndesmosis fusion in the agility total ankle replacement. A preliminary study. Foot Ankle Int. 2005;26(10):840–6.
8. Rutkowski JL, Thomas JM, Bering CL, Speicher JL, Radio NM, Smith DM, et al. Analysis of a rapid, simple, and inexpensive technique used to obtain platelet-rich plasma for use in clinical practice. J Oral Implantol. 2008;34(1): 25–33.
9. Dohan Ehrenfest DM, de Peppo GM, Doglioli P, Sammartino G. Slow release of growth factors and thrombospondin-1 in Choukroun's platelet-rich fibrin (PRF): a gold standard to achieve for all surgical platelet concentrates technologies. Growth Factors. 2009;27(1):63–9.
10. Sohn DS, Heo JU, Kwak DH, Kim DE, Kim JM, Moon JW, et al. Bone regeneration in the maxillary sinus using an autologous fibrin-rich block with concentrated growth factors alone. Implant Dent. 2011;20(5):389–95.
11. Gassling VL, Acil Y, Springer IN, Hubert N, Wiltfang J. Platelet-rich plasma and platelet-rich fibrin in human cell culture. Oral Surg Oral Med Oral Pathol Oral Radiol Endod. 2009;108(1):48–55.
12. Nurden AT, Nurden P, Sanchez M, Andia I, Anitua E. Platelets and wound healing. Front Biosci. 2008;13:3532–48.
13. Anitua E, Sanchez M, Zalduendo MM, de la Fuente M, Prado R, Orive G, et al. Fibroblastic response to treatment with different preparations rich in growth factors. Cell Prolif. 2009;42(2):162–70.
14. He L, Lin Y, Hu X, Zhang Y, Wu H. A comparative study of platelet-rich fibrin (PRF) and platelet-rich plasma (PRP) on the effect of proliferation and differentiation of rat osteoblasts in vitro. Oral Surg Oral Med Oral Pathol Oral Radiol Endod. 2009;108(5):707–13.
15. Meredith N. A review of nondestructive test methods and their application to measure the stability and osseointegration of bone anchored endosseous implants. Crit Rev Biomed Eng. 1998;26(4):275–91.
16. Salvi GE, Lang NP. Diagnostic parameters for monitoring peri-implant conditions. Int J Oral Maxillofac Implants. 2004;19(Suppl):116–27.
17. Atsumi M, Park SH, Wang HL. Methods used to assess implant stability: current status. Int J Oral Maxillofac Implants. 2007;22(5):743–54.
18. Meredith N. Assessment of implant stability as a prognostic determinant. Int J Prosthodont. 1998;11(5):491–501.
19. Sennerby L, Meredith N. Resonance frequency analysis: measuring implant stability and osseointegration. Compend Contin Educ Dent. 1998;19(5):493–8. 500, 2; quiz 4.
20. Quesada-Garcia MP, Prados-Sanchez E, Olmedo-Gaya MV, Munoz-Soto E, Gonzalez-Rodriguez MP, Valllecillo-Capilla M. Measurement of dental implant stability by resonance frequency analysis: a review of the literature. Med Oral Patol Oral Cir Bucal. 2009;14(10):e538–46.
21. Nedir R, Bischof M, Szmukler-Moncler S, Bernard JP, Samson J. Predicting osseointegration by means of implant primary stability. Clin Oral Implants Res. 2004;15(5):520–8.
22. Barewal RM, Oates TW, Meredith N, Cochran DL. Resonance frequency measurement of implant stability in vivo on implants with a sandblasted and acid-etched surface. Int J Oral Maxillofac Implants. 2003;18(5):641 51.
23. Monov G, Fuerst G, Tepper G, Watzak G, Zechner W, Watzek G. The effect of platelet-rich plasma upon implant stability measured by resonance frequency analysis in the lower anterior mandibles. Clin Oral Implants Res. 2005;16(4):461–5.
24. Huwiler MA, Pjetursson BE, Bosshardt DD, Salvi GE, Lang NP. Resonance frequency analysis in relation to jawbone characteristics and during early healing of implant installation. Clin Oral Implants Res. 2007;18(3):275–80.
25. Kroese-Deutman HC, Vehof JW, Spauwen PH, Stoelinga PJ, Jansen JA. Orthotopic bone formation in titanium fiber mesh loaded with platelet-rich plasma and placed in segmental defects. Int J Oral Maxillofac Surg. 2008; 37(6):542–9.
26. Hsu CW, Yuan K, Tseng CC. The negative effect of platelet-rich plasma on the growth of human cells is associated with secreted thrombospondin-1. Oral Surg Oral Med Oral Pathol Oral Radiol Endod. 2009;107(2):185–92.
27. Shen YX, Fan ZH, Zhao JG, Zhang P. The application of platelet-rich plasma may be a novel treatment for central nervous system diseases. Med Hypotheses. 2009;73(6):1038–40.
28. Lam WA, Chaudhuri O, Crow A, Webster KD, Li TD, Kita A, et al. Mechanics and contraction dynamics of single platelets and implications for clot stiffening. Nat Mater. 2011;10(1):61–6.
29. Gruber R, Karreth F, Kandler B, Fuerst G, Rot A, Fischer MB, et al. Platelet-released supernatants increase migration and proliferation, and decrease osteogenic differentiation of bone marrow-derived mesenchymal progenitor cells under in vitro conditions. Platelets. 2004;15(1):29–35.
30. Choi BH, Zhu SJ, Kim BY, Huh JY, Lee SH, Jung JH. Effect of platelet-rich plasma (PRP) concentration on the viability and proliferation of alveolar bone cells: an in vitro study. Int J Oral Maxillofac Surg. 2005;34(4):420–4.
31. Mooren RE, Hendriks EJ, van den Beucken JJ, Merkx MA, Meijer GJ, Jansen JA, et al. The effect of platelet-rich plasma in vitro on primary cells: rat osteoblast-like cells and human endothelial cells. Tissue Eng Part A. 2010; 16(10):3159–72.
32. Aghaloo TL, Moy PK, Freymiller EG. Investigation of platelet-rich plasma in rabbit cranial defects: a pilot study. J Oral Maxillofac Surg. 2002;60(10):1176–81.
33. Choukroun J, Diss A, Simonpieri A, Girard MO, Schoeffler C, Dohan SL, et al. Platelet-rich fibrin (PRF): a second-generation platelet concentrate. Part IV: clinical effects on tissue healing. Oral Surg Oral Med Oral Pathol Oral Radiol Endod. 2006;101(3):e56–60.
34. Prakash S, Thakur A. Platelet concentrates: past, present and future. J Maxillofac Oral Surg. 2011;10(1):45–9.
35. Rodella LF, Favero G, Boninsegna R, Buffoli B, Labanca M, Scari G, et al. Growth factors, CD34 positive cells, and fibrin network analysis in concentrated growth factors fraction. Microsc Res Tech. 2011;74(8):772–7.
36. Ademokun JA, Chapman C, Dunn J, Lander D, Mair K, Proctor SJ, et al. Umbilical cord blood collection and separation for haematopoietic progenitor cell banking. Bone Marrow Transplant. 1997;19(10):1023–8.
37. Majka M, Janowska-Wieczorek A, Ratajczak J, Ehrenman K, Pietrzkowski Z, Kowalska MA, et al. Numerous growth factors, cytokines, and chemokines are secreted by human CD34(+) cells, myeloblasts, erythroblasts, and megakaryoblasts and regulate normal hematopoiesis in an autocrine/ paracrine manner. Blood. 2001;97(10):3075–85.
38. Kim TH, Kim SH, Sandor GK, Kim YD. Comparison of platelet-rich plasma (PRP), platelet-rich fibrin (PRF), and concentrated growth factor (CGF) in rabbit-skull defect healing. Arch Oral Biol. 2014;59(5):550–8.
39. Takeda Y, Katsutoshi K, Matsuzaka K, Inoue T. The effect of concentrated growth factor on Rat bone marrow cells in vitro and on calvarial bone healing in vivo. Int J Oral Maxillofac Implants. 2015;30(5):1187–96.
40. Kim SG, Chung CH, Kim YK, Park JC, Lim SC. Use of particulate dentin-plaster of Paris combination with/without platelet-rich plasma in the treatment of bone defects around implants. Int J Oral Maxillofac Implants. 2002;17(1):86–94.

19

Clinical outcome of alveolar ridge augmentation with individualized CAD-CAM-produced titanium mesh

K. Sagheb[1†], E. Schiegnitz[1*†], M. Moergel[1], C. Walter[1,2], B. Al-Nawas[1] and W. Wagner[1]

Abstract

Background: The augmentation of the jaw has been and continues to be a sophisticated therapy in implantology. Modern CAD-CAM technologies lead to revival of old and established augmentation techniques such as the use of titanium mesh (TM) for bone augmentation. The aim of this retrospective study was to evaluate the clinical outcome of an individualized CAD-CAM-produced TM based on the CT/DVT-DICOM data of the patients for the first time.

Methods: In 17 patients, 21 different regions were augmented with an individualized CAD-CAM-produced TM (Yxoss CBR®, Filderstadt, Germany). For the augmentation, a mixture of autologous bone and deproteinized bovine bone mineral (DBBM) or autologous bone alone was used. Reentry with explantation of the TM and simultaneous implantation of 44 implants were performed after 6 months. Preoperative and 6-month postoperative cone beam computed tomographies (CBCT) were performed to measure the gained bone height.

Results: The success rate for the bone grafting procedure was 100%. Thirty-three percent of cases presented an exposure of the TM during the healing period. However, premature removal of these exposed meshes was not necessary. Exposure rate in augmentations performed with mid-crestal incisions was higher than in augmentations performed with a modified poncho incision (45.5 vs. 20%, $p = 0.221$). In addition, exposure rates in the maxilla were significantly higher than in the mandible (66.7 vs. 8.3%, $p = 0.009$). Gender, smoking, periodontal disease, gingiva type, used augmentation material, and used membrane had no significant influence on the exposure rate ($p > 0.05$). The mean vertical augmentation was 6.5 ± 1.7 mm, and the mean horizontal augmentation was 5.5 ± 1.9 mm. Implant survival rate after a mean follow-up of 12 ± 6 months after reentry was 100%.

Conclusion: Within the limits of the retrospective character of this study, this study shows for the first time that individualized CAD-CAM TM provide a sufficient and safe augmentation technique, especially for vertical and combined defects. However, the soft tissue handling for sufficient mesh covering remains one of the most critical steps using this technique.

Keywords: CAD-CAM , Titanium mesh, Augmentation, Bone atrophy, Bone regeneration, PRF

Background

Dental implant placement is an effective treatment method for the replacement of lost teeth with high survival rates after long-term follow-up [1–3]. However, the long-term success and stability of implants in function are directly correlated with the quality and quantity of the available bone at the prospective implant site [4, 5]. Despite the development of various techniques and augmentation materials, the reestablishment of an adequate amount of bone especially in the vertical direction remains challenging. Many different augmentation procedures, depending on location and size of the defect, were described and have been studied extensively in human and animal studies by evaluating healing events via histological, radiological, and clinical outcomes [6].

The use of conventional titanium meshes (TM) was first described for the reconstruction of osseous-maxillo-facial defects and secondarily introduced for osseous restoration

* Correspondence: schiegnitz@gmx.com
[†]Equal contributors
[1]Department of Oral and Maxillofacial Surgery, Plastic Surgery, University Medical Centre of the Johannes Gutenberg-University Mainz, Mainz, Germany
Full list of author information is available at the end of the article

of deficient edentulous maxillary ridges [7–9]. In addition, they were used for localized alveolar ridge augmentation of ridge defects with simultaneous and secondary implant insertion [10–12]. Further clinical studies showed predictable results for both lateral and vertical bone reconstruction with this titanium mesh technique [13]. These conventional TM are designed as planar plates. Therefore, intraoperative manual shaping and bending of the premade TM according to the individual defect is necessary, which is manually challenging and time-consuming [14, 15]. Furthermore, the corners and edges of these cut and bended meshes possibly provoke damages to the gingiva and mesh exposure. The CAD-CAM technology provides a sufficient solution for these disadvantages. Based on the cone beam computed tomography (CBCT) scan data of the bony defect and a digital work flow system, individualized titanium mesh cages can be created that it can fit perfectly over the bone defect of the augmentation site. However, due to the stiffness of the TM with mechanical irritation to the mucosal flap, the risk of flap dehiscence with exposure of the graft and possible particular or even complete loss of the graft material remains [16, 17].

The aim of this clinical study was to present the clinical outcome of individualized CAD-CAM-produced TM in combination with particulate autogenous bone mixed with deproteinized bovine bone mineral (DBBM) used to augment horizontal and/or vertical bony defects in both maxillary and mandibular arches, within a two-stage technique. Furthermore, gained horizontal and vertical bone height and the influence of incision technique, location, and reason of bone defect on dehiscence rate and augmentation success were evaluated.

Methods

Study design

In a retrospective study, the clinical outcome of an individualized CAD-CAM-produced TM (Yxoss CBR®, Filderstadt, Germany) inserted by experienced surgeons in the Department of Oral and Maxillofacial Surgery of the University Medical Centre Mainz, Germany, between December 2014 and January 2017, was analyzed. Therefore, all patients with this CAD-CAM mesh augmentation and reentry operation for implant insertion in this time period were included in this study. There were no patients excluded from this study. The retrospective data analysis was conducted in accordance with the Helsinki Declaration of 1975, as revised in 2008, and all patients signed an informed consent. After consulting the local ethic committee, the decision was that due to the retrospective character of this study with no additional data acquisition, no ethical approval was needed according to the hospital laws of the appropriate state (Landeskrankenhausgesetz Rhineland Palatinate, Germany).

Surgical procedure

With the Customized Bone Regeneration (CBR®) technology, the manufacturing of custom-molded protective TM is achieved. Using the DICOM data of the CBCT scan of the defect region, an individualized mesh was produced using the CAD-CAM technology by ReOss Ltd. (Filderstadt, Germany). The meshes were produced using three-dimensional printing. Surgeries were performed under local or anesthesia or in general anesthesia. Depending on the defect configuration, a mid-crestal or a modified poncho incision was performed. For the modified poncho, the incision was made in the vestibulum parallel to the alveolar ridge by a tunneling preparation (Fig. 1). This poncho technique was preferred in pronounced vertical defects. After incision, preparation of a mucoperiosteal flap, debridement of scar tissue, and exposure of the defect were conducted. Then, a passive tension-free fit of the TM was verified. Autologous bone was harvested with bone scraper from the intraoral regions, such as the tuber maxillae, the symphysis, the mandibular body, and the retromolar pad region (Safescraper®, Zimmer Biomet, Germany) or from the iliac crest. The TM was loaded with an equal mixture of deproteinized bovine bone mineral (Bio-Oss®, Geistlich Biomaterials, Switzerland) and autologous bone or autologous bone alone and fitted to the defect. The rationale of mixing autogenous bone with DBBM is to combine the scaffold properties of the xenograft with the osteogenic and osteoinductive properties of the autograft [18–20]. To fix the TM in place, two bone screws were used. TM were covered in situ with nothing, a resorbable collagen membrane (Bio-Gide®, Geistlich Biomaterials, Switzerland) alone, or a resorbable collagen membrane, followed by platelet-rich fibrin (PRF) membranes (Choukroun A-PRF™) in a double-layer technique. The PRF membranes were produced according to the manufacturer's protocol. All patients underwent an oral antibiotic therapy with amoxicillin 1000 mg (1 to 0–1) for 5 days starting at the operation day. Reentry with explantation of the TM and simultaneous implantation were performed after a 6-month healing period. Figures 2, 3, 4, 5, 6, 7, and 8 present a clinical case.

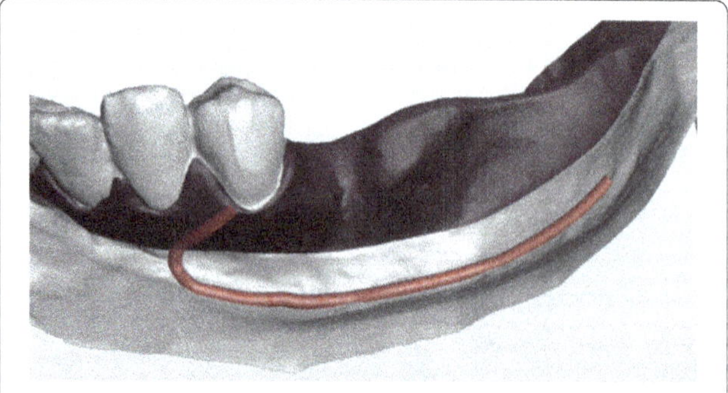

Fig. 1 Schematic drawing of the poncho flap approach

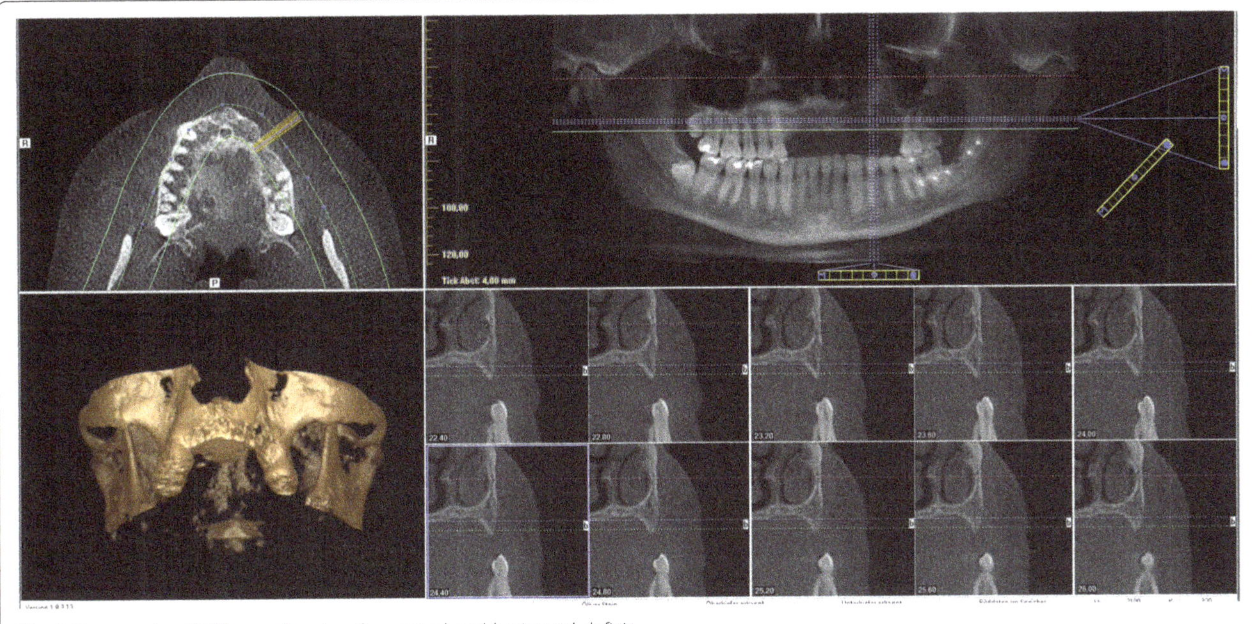

Fig. 2 Preoperative CBCT scan showing the vertical and horizontal deficit

Radiographic analysis

Cone beam computed tomography (CBCT) of the treated sites was performed before augmentation procedure and 6 months postoperatively at time of reentry. Craniofacial bone and TM showed different radio-opacity, which allowed their easy differentiation on the scans after regulating the brightness and contrast. In our department, two different CBCTs were available (Accuitomo, J. Morita Corporation, Japan and 3D eXamVision, Kavo Dental GmbH, Germany). For large defects and in existence of possible other indications (e.g., sinus maxillary diagnostic), the 3D eXamVision was used. Small locoregional defects were imaged with the Accuitomo. Gained bone height and width was quantified using the KaVo-eXam Vision software (Kavo Dental GmbH, Germany) and One Volume Viewer software (J. Morita Corporation, Japan) on one descriptive slide of the CBCT scan [21]. Therefore, the margins of the basal and grafted bone and the rim of the TM were defined, and linear measurements for vertical and horizontal bone augmentation were made on one descriptive coronal section in a midalveolar position (Fig. 9). For horizontal bone augmentation, the widest horizontal distance in midalveolar position was evaluated. However, this evaluation technique has to be assessed critically as it is hard to distinguish between graft material and real new bone. A layer of soft tissue with some embedded granules underneath the mesh, which is usually removed at the time of implant insertion and mesh removal, could not be subtracted from the augmentation bone gain regularly.

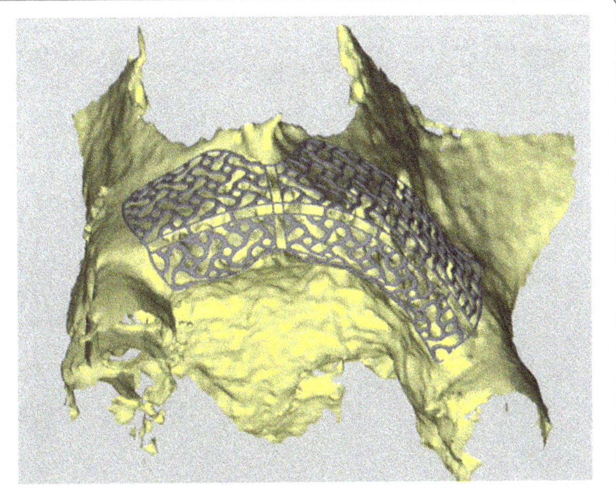

Fig. 3 3D design of the CAD-CAM-based individualized TM by ReOss®

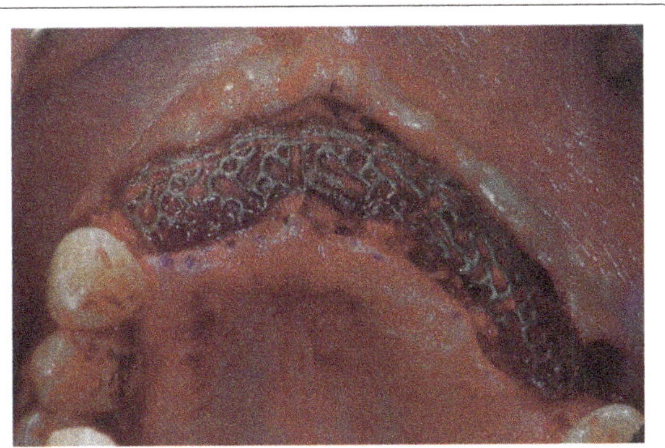

Fig. 4 Intraoperative clinical picture after insertion of CAD-CAM mesh

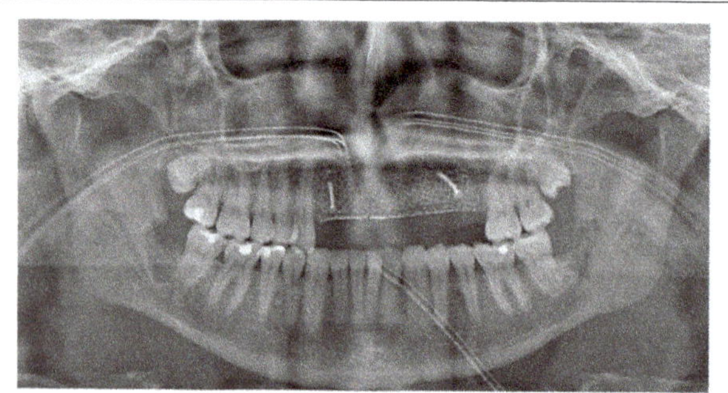

Fig. 5 Orthopantomogram after augmentation

Statistics

The statistical analysis was performed using the IBM® SPSS® Statistics version 23.0 for Windows®. We report descriptive *p* values of tests, and no adjustment to multiple testing due to the low case number was performed. Chi-quadrat-test was performed to identify potential influencing factors for a higher risk of exposure of the TM.

Results

Patient data

In the investigated time period, 17 patients received 21 TM augmentations. Fourteen of these patients were women and three men. Mean age at the time of augmentation was 37 ± 15 years (17–64 years). Twelve of the patients were non-smoker, and 5 patients were smoker. In 8 patients, a steady periodontal disease could be detected. Sixty-five percent (n = 11) of the patients presented a thin gingival morphotype A and 35% (n = 6) of the patients a thick gingival morphotype B. Fifty-seven percent (n = 12) of the augmented regions were located in the mandible and 43% (n = 9) in the maxilla. The length of the defects ranged from a minimum of one to a maximum of nine teeth (mean 3 ± 2 teeth). A mid-crestal incision was performed in 11 augmentation sides (52%), and a modified poncho incision was applied in 10 augmentation sides (48%). In 19 augmented sites, a mixture of deproteinized bovine bone mineral and autologous bone was used. In two augmented sites, autologous bone alone was inserted. In two cases, no membrane for covering the TM was used, in six cases, a resorbable collagen membrane, and in 13 cases, a double layer of collagen membrane, and PRF membranes were inserted.

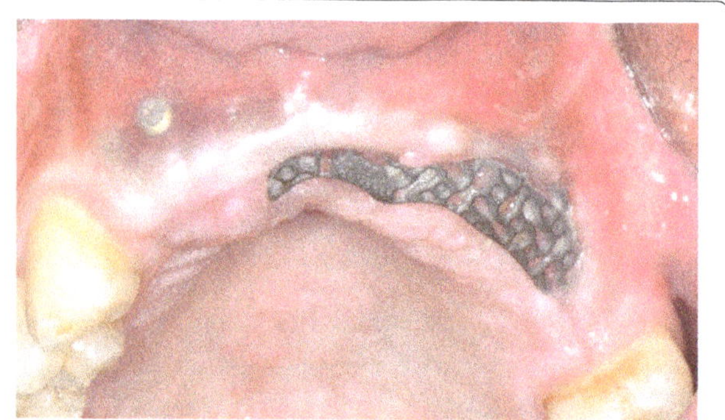

Fig. 6 Clinical picture after 6 months showing an exposure of the mesh

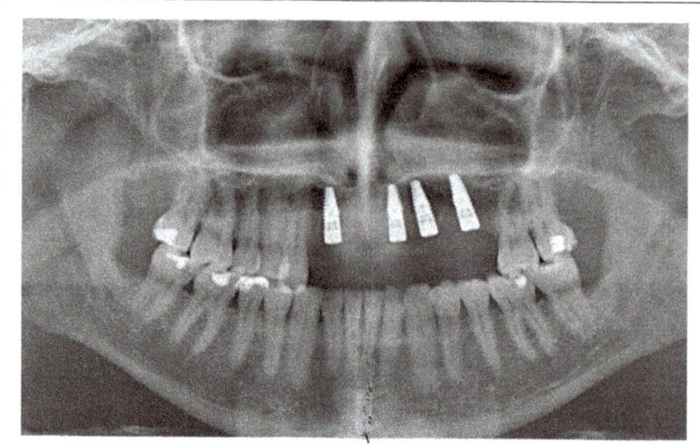

Fig. 7 Orthopantomogram after implant insertion

Clinical and radiological outcome

In all cases, the individualized TM could easily be placed into the planned area of augmentation. The postoperative healing was uneventful in 14 cases (67%) during the follow-up time of 6 months until reentry. In seven cases (33%), an exposure of the TM after a period ranging from 5 to 12 weeks from first-stage surgery was seen. All the dehiscences appeared in the area of the suture. Patients with TM exposure were treated with chlorhexidine mouthwash rinse. The premature removal of the TM after exposure was necessary in none of the cases, and all the preoperatively planed implantations could be carried out. Therefore, exposure of the TM had no negative influence on the clinical outcome of the augmentation procedure and success of the bone grafting procedure was 100%. Exposure rate in augmentations performed

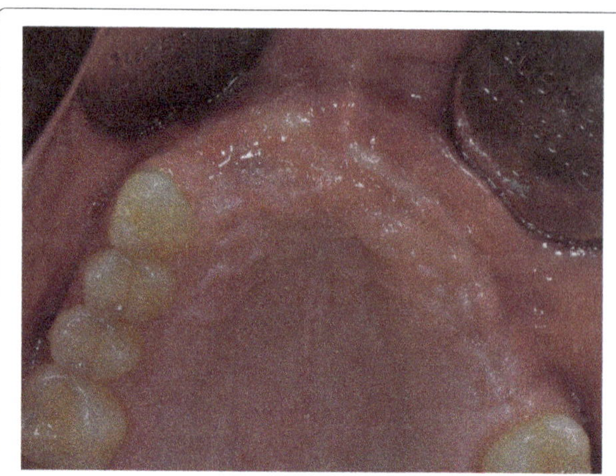

Fig. 8 Clinical picture after implant insertion

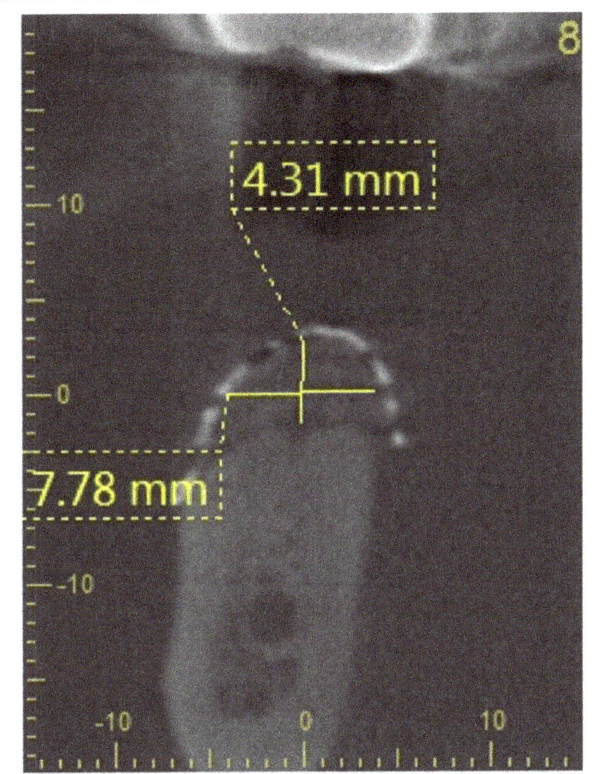

Fig. 9 Representative picture of analysis of vertical and horizontal bone augmentation on CBCT scan

with mid-crestal incisions (45.5%) was higher than in augmentations performed with a modified poncho incision (20%), however, not statistically significant ($p = 0.221$). In addition, exposure rates in the maxilla were significantly higher than in the mandible (66.7 vs. 8.3%, $p = 0.009$). Gender, smoking, periodontal disease, gingiva type, used augmentation material, and used membrane had no significant influence on exposure rates ($p > 0.05$). Comparing the preoperative and 6-month postoperative cone beam computed tomography (CBCT), a mean vertical augmentation of 6.5 ± 1.7 mm and a mean horizontal augmentation of 5.5 ± 1.9 mm was achieved (Fig. 10). After a mean follow-up of 12 ± 6 months after second-stage surgery, none of the 44 inserted implants was lost, indicating a survival rate of 100%.

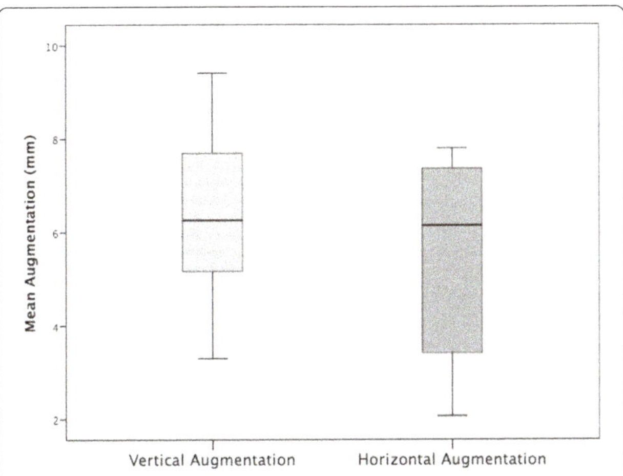

Fig. 10 Mean vertical and horizontal augmentation height (mm)

Discussion

The vertical and horizontal regeneration of resorbed alveolar ridges remains a challenging surgical procedure, especially in the case of extensive bone atrophy. During the past years, different augmentation techniques have been proposed to restore an adequate bone volume. The aim of this study was to evaluate a technique for ridge augmentation in the maxilla and mandible using an individualized CAD-CAM-produced titanium mesh.

In our study, titanium mesh exposure occurred in 33% of the augmented sites. However, a premature removal of these exposed meshes was not necessary in any of these cases. In addition, exposure of the mesh did not affect the final outcome of the augmentation as implant insertion was possible in all cases in the desired position, indicating a success rate of 100% for the augmentation technique. The titanium mesh exposure is a common complication, with reported exposure rates between 0 and 80% in the international literature [11, 17]. Sumida et al. investigated custom-made titanium devices for bone augmentation compared to conventional titanium meshes in 26 patients [15]. Mucosal rupture occurred in a patient in the custom-made group (7.7%) and 3 in the conventional group (23.1%), indicating better results for the individualized mesh, however, neither statistically nor clinically significant. In a further clinical study investigating a conventional titanium mesh, exposure occurred in 6 of the 17 patients (35%) [22]. Two of them were early exposures (within 2 weeks) and 4 of them late exposures. Corinaldesi et al. showed an exposure rate of 14.8% [23]. These cases necessitated premature removal of the titanium mesh. In these exposed sites, reduction in mean bone regeneration was observed compared to mesh-retained sites in patients who received simultaneous augmentation and implant placement. A critical point discussed in the international literature is the time elapsed between augmentation procedure and exposure. An early exposure within the first weeks showed a negative impact on bone regeneration in contrast to a late exposure [12, 23–25]. To prevent such an exposure, an accurate soft tissue handling in terms of tension-free flaps over the mesh is mandatory.

In our study, PRF membranes were additionally to collagen membranes used to cover the CAD-CAM mesh. The aim of this clinical approach was to improve and accelerate wound healing. The results with the low exposure rates and the sufficient augmentation heights indicated that these

PRF membranes are a promising technique. However, due to low case number in the control group without a PRF membrane, definitive conclusions are not possible. The positive effects of PRF regarding wound healing may be explained by the contents of the PRF clot. These clots contain stem cells, fibrin, platelets, and leucocytes [26, 27]. Furthermore, PRF membranes have a sustained release of high quantities of the growth factors TGFbeta-1, PDGF-AB, and VEGF and coagulation matricellular glycoprotein (thrombospondin-1, TSP-1) during 7 days [27]. Therefore, PRF is a biodegradable scaffold that promotes the development of microvascularization and epithelial cell migration to its surface [28, 29]. There are several clinical studies and systematic reviews that show the promising potential of PRF for bone and soft tissue regeneration [28, 30, 31]. Torres et al. examined the effect of platelet-rich plasma in preventing mesh exposure by using it to cover conventional meshes [32]. In this study, 43 alveolar bone augmentations with the mesh technique using anorganic bovine bone as graft material were performed. In half of the patients, the meshes were covered with platelet-rich plasma, whereas in the other half, the meshes were not. The results showed that mesh exposure was significantly less in the platelet-rich plasma group as well as that bone augmentation was higher in the platelet-rich plasma group than in the control group. In conclusion, these results promote the use of PRP/PRF in augmentation procedures.

Besides the use of membranes, the application of a sufficient incision technique is crucial to avoid dehiscences. In our study, augmentations performed with a modified poncho incision had lower exposure rates than augmentations performed with a mid-crestal incision. All the dehiscences appeared in the area of the suture. Therefore, positioning the margin of the wound in the vestibulum and in distance to the mesh seems to reduce the risk for an exposure of the TM as the margin of a wound represents the most important nutritional structure for survival and the basis for reliable wound healing [33, 34]. In addition, exposure rate in the maxilla was significantly higher than in the mandible. This could be explained with the higher augmentations in the maxilla in our study. In our study, both craniofacial and iliac crest bones were used for augmentation procedures. This may influence later bone resorption and long-term stability. However, a recent influence of the used material on augmentation success was not seen.

The results showed that in all 21 augmented sites, a significant ridge augmentation was achieved, with a mean vertical augmentation of 6.5 ± 1.7 mm and a mean horizontal augmentation of 5.5 ± 1.9 mm. To our best knowledge, this is the first study investigating these parameters in individualized CAD-CAM-produced titanium meshes. For conventional titanium meshes, several studies were published. Torres et al. investigated the effectiveness of anorganic bovine bone in alveolar bone augmentation with the titanium mesh technique [32]. The average bone height gained was 3.3 ± 0.2 mm and the average bone width 3.9 ± 0.2 mm. Corinaldesi et al. indicated in 24 patients with 27 micromeshes a mean vertical bone augmentation of 5.4 ± 1.81 mm [23]. Pieri et al. examined the clinical and radiographic parameters of implants placed in augmented ridges using a 70:30 mixture of autogenous bone and bovine bone mineral in association with titanium meshes [21]. Radiographic assessment showed a mean vertical augmentation of 3.71 ± 1.24 mm and mean horizontal augmentation of 4.16 ± 0.59 mm. Proussaefs and Lozada applied a titanium mesh for localized alveolar ridge augmentation with an equal mixture of autogenous bone and bovine bone mineral [22]. Radiographic evaluation indicated a mean vertical ridge augmentation of 2.56 ± 1.32 mm and a mean horizontal ridge augmentation of 3.75 ± 1.33. In total, the mesh technique is a predictable procedure with sufficient horizontal and vertical bone gain.

Conclusions

Within the limitations of this study, being retrospective and having no control group, the results show that individualized CAD-CAM-produced titanium meshes are a safe and predictable procedure for large vertical and horizontal ridge augmentations. The soft tissue covering remains one of the most critical steps using this technique. However, exposure of the mesh does not result in complete loss of the augmentation.

Authors' contributions

KS, ES, MM, CW, BA-N, and WW made substantial contributions to the conception or design of the work, or the acquisition, analysis, or interpretation of the data for the work, and drafted the work or revised it critically for important intellectual content. KS, ES, MM, CW, BA-N, and WW had an agreement to be accountable for all the aspects of the work in 'ensuring that questions related to the accuracy or integrity of any part of the work are appropriately investigated and resolved. All authors gave final approval of the version to be published.

Competing interests

Keyvan Sagheb reports personal fees and grants from Dentsply, Geistlich, and Nobel Biocare outside the submitted work. Eik Schiegnitz reports personal fees and grants from Septodont, Dentsply, Geistlich, and Straumann outside the submitted work. Maximilian Moergel reports grants from Camlog outside the submitted work. Christian Walter reports grants and personal fees from Straumann outside the submitted work. Bilal Al-Nawas reports grants and personal fees from Camlog, Dentsply, Geistlich, Nobel Biocare, and Straumann outside the submitted work. Wilfried Wagner reports grants and personal fees from Camlog, Dentsply, Geistlich, Nobel Biocare, Straumann, and Zimmer outside the submitted work.

Author details

[1]Department of Oral and Maxillofacial Surgery, Plastic Surgery, University Medical Centre of the Johannes Gutenberg-University Mainz, Mainz, Germany. [2]Mediplus, Oral and Maxillofacial Surgery, Private Praxis, Mainz, Germany.

References

1. Moraschini V, Poubel LA, Ferreira VF, Barboza ES. Evaluation of survival and success rates of dental implants reported in longitudinal studies with a follow-up period of at least 10 years: a systematic review. Int J Oral Maxillofac Surg. 2015;44(3):377–88. PubMed PMID: 25467739
2. Al-Nawas B, Kammerer PW, Morbach T, Ladwein C, Wegener J, Wagner W. Ten-year retrospective follow-up study of the TiOblast dental implant. Clin Implant Dent Relat Res. 2012;14(1):127–34. PubMed PMID: 20156231
3. Schiegnitz E, Al-Nawas B, Tegner A, Sagheb K, Berres M, Kammerer PW, et al. Clinical and radiological long-term outcome of a tapered implant system with special emphasis on the influence of augmentation procedures. Clin Implant Dent Relat Res. 2016;18(4):810–20. PubMed PMID: 25810365
4. Al-Nawas B, Schiegnitz E. Augmentation procedures using bone substitute materials or autogenous bone—a systematic review and meta-analysis. European journal of oral implantology. 2014;7(Suppl 2):S219–34. PubMed PMID: 24977257
5. Aghaloo TL, Moy PK. Which hard tissue augmentation techniques are the most successful in furnishing bony support for implant placement? Int J Oral Maxillofac Implants. 2007;22(Suppl):49–70. PubMed PMID: 18437791
6. Kammerer PW, Palarie V, Schiegnitz E, Nacu V, Draenert FG, Al-Nawas B. Influence of a collagen membrane and recombinant platelet-derived growth factor on vertical bone augmentation in implant-fixed deproteinized bovine bone—animal pilot study. Clin Oral Implants Res. 2013;24(11):1222–30. PubMed PMID: 22762383
7. Boyne PJ. Restoration of osseous defects in maxillofacial casualities. J Am Dent Assoc. 1969;78(4):767–76. PubMed PMID: 4975262
8. Boyne PJ, Cole MD, Stringer D, Shafqat JP. A technique for osseous restoration of deficient edentulous maxillary ridges. J Oral Maxillofac Surg. 1985;43(2):87–91. PubMed PMID: 3881576
9. Gongloff RK, Cole M, Whitlow W, Boyne PJ. Titanium mesh and particulate cancellous bone and marrow grafts to augment the maxillary alveolar ridge. Int J Oral Maxillofac Surg. 1986;15(3):263–8. PubMed PMID: 3088153
10. von Arx T, Hardt N, Wallkamm B. The TIME technique: a new method for localized alveolar ridge augmentation prior to placement of dental implants. Int J Oral Maxillofac Implants. 1996;11(3):387–94. PubMed PMID: 8752560
11. von Arx T, Kurt B. Implant placement and simultaneous peri-implant bone grafting using a micro titanium mesh for graft stabilization. Int J Periodontics Restorative Dent. 1998;18(2):117–27. PubMed PMID: 9663090
12. von Arx T, Kurt B. Implant placement and simultaneous ridge augmentation using autogenous bone and a micro titanium mesh: a prospective clinical study with 20 implants. Clin Oral Implants Res. 1999;10(1):24–33. PubMed PMID: 10196787
13. Rasia-dal Polo M, Poli PP, Rancitelli D, Beretta M, Maiorana C. Alveolar ridge reconstruction with titanium meshes: a systematic review of the literature. Med Oral Patol Oral Cir Bucal. 2014;19(6):e639–46. PubMed PMID: 25350597. Pubmed Central PMCID: 4259384
14. Ciocca L, Ragazzini S, Fantini M, Corinaldesi G, Scotti R. Work flow for the prosthetic rehabilitation of atrophic patients with a minimal-intervention CAD/CAM approach. J Prosthet Dent. 2015;114(1):22–6. PubMed PMID: 25862269
15. Sumida T, Otawa N, Kamata YU, Kamakura S, Mtsushita T, Kitagaki H, et al. Custom-made titanium devices as membranes for bone augmentation in implant treatment: clinical application and the comparison with conventional titanium mesh. J Craniomaxillofac Surg. 2015;43(10):2183–8. PubMed PMID: 26603108
16. Boudet C. Platelet-rich fibrin in mesh exposure repair. Dentistry today. 2014; 33(1):112–3. PubMed PMID: 24660440
17. Lizio G, Corinaldesi G, Marchetti C. Alveolar ridge reconstruction with titanium mesh: a three-dimensional evaluation of factors affecting bone augmentation. Int J Oral Maxillofac Implants. 2014;29(6):1354–63. PubMed PMID: 25397798
18. Poli PP, Beretta M, Cicciu M, Maiorana C. Alveolar ridge augmentation with titanium mesh. A retrospective clinical study. Open Dent J. 2014;8:148–58. PubMed PMID: 25317209. Pubmed Central PMCID: 4192861
19. Yildirim M, Spiekermann H, Handt S, Edelhoff D. Maxillary sinus augmentation with the xenograft bio-Oss and autogenous intraoral bone for qualitative improvement of the implant site: a histologic and histomorphometric clinical study in humans. Int J Oral Maxillofac Implants. 2001;16(1):23–33. PubMed PMID: 11280359
20. Misch CE, Dietsh F. Bone-grafting materials in implant dentistry. Implant Dent. 1993;2(3):158–67. PubMed PMID: 8142935
21. Pieri F, Corinaldesi G, Fini M, Aldini NN, Giardino R, Marchetti C. Alveolar ridge augmentation with titanium mesh and a combination of autogenous bone and anorganic bovine bone: a 2-year prospective study. J Periodontol. 2008;79(11):2093–103. PubMed PMID: 18980518
22. Proussaefs P, Lozada J. Use of titanium mesh for staged localized alveolar ridge augmentation: clinical and histologic-histomorphometric evaluation. The Journal of oral implantology. 2006;32(5):237–47. PubMed PMID: 17069168
23. Corinaldesi G, Pieri F, Sapigni L, Marchetti C. Evaluation of survival and success rates of dental implants placed at the time of or after alveolar ridge augmentation with an autogenous mandibular bone graft and titanium mesh: a 3- to 8-year retrospective study. Int J Oral Maxillofac Implants. 2009; 24(6):1119–28. PubMed PMID: 20162118
24. Artzi Z, Dayan D, Alpern Y, Nemcovsky CE. Vertical ridge augmentation using xenogenic material supported by a configured titanium mesh: clinicohistopathologic and histochemical study. Int J Oral Maxillofac Implants. 2003;18(3):440–6. PubMed PMID: 12814321
25. Watzinger F, Luksch J, Millesi W, Schopper C, Neugebauer J, Moser D, et al. Guided bone regeneration with titanium membranes: a clinical study. Br J Oral Maxillofac Surg. 2000;38(4):312–5. PubMed PMID: 10922157
26. Joseph VR, Sam G, Amol NV. Clinical evaluation of autologous platelet rich fibrin in horizontal alveolar bony defects. Journal of clinical and diagnostic research : JCDR. 2014;8(11):ZC43–7. PubMed PMID: 25584315. Pubmed Central PMCID: 4290326
27. Dohan DM, Choukroun J, Diss A, Dohan SL, Dohan AJ, Mouhyi J, et al. Platelet-rich fibrin (PRF): a second-generation platelet concentrate. Part III: leucocyte activation: a new feature for platelet concentrates? Oral Surg Oral Med Oral Pathol Oral Radiol Endod. 2006;101(3):e51–5. PubMed PMID: 16504851
28. Borie E, Olivi DG, Orsi IA, Garlet K, Weber B, Beltran V, et al. Platelet-rich fibrin application in dentistry: a literature review. Int J Clin Exp Med. 2015; 8(5):7922–9. PubMed PMID: 26221349. Pubmed Central PMCID: 4509294
29. Li Q, Pan S, Dangaria SJ, Gopinathan G, Kolokythas A, Chu S, et al. Platelet-rich fibrin promotes periodontal regeneration and enhances alveolar bone augmentation. Biomed Res Int. 2013;2013:638043. PubMed PMID: 23586051. Pubmed Central PMCID: 3622372
30. Ali S, Bakry SA, Abd-Elhakam H. Platelet-rich fibrin in maxillary sinus augmentation: a systematic review. The Journal of oral implantology. 2015;41(6):746–53. PubMed PMID: 25536095
31. Moraschini V, Barboza ES. Effect of autologous platelet concentrates for alveolar socket preservation: a systematic review. Int J Oral Maxillofac Surg. 2015;44(5):632–41. PubMed PMID: 25631334
32. Torres J, Tamimi F, Alkhraisat MH, Manchon A, Linares R, Prados-Frutos JC, et al. Platelet-rich plasma may prevent titanium-mesh exposure in alveolar ridge augmentation with anorganic bovine bone. J Clin Periodontol. 2010; 37(10):943–51. PubMed PMID: 20796106
33. Kleinheinz J, Buchter A, Kruse-Losler B, Weingart D, Joos U. Incision design in implant dentistry based on vascularization of the mucosa. Clin Oral Implants Res. 2005;16(5):518–23. PubMed PMID: 16164456
34. Arnold F, West DC. Angiogenesis in wound healing. Pharmacol Ther. 1991; 52(3):407–22. PubMed PMID: 1726477

20

Bioactive–hybrid–zirconia implant surface for enhancing osseointegration: an in vivo study

Dawlat Mostafa and Moustafa Aboushelib*

Abstract

Background: Zirconia is characterized by a hard, dense, and chemically inert surface which requires additional surface treatments in order to enhance osseointegration. The proposed hypothesis of the study was that combination of a nano-porous surface infiltrated with a bioactive material may enhance osseointegration of zirconia implants.

Methods: Custom-made zirconia implants (3.7 mm × 8 mm) were designed, milled, and sintered according to manufacturer recommendations. All implants received selective infiltration etching (SIE) technique to produce a nano-porous surface. Surface porosities were either filled with nano-hydroxy apatite particle- or platelet-rich plasma while uncoated surface served as a control ($n = 12$, $\alpha = 0.05$). New surface properties were characterized with mercury porosimetry, XRD analysis, SEM, and EDX analysis. Implants were inserted in femur head of rabbits, and histomorphometric analysis was conducted after healing time to evaluate bone–implant contact percentage (BIC%).

Results: Selective infiltration etching produced a nano-porous surface with interconnected surface porosities. Mercury porosimetry revealed a significant reduction in total porosity percent after application of the two coating materials. XRD patterns detected hexagonal crystal structure of HA superimposed on the tetragonal crystal phase of zirconia. Histomorphometric analysis indicated a significantly higher ($F = 14.6$, $P < 0.001$) BIC% around HA–bioactive–hybrid surface (79.8 ± 3%) and PRP-coated surface (71 ± 6 %) compared to the control (49 ± 8%).

Conclusions: Bioactive–hybrid–zirconia implant surface enhanced osseointegration of zirconia implants.

Keywords: Zirconia implants, Selective etching, Hybrid ceramic surface, SEM

Background

Dental implants became one of the most reliable techniques used to restore missing teeth [1, 2]. Material composition and surface topography play a fundamental role in osseointegration [3]. Therefore, various chemical and physical surface modifications have been developed to improve osseous healing around the inserted implants. Two main approaches have been suggested to improve surface properties of dental implants either by optimizing its micro-roughness or through applying bioactive coatings [4–6].

Hydroxyapatite (HA) is the most widely used bioactive-ceramic material in the field of bone regeneration and augmentation because of its unique bioactivity and stability [7]. Hydroxyapatite promotes growth of bone tissue directly on its surface; hence, HA coatings have been applied to implant fixtures to produce a bioactive surface that stimulates faster bone formation and reduced healing time [8–10]. HA promotes cell attachment and proliferation of a variety of cells including fibroblasts, osteoblasts, and periodontal ligament cells [7].

Platelet-rich plasma (PRP) growth factors loaded onto titanium implant surface were tested in animal models as potential agents to enhance osseointegration. PRP protein coat has two important properties that contribute to optimizing and accelerating the osseointegration process: the osteo-conductive properties attributed to fibrin and the recognized osteo-inductive activities of the growth factors, thereby creating a new dynamic implant surface [11].

* Correspondence: bluemarline_1@yahoo.com; moustafaaboushelib@gmail.com
Dental Biomaterials, Faculty of Dentistry, Alexandria University, Champolion St., Azarita, Alexandria, Egypt

All-ceramic dental implants gained lots of attention offering a solution to the potential immunologic and possible esthetic compromises observed with titanium implants [12, 13]. The superior mechanical properties of zirconia made it a material of choice for fabrication of dental implants [14]. Zirconia has an exceptional biocompatibility, chemical stability, and high toughness compared to other metallic materials [15, 16]. Zirconia has an opaque whitish color which prevents grayish discoloration observed with thin gingival biotypes [17–20]. Moreover, the inflammatory response and bone resorption induced by released ceramic particles are much less compared to those induced by titanium particles [21, 22]. On the other hand, zirconia is characterized by a hard, dense, and chemically inert surface that does not react readily to etching even by aggressive chemical agents [23]. Poor surface properties resulted in adhesion problems and caused deboning of coating materials [24].

Different surface modifications of zirconia were tested to increase its surface roughness, wetting capacity, and surface energy [25]. Such approaches mainly include topographical modifications via milling, particle abrasion, hot acid etching [25, 26], or laser micro-etching [27, 28]. Improved surface properties enhanced the performance of zirconia implants [29].

In 2007, Aboushelib and Feilzer introduced a surface treatment method known as selective infiltration etching (SIE) technique that uses the principles of heat-induced maturation and grain boundary diffusion to transform the relatively dense and smooth (non-bonding) surface of zirconia into a highly retentive nano-porous surface which greatly enhanced wetting and bonding capacity to zirconia [24]. This principle could also be used to increase retention of bioactive coatings on the surface of selective infiltration etching zirconia implants where the created nano-pores could be filled with the desired coating material creating a novel bioactive–hybrid ceramic surface without the risk of delamination of the coated material. The only consideration is that the filling particles should be smaller in diameter than the average pore diameter to insure proper pore filling.

For a bioactive coat to achieve its intended functions successfully, several factors must be considered; implant surface treatment (either mechanically or chemically), the thickness of the coated film (thicker films have higher tendency to delaminate), and the properties of the coated film (chemical structure, crystal structure, and surface topography) [30]. The aim of this study was to evaluate the influence of novel bioactive–hybrid–zirconia implant surfaces on osseointegration in a rabbit model. The proposed hypothesis was that the bioactive–hybrid surfaces would enhance osseointegration in the tested animal model.

Methods

Preparation of zirconia implants

CAD/CAM zirconia milling blocks (NobelBiocare, Göteborg, Sweden) were used for preparation of zirconia implants (cylinders 3.7 mm × 8 mm). The milled implants were sintered according to manufacturer recommendations (1350 °C for 6 h) [24]. To produce a nano-porous surface, all specimens were subjected to selective infiltration etching (SIE) technique to modify their surface topography through the creation of a nano-porous zirconia surface that extends few microns deep below the surface. Further details are mentioned elsewhere [31]. The prepared implants were divided into two groups ($n = 12$), according to the coating used to fill surface porosities, while uncoated surface served as a control.

Characterization of zirconia surface

Several surface characterization techniques were implemented to study the proposed hypothesis. Mercury porosimetry was performed for testing the surface nanoporosity and its relevant parameters including the total porosity percent and the average pore diameter in nanometers. Poresizer (Porosimeter, Micromeritics 9320, USA) was used for testing the nano-porosity created on the surface covering pore diameter range from approximately 0.006 to 360 µm. Atomic force microscopy (AFM) was used to confirm surface topography on the nano-scale. High-resolution X-ray diffraction analysis (XRD) for thin coats (PANalytical, X Pert PRO) with Cu target ($\lambda = 1.54°$A), 45 kV, 40 mA, and 2 (10°–80°) was performed to investigate the crystallographic structure of the implants. Zirconia implants were gold sputter-coated (fine coat, JEOL JFC-1100E, Japan) before scanning electron microscopic examination (JEOL, JSM, 5410, Japan) at an accelerating voltage of 25 kV. Energy dispersive X-ray analysis (EDX) was used (INCA Penta FETX3, OXFORD Instruments, Model 6583, England) to study the elemental composition of the specimens.

Preparation of HA coating material

Natural hydroxyapatite was extracted from femoral bones of line V Spain white rabbits (the animal models of the experimental study) through two stages: the first stage was the deproteinization process that was conducted to eliminate all organic and protein components of bone, followed by a heat treatment (calcination) process of the inorganic bone salts for elimination of all phases other than HA [32]. EDX and XRD analysis were accomplished to characterize the extracted natural HA for its chemical and crystal phase purity. The prepared powder was firstly ground to reduce its particle size to the sub-micron scale using ultrasonic vibration (ESPE. CAPMIX 410630, W-Germany) with a ceramic ball.

Afterwards, high-energy ball milling (8000 M Mixer/Mill, SPEX Sample Prep, USA) was used for grinding of the produced micro-particles to reduce their size to the nano-scale (100 nm). The produced nano-particles were collected using high-speed centrifugal unit.

A hydroxyapatite suspension was prepared by weighing 0.2 g of the milled nano-particles using a calibrated digital balance (OHAUS, CT 1200-S, USA) and adding them to 20 ml absolute ethyl alcohol, followed by shaking the suspension in ultrasonic shaker for 5 min to achieve even distribution at room temperature. Immersion coating was performed by completely immersing the prepared implants in the suspension for 3 min, followed by heat drying at 150 °C for 10 min (Nuova II, Sybron/Thermolyne, Spain). This immersion cycle was repeated three times. Finally, all specimens were heated at 850 °C for 3 h to fuse the particles with the surface of zirconia.

Preparation of platelet-rich plasma coating material

This study was approved by the ethics committee of Science and Technology Development Fund (STDF-389, the academy of scientific research) regarding using animals in research studies. Autologous platelet-rich plasma (PRP) was freshly prepared from each animal independently just before insertion of zirconia implants into the rabbit femurs. Protocol of blood collection from rabbits was approved by the ethics committee of Alexandria University for studies involving animal models [33]. The collected blood was centrifuged at 4000 rpm for 8 min at room temperature. The centrifuged blood was separated into platelet-poor plasma (PPP), PRP (buffy coat), and the more dense red blood cells. The PRP-coating solution was prepared by collecting the buffy coat in another sterile graduated tube, and 0.5 ml of 10% *w*/*v* calcium chloride was added to each 0.1 ml of separated PRP [34]. Each zirconia implant was completely immersed into the prepared PRP solution for 10 min at room temperature immediately before its insertion into its surgically prepared socket that was completely filled with the prepared PRP solution.

Surgical phase

Twenty-four male line V Spain white rabbits were obtained from the Poultry Research Center, Faculty of Agriculture, Alexandria University (6 months old and 3 kg), in good health. The rabbits were kept at the animal house and provided soft diet enriched with vitamins (General Pharma Group, Egypt) and selenium (Mchandes Pharma Veterinary, Egypt) which were added to the drinking water with dose of 1 ml/l for about 2 weeks before surgery. All surgical procedures were performed under general anesthesia and aseptic conditions; the same surgeon completed all surgical procedures. Animals were randomly divided into two groups (n = 12), in each group; each animal received one hybrid–zirconia implant surface coated with either HA or PRP in the right femur head while the left side received uncoated zirconia implant used as a control.

Before surgery, surgical sites were shaved to expose the skin that was coated with antiseptic iodine-based solution. Rabbits were anesthetized with intramuscular injection of ketamine in combination with xylazine at a dose of 35 and 5 mg/kg of body weight respectively. Surgical flap was made and reflected to expose the distal head of the femur; then, sequential drilling of implant socket was carried out under sufficient cooling at room temperature and with an absolute minimum amount of trauma; and afterwards, the implant was inserted into its created socket. Finally, the surgical flap was repositioned and sutured. Postoperative intramuscular injection of broad-spectrum antibiotic (Cefotax 250 mg; Egyptian INT; Pharmaceutical Industrial Co., Egypt) and analgesic (Voltaren 75 mg/3 ml; Novartis Pharma S.A.E. Egypt) were administrated daily for 10 days to avoid any infection and to relief pain. Rabbits were monitored daily for weight gain and cage behavior. The wounds were allowed to heal for 6 weeks before sacrifice by injection of an over dose of intravenous anesthetic agent [35, 36].

Histomorphometric analysis

Six weeks after insertion of the implants, bone blocks were collected, subjected to fixation and dehydration, imbedded in transparent methyl methacrylate monomer, and finally sectioned in a precision cutting machine using a diamond-coated disc producing 150-µm-thick sections. Sections were polished using silicon carbide and stained using Stevenel's Blue and van Gieson picrofuchsin. Histomorphometric analysis and determination of bone-to-implant contact percentage (BIC%) was performed on the mid section of each implant using digital images obtained from a stereo stereomicroscope (Olympus imaging digital camera, model E.330 DC 7. 4 V, Japan). The images were then analyzed using computer software program (Olypus. Cell ˆA). Mature bone stained red in contact with implant diameter was measure as a percentage of the entire implant diameter to calculate bone implant contact percent of each test group. Data were fed to a statistical software (SPSS 14.0, SPSS Inc). One-way analysis of variance (ANOVA) and Bonferroni post hoc tests were used to analyze the data based on power analysis test [37, 38].

Results

Mercury porosimetry revealed comparable ($F = 0.047$, $P < 0.9$) average pore diameter (136.43 ± 2.76 nm) for all the prepared specimens in all groups (Fig. 1a). There was a significant reduction in total porosity percent ($F = 848.960$, $P < 0.001$) after application of

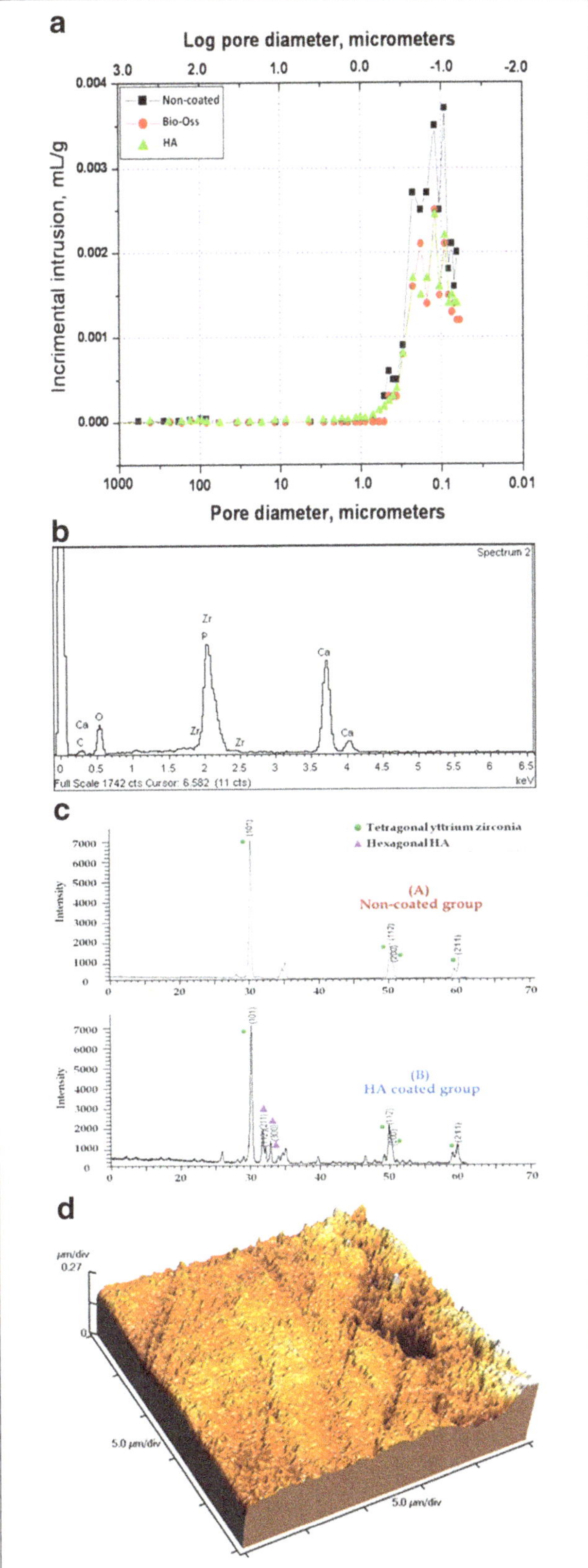

Fig. 1 **a** Mercury porosimetry and the average pore diameter of the prepared implants. **b** EDX analysis of hybrid–zirconia surface showing peaks of zirconia, calcium, and phosphate. Ca/P ratio is 1.67. **c** XRD peaks of uncoated and bioactive implants showing characteristic peaks specific for tetragonal yttrium zirconium oxide crystal system represented by (101), (112), (200), and (211) and hybrid implants showing characteristic peaks specific for hexagonal HA crystal system. **d** Atomic force microscope of selective infiltration etching zirconia surface demonstrating subsurface porosities

coating materials: 9 ± 2% for HA–hybrid surface and 4 ± 1% for PRP-coated surface. EDX analysis of the extracted natural HA revealed that calcium phosphate ratio was 1.67 indicating successful extraction of pure hydroxyapatite (Fig. 1b). XRD pattern revealed the characteristic peaks specific for the hexagonal HA crystal phase represented by (211), (112), and (300 peaks), which proved the phase purity of the extracted HA. High-resolution XRD of uncoated specimen detected only one crystal phase, the tetragonal phase. HA peaks were detected on the hybrid-coated surface (Fig. 1c). EDX detected standard chemical composition of zirconia and HA particles. Atomic force microscopy revealed nano-porosity created as a result of selective infiltration etching surface treatments (Fig. 1d). SEM images of uncoated specimens revealed the presence of three-dimensional networks of nano-pores on the treated surface. Images of the hybrid–zirconia surfaces revealed the presence of agglomeration of HA nano-particles filling the porous surface (Fig. 2). Examination of histological sections indicated significantly higher ($F = 14.6$, $P < 0.001$) amount of newly formed bone (BIC%) around HA–bioactive–hybrid surfaces (79.8 ± 3%) and PRP-coated surfaces (71 ± 6%) compared to the uncoated surfaces (49 ± 8%) (Fig. 3).

Discussion

Several techniques were previously tested for coating hydroxyl apatite particles in the surface of implants as the following: thermal (plasma) spraying [39], dipping coating [30], electrochemical deposition [40], sputter coating [41], pulsed laser deposition [42], and sol-gel technique [43]. Many parameters determined the performance of HA coating both in vitro and in vivo, including chemical composition, crystallinity and purity, surface morphology, porosity, and thickness. These parameters differ from one technique to the another not to mention the effect of varying the operating parameters of each technique [39]. In this study, HA particles were ground to the nano-scale (100 nm) to be incorporated into the three-dimensional nano-pores, with average diameter of 136.43 ± 2.76 nm, thus using the modified zirconia

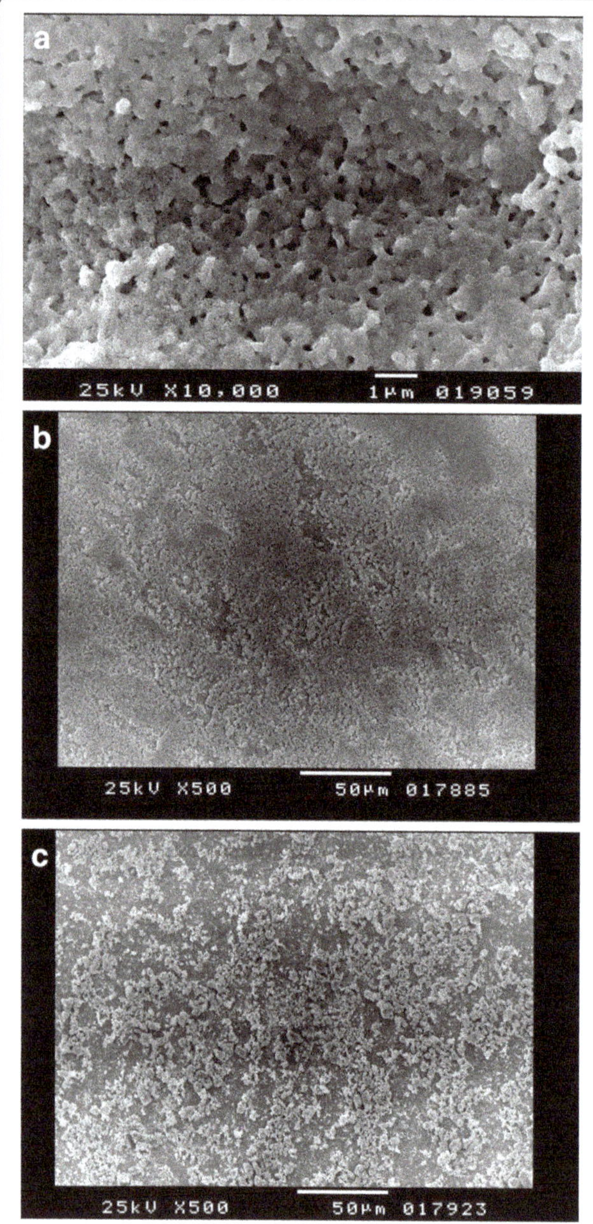

Fig. 2 a SEM image, ×10,000, demonstrating the characteristic porous surface of selective infiltration etching surface of zirconia. **b** SEM image, ×500, demonstrating deposition of PRP coat and complete filling of the porous surface. **c** SEM image, ×500, demonstrating filling of the porous surface with particles of HA

surface as a carrier to the bioactive particles either hydroxy apatite or platelet-rich plasma.

Immersion of a nano-porous zirconia implant in a solution of bioactive materials either HA or PRP created a unique bioactive–hybrid ceramic surface that enhanced the tissue interaction and healing mechanism around the inserted implants. The advantage of this hybrid ceramic surface is that the coated layer is adsorbed few microns beneath the surface, thus reducing any chance of

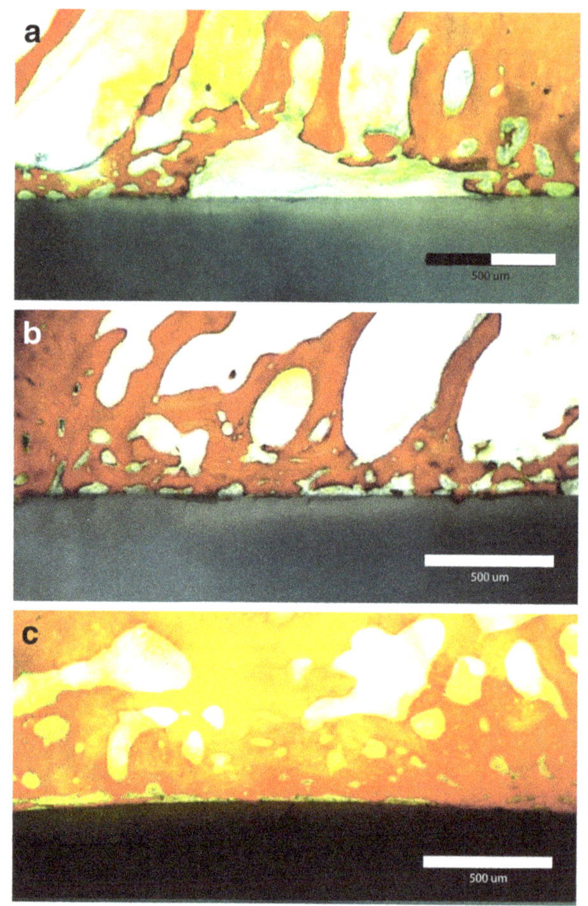

Fig. 3 a Stained histomorphometric section demonstrating bone implant contact of uncoated zirconia implant. **b** Stained histomorphometric section demonstrating bone implant contact of HA–hybrid–zirconia surface. **c** Stained histomorphometric section demonstrating bone implant contact of PRP–hybrid–zirconia surface

delamination and debonding. Moreover, a nano-rough surface is known to enhance implant stability and facilitate improved implant–bone contact, which was directly observed in this study. The proposed hypothesis was accepted.

Histomorphometric analysis are in accordance with many studies, which reported similar findings [44–48]. A histological study used partially stabilized zirconia (Y-TZP) coated with a thin carbonate-containing hydroxyapatite (CA) showed a significantly higher bone-to-implant contact ratio and more bone mass after insertion in the femoral trabecular bone of rabbits [49]. Also, in 2015, it was reported that pre-osteoblast cells exhibited higher proliferation rate on HA-coated zirconia than those grown on uncoated zirconia plants, while gene expression analysis indicated good osteogenic responses on HA-coated [50]. Similar successful findings were observed using PRP coating [51–57]. It was suggested that PRP alone could not induce new bone formation until 6 weeks after implantation,

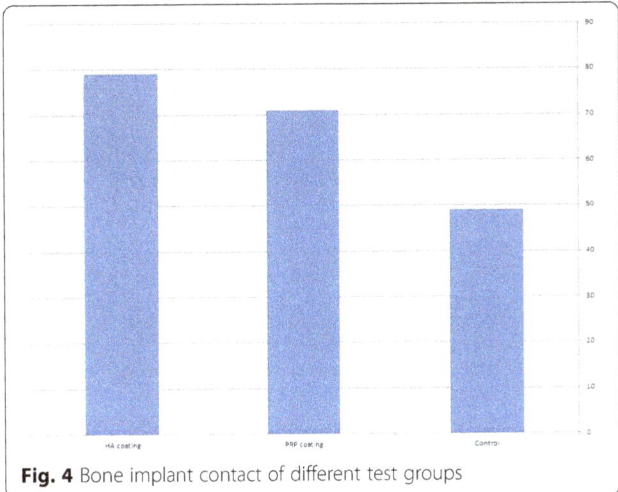

Fig. 4 Bone implant contact of different test groups

while PRP/HA composite activated osteogenic cells, resulting in enhanced bone formation [58] (Fig. 4).

On the other hand, although both the extracted natural HA and PRP bioactive coatings were autologous in nature, the hybrid–HA–zirconia implants showed a higher BIC% than the hybrid–PRP implants, which is directly related to the ability of bioactive HA to promote attachment and proliferation of matrix producing bone cells on its carbonated apatite surface, which has the same surface chemistry as natural bone [7, 8, 59]. Moreover, PRP has a limited time of effectiveness as it acts only in the early phase of clot formation and healing process while the effect of HA particles could be extended over several months.

It is worth mentioning that this significant enhancement in the peri-implant bone healing and osseointegration proves successful incorporation and absorption of the HA nano-particles and the PRP solutions into the nano-porous surfaces of the zirconia implants, thus creating a unique bioactive–hybrid surface, which contributes to enhancing the biological responses at the bone–implant interface and consequently optimizing the overall success rate of the coated implants. Being few microns thick, there is no fear of delamination or detachment observed with other coating techniques. Further studies are needed to optimize the design and performance of these hybrid surfaces.

Conclusions

Within the limitations of this study, hybrid–zirconia surface enhanced osseointegration in rabbit model. The proposed hypothesis was accepted.

Acknowledgements

The authors would like to thank the Science and Technology Development Fund (STDF-389).

Clinical relevance

Hybrid-zirconia-bioactive surface could enhance clinical performance of zirconia implants and improve wound healing.

Funding

No funding conflicts are related to the study.

Authors' contributions

Author DM prepared the specimens, performed the histomophometric analysis of collected sections, and shared in the preparation of the manuscript. Author MA performed the animal surgeries, conducted the laboratory tests, and wrote the draft of the manuscript. Both authors read and approved the final manuscript.

Competing interests

Dawlat Mostafa and Moustafa Aboushelib declare that they have no competing interests.

References

1. Pye AD, Lockhart DEA, Dawson MP, et al. A review of dental implants and infection. J Hosp Infect. 2009;72:104–10.
2. Heydecke G, Thomason JM, Lund JP, Feine JS. The impact of conventional and implant supported prostheses on social and sexual activities in edentulous adults: results from a randomized trial 2 months after treatment. J Dent. 2005;33:649–57.
3. Albrektsson T, Branemark PI, Hansson HA, Lindstrom J. Osseointegrated titanium implants: requirements for ensuring a long-lasting, direct bone-to-implant anchorage in man. Acta Orthop Scand. 1981;52:155–70.
4. Albrektsson T, Wennerberg A. Oral implant surfaces: part I—review focusing on topographic and chemical properties of different surfaces and in vivo responses to them. Int J Prosthodont. 2004a;17:536–43.
5. Albrektsson T, Wennerberg A. Oral implant surfaces: part II—review focusing on clinical knowledge of different surfaces. Int J Prosthodont. 2004b;17:544–64.
6. Langhoff JD, Voelter K, Scharnweber D, Schnabelrauch M, Schlottig F, Hefti T, et al. Comparison of chemically and pharmaceutically modified titanium and zirconia implant surfaces in dentistry: a study in sheep. Int J Oral Maxillofac Surg. 2008;37:1125–32.
7. Ciobanu G, Ignat D, Luca C. Polyurethane–hydroxyapatite bionanocomposites: development and characterization. Chem Bull. 2009;54:1.
8. Koklubo T, Kim HM, Kawashita M. Novel bioactive materials with different mechanical properties. Biomaterials. 2003;13:2161–75.
9. Johansson P, Jimbo R, Kozai Y, Sakurai T, Kjellin P, Currie F, Wennerberg A. Nanosized hydroxyapatite coating on PEEK implants enhances early bone formation: a histological and three-dimensional investigation in rabbit bone. Materials. 2015;8:3815–30.
10. He Y, Zhang Y, Zhang J, Jiang Y, Zhou R. Fabrication and characterization of Ti-13Nb-13Zr alloy with radial porous Ti-HA coatings for bone implants. Mater Lett. 2017;209:543–6. Elsevier B.V
11. Zechner W, Tangi S, Tapper G, Fürst G, Bernhart T, Haas R, et al. Influence of platelet rich plasma on osseous healing of dental implants: a histological and histomorphometry study in minipigs. Int J Oral Maxillofac Implants. 2003;18:15–22.
12. Bianco PD, Ducheyne P, Cuckler JM. Local accumulation of titanium released from a titanium implant in the absence of wear. J Biomed Mater Res. 1996;31:227–34.
13. Stejskal J, Stejskal VDM. The role of metals in autoimmunity and the link to neuroendocrinology. Neuroendocrinol Lett. 1999;20:351–64.
14. Bosshardt DD, Chappuis V, Buser D. Osseointegration of titanium, titanium alloy and zirconia dental implants: current knowledge and open questions. Periodontol. 2017;73:22–40.
15. Hayashi K, Inadome T, Tsumura H, et al. Bone-implant interface mechanics of in vivo bio-inert ceramics. Biomaterials. 1993;14:1173–9.
16. Andreiotelli M, Kohal RJ. Fracture strength of zirconia implants after artificial aging. Clin Implant Dent Relat Res. 2009;11:158–66.
17. Andreiotelli M, Wenz HJ, Kohal RJ. Are ceramic implants a viable alternative to titanium implants? A systematic literature review. Clin Oral Implants Res. 2009;20:32–47.
18. Depprich R, Zipprich H, Ommerborn M, et al. Osseointegration of zirconia implants compared with titanium: an in vivo study. Head Face Med. 2008;4:30.
19. Özkurt Z, Kazazoğlu E. Zirconia dental implants: a literature review. J Oral Implantol. 2011;37:367–76.
20. Lyon D, Chevalier J, Gremillard L, Cam CAD. Zirconia as a biomaterial. Compr Biomater. 2011;20:95–108.

21. Ichikawa Y, Akagawa Y, Nikai H, Tsuru H. Tissue compatibility and stability of a new zirconia ceramic in vivo. J Prosthet Dent. 1992;68(2):322–6.
22. Warashina H, Sakano S, Kitamura S, et al. Biological reaction to alumina, zirconia, titanium and polyethylene particles implanted onto murine calvaria. Biomaterials. 2003;24:3655–61.
23. Obradovic-Djuricic K, Medić V, Dodić S, et al. Dilemmas in zirconia bonding: a review. Srp Arh Celok Lek. 2013;141:395–401.
24. Aboushelib MN, Kleverlaan CJ, Feilzer AJ. Selective infiltration-etching technique for a strong and durable bond of resin cements to zirconia-based materials. J Prosthet Dent. 2007;98:379–88.
25. Noro A, Kaneko M, Murata I, Yoshinari M. Influence of surface topography and surface physicochemistry on wettability of zirconia (tetragonal zirconia polycrystal). J Biomed Mater Res B Appl Biomater. 2013;101(B):355–63.
26. Aboushelib MN, Matinlinna JP, Salameh Z, Ounsi HF. Innovations in bonding to zirconia-based materials: part I. Dent Mater. 2008;24:1268–72.
27. Conrad HJ, Seong W-J, Pesun IJ. Current ceramic materials and systems with clinical recommendations: a systematic review. J Prosthet Dent. 2007;98: 389–404.
28. Chevalier J, Gremillard L. Ceramics for medical applications: a picture for the next 20 years. J Eur Ceram Soc. 2009;29:1245–55.
29. Saulacic N, Erdosi R, Bosshardt DD, Gruber R, Buser D. Acid and alkaline etching of sandblasted zirconia implants: a histomorphometric study in miniature pigs. Clin Implant Dent Relat Res. 2014;16:313–22.
30. Gottlander M, Albrektsson T. Histomorphometric studies of hydroxyapatite-coated and uncoated CP titanium threaded implants in bone. Int J Oral Maxillofac Implants. 1991;6:399–404.
31. Aboushelib M, Feilzer A. New surface treatment for zirconia based materials. European patent application, no 050773969; 2006.
32. Gören S, Gökbayrak H, Altıntaş S. Production of Hydroxylapatite from animal bone. Key Eng Mater. 2004;264-8:1949–52.
33. Parasuraman S, Raveendran R, Kesavan R. Blood sample collection in small laboratory animals. J Pharmacol Pharmacother. 2010;1:87–93.
34. Anitua EA. Enhancement of osseointegration by generating a dynamic implant surface. J Oral Implantol. 2006;32:72–6.
35. Takayuki M, Salvi GE, Offenbacher S, Felton DA, Cooper LF. Cell and matrix reactions at titanium implants in surgically prepared rat tibiae. Int J Oral Maxillofac Implants. 1997;12:472–85.
36. Buser D, Schenk RK, Steinemann S, Fiorellini JP, Fox CH, Stich H. Influence of surface characteristics on bone integration of titanium implants. A histomorphometric study in miniature pigs. J Biomed Mater Res. 1991;25:889–902.
37. Leslie E, Geoffrey J, James M. Statistical analysis. Interpretation and uses of medical statistics. Oxford: Scientific Publications; 1991. p. 411–6.
38. Kirkpatrick LA, Feeney BC. A simple guide to IBM SPSS statistics for version 20.0. Student ed. Belmont: Wadsworth, Cengage Learning; 2013. p. 115.
39. Sun L, Berndt CC, Gross KA, Kucuk A. Material fundamentals and clinical performance of plasma-sprayed hydroxyapatite coatings: a review. J Biomed Mater Res. 2001;58:570–92.
40. Ban S, Hasegawa J. Morphological regulation and crystal growth of hydrothermal-electrochemically deposited apatite. Biomaterials. 2002;23: 2965–72.
41. Wolke JG, van Dijk K, Schaeken HG, de Groot K, Jansen JA. Study of the surface characteristics of magnetron-sputter calcium phosphate coatings. J Biomed Mater Res. 1994;28:1477–84.
42. Lo WJ, Grant DM, Ball MD, Welsh BS, Howdle SM, Antonov EN, et al. Physical, chemical, and biological characterization of pulsed laser deposited and plasma sputtered hydroxyapatite thin films on titanium alloy. J Biomed Mater Res. 2000;50:536–45.
43. Milella E, Cosentino F, Licciulli A, Massaro C. Preparation and characterisation of titania/hydroxyapatite composite coatings obtained by sol-gel process. Biomaterials. 2001;22:1425–31.
44. Weinlander M, Kenney EB, Lekovic V, Beumer J, Moy PK, Lewis S. Histomorphometry of bone apposition around three types of endosseous dental implants. Int J Oral Maxillofac Implants. 1992;7:491–6.
45. Gottlander M, Albrektsson T, Carlsson V. A histomorphometric study of unthreaded HA-coated and titanium-coated implants in rabbit bone. Int J Oral Maxillofac Implants. 1992;7:485–90.
46. Wong M, Eulenberger J, Schenk R, Hunziker E. Effect of surface topology on the osseointegration of implant materials in trabecular bone. J Biomed Mater Res. 1995;29:1567–75.
47. Takashi S, Shunsuke F, Yasuaki N, Iwao N, Takashi N. Ability of zirconia double coated with titanium and hydroxyapatite to bond to bone under load-bearing conditions. Biomaterials. 2006;27:996–1002.
48. Bigi A, Fini M, Bracci B, Boanini E, Torricelli P, Giavaresi G, et al. The response of bone to nanocrystalline hydroxyapatite-coated Ti13Nb11Zr alloy in an animal model. Biomaterials. 2008;29:1730–6.
49. Hirota M, Hayakawa T, Ohkubo C, Sato M, Hara H, Toyama T, Tanaka Y. Bone responses to zirconia implants with a thin carbonate-containing hydroxyapatite coating using a molecular precursor method. J Biomed Mater Res B Appl Biomater. 2014;102(6):1277–88.
50. Cho Y, Hong J, Ryoo H, Kim D, Park J, Han J. Osteogenic responses to zirconia with hydroxyapatite coating by aerosol deposition. J Dent Res. 2015;94(3):491–9.
51. Stefani CM, Machado MA, Sallum EA, Sallum AW, Toledo S, Nociti H Jr. Platelet-derived growth factor/insulin like growth factor-1 combination and bone regeneration around implants placed into extraction sockets: a histometric study in dogs. Implant Dent. 2000;9:126–30.
52. St John TA, Vaccaro AR, Sah AP, Schaefer M, Berta SC, Albert T, et al. Physical and monetary costs associated with autogenous bone graft harvesting. Am J Orthop. 2003;32:18–23.
53. Tayapongsak P, O'Brien DA, Monteiro CB, Arceo DL. Autologous fibrin adhesive in mandibular reconstruction with particulate cancellous bone and marrow. J Oral Maxillofac Surg. 1994;52:161–5.
54. Slater M, Patava J, Kingham K, Mason RS. Involvement of platelets in stimulating osteogenic activity. J Orthop Res. 1995;13:655–63.
55. Wang HJ, Wan HL, Yang TS, Wang DS, Chen TM, Chang DM. Acceleration of skin graft healing by growth factors. Burns. 1996;22:10–4.
56. Steed DL. The role of growth factors in wound healing. Surg Clin North Am. 1997;77:575–86.
57. Garcia RV, Gabrielli MA, Hochuli-Vieira E, Spolidorio LC, Filho JG, Neto FA, de Cardoso LA, Shibli JA. Effect of platelet-rich plasma on peri-implant bone repair: a histologic study in dogs. J Oral Implantol. 2010;36(4):281–90.
58. Ohba S, Wang W, Itoh S, Takagi Y, Nagai A, Yamashita K. Acceleration of new bone formation by an electrically polarized hydroxyapatite microgranule/ platelet-rich plasma composite. Acta Biomater. 2012;8:2778–87.
59. Siebers MC, ter Brugge PJ, Walboomers XF, Jansen JA. Integrins as linker proteins between osteoblasts and bone replacing materials. A critical review. Biomaterials. 2005;26:137–46.

The effect of membrane exposure on lateral ridge augmentation

Mehmet A. Eskan[1,5*], Marie-Eve Girouard[2], Dean Morton[3] and Henry Greenwell[4]

Abstract

Background: The effect of membrane exposure on guided bone regeneration (GBR) for lateral ridge augmentation has been poorly addressed. This case-controlled study aimed to investigate potential effect of membrane exposure lateral ridge augmentation and subsequent implant placement.

Methods: A total of 14 patients that did receive lateral ridge augmentation procedure using allogeneic cancellous graft particulate in combination with an alloplastic bioresorbable matrix barrier were retrospectively selected for this study. Bone width was measured at the crest with a digital caliper before bone augmentation and at the reopening for implant placement 4 months later for all patients. Cases where primary flap closure was achieved and the barrier did not expose throughout the time until implant placement were assigned to the control group ($n = 7$). Cases where primary closure could not be achieved or a barrier exposure happened within the first week following the initial surgery were assigned to the test group.

Results: The measured alveolar ridge width before surgery as well as after GBR procedure were not statistically significant different between the two groups ($p > 0.05$). Both groups showed a significant ($p < 0.05$) increase in their mean alveolar ridge width 4 months after later augmentation procedure, from 3.4 ± 1.2 to 6.0 ± 1.1 mm in the control group and from 3.6 ± 1.0 to 5.0 ± 1.4 mm in the test group. However, the mean alveolar ridge gain was significantly greater in the control group than in the test group ($p < 0.05$). Consequently, the reduction of the augmented alveolar ridge was significantly higher in the test group averaging to 4.7 mm than for the control group showing a loss of 3.1 mm after 4 months, respectively. However, in all 14 cases, successful implant placement was achieved after 4 months.

Conclusions: Within the limit of this study, it can be concluded that early exposure of a bioresorbable matrix barrier during lateral ridge augmentation may compromise the results of the GBR procedure but may still result in a favorable alveolar ridge width gain that allows for the placement of dental implants.

Keywords: Graft loss, Lateral ridge augmentation, Matrix barrier, Membrane exposure

Background

It has been reported that unpreserved alveolar ridges can show substantial horizontal and/or vertical ridge deficiency [1, 2] that lack the sufficient alveolar ridge dimensions to allow the ideal positioning of the implant and enhance long-term prognosis of the clinical outcomes [3]. Guided bone regeneration (GBR) is a predictable technique for augmenting the alveolar ridge width that has been used for more than two decades, and osseointegration and long-term implant survival rate have been reported to be similar in grafted areas than in native bone [4, 5].

One of the main components in GBR procedures is the use of a resorbable or non-resorbable barrier membranes that stabilize the bone grafting material and protect it from the ingrowth of surrounding soft tissues [6, 7]. Therefore, non-resorbable PTFE membranes have been developed for GBR that present an inner occlusive surface

* Correspondence: makifeskan@gmail.com
[1]Sisli, Istanbul, Turkey
[5]Clinic Eska, Terrace Fulya, Tesvikiye Mah., Hakki Yeten Cad, Sisli, Istanbul, Turkey
Full list of author information is available at the end of the article

to prevent migration of epithelial and fibroblast cells into the defect and to maintain adequate space for bone formation and wound stabilization [8]. However, PTFE membrane might lead to compromised vascular supply of the flaps [9] and exhibited a higher incidence of premature membrane exposures [8, 10, 11] as well as gingival recession [12], which might cause an esthetic problems in the anterior regions.

It is well know that primary closure is increasing the clinical outcome of the GBR procedures [6]. To overcome membrane exposure, it has been suggested to perform a periosteal releasing incision [13]. However, periosteal releasing incisions might cause more swelling, bleeding, and patient discomfort. Importantly, they also may compromise blood circulation [14], and re-positioning flap coronally can result in a misaligned mucogingival line (MGL) if not properly performed [13]. This misaligned MGL might also cause esthetic problems especially in the anterior regions. Therefore, the use of resorbable membrane in the patients might be beneficial, especially in patients with thin soft tissue biotypes.

Various resorbable membranes exist in the market composing of dura mater, poly-lactic acid, polyglycolic acid, polyurethane, or mostly collagen. Still, even resorbable membranes show frequent events of membrane exposures after GBR procedures. For example, between 22 and 32% of early membrane exposure have been reported for collagen membrane by several authors [15–18]. A major drawback of collagen membrane might be that lose their integrity in 1 week [18] when exposed to the proteolytic environment of the oral cavity that leaves the graft material unprotected and can lead to graft loss.

Alloplastic barriers have been proposed as dental membranes for regenerative dentistry that show slower degradation but still good biocompatibility [19–21]. Among those, bioresorbable matrix barrier has been developed for periodontal regeneration and showed effectiveness to reduce epithelial down-growth while promoting the formation of periodontal ligament and alveolar bone in various clinical studies [19, 22–25]. However, the documentation of the performance of bioesorbable matrix barrier in GBR procedures is spares [26–29] and their performance in the case of matrix exposure remains elusive.

Therefore, this case-controlled study aims to investigate the effectiveness of GUIDOR *bioresorbable matrix barrier* for lateral bone augmentation procedures and the effect of exposures on its performance.

Methods

Fourteen subjects were retrospectively recruited for this case-controlled study. In test group (seven patients), primary closure was not achieved and membrane was left exposed at the initial surgery or it became exposed during the first week of healing. In the control group (seven patients), primary wound closure was achieved and no exposure of the membrane occurred until the placement of a dental implant 4 months after augmentation. Each patient received a particulate cancellous allograft (500 to 800 µm, RegenerOss, BioMet 3i), and then, the grafted defect area was covered with a bioresorbable matrix membrane (Sunstar, Suisse SA, Etoy, Switzerland). Longer span edentulous spaces were divided into individual sites based on a 10–12-mm width per site, and each site was bordered by at least one tooth. The subject inclusion criteria included a treatment that was planned to receive a dental implant in the future. At least 18-year-old males and females were included in this study. All subjects signed an informed consent approved by the University of Louisville Institutional Review Board in July 2010. Exclusion criteria excluded patients with uncontrolled diabetes, who are smokers, and with immune diseases or other systemic diseases that significantly affect the periodontium; patients with an allergy to any material or medication used in this study; and patients who need prophylactic antibiotics, previous head and neck radiation therapy, and chemotherapy in the previous 12 months and with severe psychological problems.

Surgical treatment

All surgical procedures were done by one surgeon (ME). The surgical procedure consisted of the reflection of a full thickness flap to expose the residual alveolar ridge. Following complete exposure of the defect area, horizontal ridge width was measured with a digital caliper at the midridge crestal level. Horizontal ridge measurements (at the crestal level) included initial ridge, initial augmented ridge (residual ridge plus graft), and the ridge at the re-entry after the 4-month healing time. All measurements were performed by a masked examiner (MEG), who was unaware of the treatments. Cortical perforations were performed with a ½ round bur to increase vascularization in the defect area [30]. The bone screws (Salvin Dental Specialties, Charlotte, NC) and cancellous particulate allograft were placed to allow for augmentation to achieve 8 mm horizontal width available for implant placement. Horizontal measurements were again taken with the same caliper. Then, the grafted area was covered with a bioresorbable matrix barrier. In the buccal surface, the graft material was completely covered by the membrane. However, in the lingual or palatal surface, the membrane was tucked least 5 mm between the alveolar bone and gingival tissue. Periosteal releasing incisions were performed when needed, and all wound was tried to close primarily and flap re-positioned coronally without compromising MGL. In the test group, the membrane could not be closed primarily (Fig. 1a) or became exposed to the oral environment in 1 week after primary closure was achieved during surgery (Fig. 1b). In the control group, primary closure was achieved with a monofilament suture (Cytoplast, PTFE Suture, Osteogenics Biomedical, Lubbock, TX) (Fig. 1c). The patients were prescribed doxycycline hyclate 50 mg once a day for 2 weeks and hydrocodone when needed. Sutures were removed in 10 days. The subjects were seen every other week to clean the area with hydrogen peroxide.

Statistical analysis

Means ± SD was calculated for all parameters. The statistical significance difference of means between the groups was tested using an exact two-sample Fisher-Pitman permutation test; since the sample size seemed too small to test for normality, $p < 0.05$ was considered to be significant.

Results

The effect of early membrane exposure on alveolar ridge width changes

To assess if the baseline situations of the patients in the two treatment groups were comparable and well balanced, the distribution of gender, age, and the initial ridge measurements were compared. There were three women and four men in each group. The median age for the test and control group was 50 and 62 years old, respectively (Table 1). The initial alveolar mean ridge widths before lateral augmentation in the test and control group were 3.6 ± 1.0 and 3.4 ± 1.2 mm, respectively (Table 2). Therefore, the baseline situation of the two groups was comparable ($p > 0.05$).

Table 1 Patient population and demographics and sites

Groups	Subject no.	Sex	Site	Age
Exposed (test) group	1	Female	13	74
	2	Male	6	62
	3	Female	29	62
	4	Male	12	62
	5	Male	8	59
	6	Male	19	29
	7	Female	9	23
Non-exposed (control) group	8	Female	11	60
	9	Female	30	68
	10	Male	30	68
	11	Male	9	50
	12	Male	25	42
	13	Female	10	39
	14	Male	9	25

In the control (non-membrane exposure) and test group (membrane exposure), the subject's age, sex, and defect areas are presented

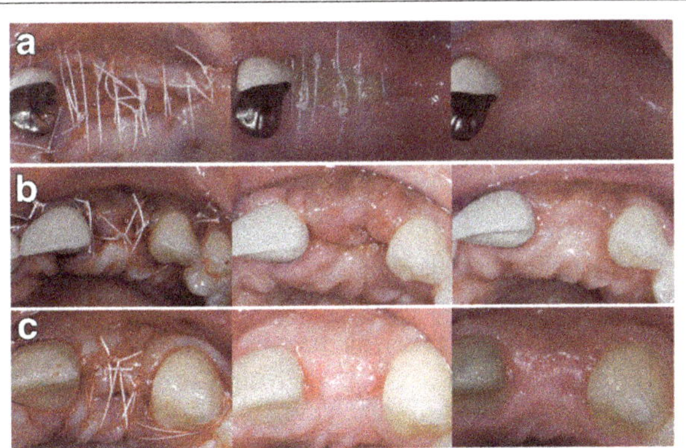

Fig. 1 Clinical photographs of the both treatment groups after the initial surgery, 1 week post-op and at the re-entry. **a)** In the test group, no primary wound closure was achieved (*left*) and the barrier was left exposed for secondary intention healing. After 1 week, the matrix remained exposed (*middle*) showing no signs of infection. For months later, the exposed area was covered by a keratinized tissue (*right*). **b)** In the test group, primary wound closure was achieved at surgery (*left*). However, the barrier became exposed after 1 week of healing (*middle*). For months later, exposed area was covered with a keratinized tissue (*right*). **c)** In the control group, primary wound closure was achieved (*left*). After 1 week (*middle*), primary healing happened without any signs of membrane exposure. For months later, the site healed uneventfully (*right*)

No infection, discomfort, or suppuration was reported for neither of the two groups throughout the study, and all surgical sites did heal uneventfully. The initial mean ridge width before lateral augmentation of the control group increased from 3.4 ± 1.2 to 6.0 ± 1.1 mm at the 4-month re-entry (Table 2). The initial mean ridge width before lateral augmentation increased from 3.6 ± 1.0 to 5.0 ± 1.4 mm at the 4-month re-entry in the test group (Table 2). This led to an alveolar mean ridge gain of 1.4 ± 1.0 mm in the test group and 2.6 ± 1.0 mm in the control group. Both groups did show a statistically significant ($p < 0.05$) ridge width gain between baseline and at the 4-month re-entry (Table 2). However, the results showed that early exposure (test group) resulted in significant ($p < 0.05$) less gain of the alveolar ridge width than when the membrane was not exposed (Table 2).

The effect of early membrane exposure on graft reduction

Furthermore, the reduction of the augmented ridge width right after the lateral augmentation (baseline) to implant placement (after 4 months) was assessed in each subjects. The mean ridge width after lateral ridge augmentation procedure was 9.7 ± 0.9 mm for the test group and 9.1 ± 0.8 mm for the control group (Table 3). The difference between the groups were not statically significant (Table 3). Therefore, baseline situations of the two groups were comparable. Regardless the membrane exposure, there was a significant ($p > 0.05$) reduction of

Table 2 Baseline and re-entry measurement of the alveolar ridge width

Groups	Initial ridge width (mm)	Ridge width at re-entry (mm)	Ridge width gain (mm)
Exposed (tests)	3.6 ± 1.0	5.0 ± 1.4	1.4 ± 1.0
Non-exposed (control)	3.4 ± 1.2	6.0 ± 1.1	2.6 ± 1.0
Fisher-Pitman permutation	$p = 1.00$	$p = 0.168$	$p = 0.047$

At the entry and re-entry, the alveolar ridge width was measured using a digital caliper at the crestal level in both groups. In the control group (non-exposure), the mean ridge width was 3.4 mm and changed to 6.0 mm ($p < 0.01$). In the test group, the mean of ridge was 3.6 mm and changed to 5.0 mm. p values that were calculated for between mean groups analysis are displayed. Alveolar ridge gain was calculated by subtracting re-entry measurement from the entry measurement for each patient at the crestal level using a digital caliper. In the control group, the mean of the gain was 2.6 mm, while it was 1.4 mm in the test group. p values for between-groups analysis are displayed

the initial later ridge augmentation in the both groups after the 4-month healing time. However, the augmented ridge width reduction of 4.7 ± 1.4 mm in the test group was significantly higher ($p < 0.05$) than the 3.1 ± 0.9 mm assessed for the control group (Table 3). The percentage of ridge width reduction was 48 ± 13% in the test group compared to 33 ± 10% in the control group. Therefore, early membrane exposure resulted in higher reduction of the augmented ridge.

Discussion

Although numerous studies in the literature show successful outcomes of the GBR procedure [6, 31], the most common clinical complication in GBR procedures is early membrane exposure [9]. There is a general clinical impression that the ridge augmentation results are compromised in the case of early membrane exposures [32, 33]. In this case-controlled study, which was based on a patient subset from our previous randomized clinical trial, the clinical effect of exposure of a bioresorbable matrix membrane was evaluated [27]. Based on clinical ridge width dimension measurements, a mean ridge width gain of 1.4 and 2.6 mm were calculated for the test and the control group, respectively. On the other hand, a reduction of 4.7 and 3.1 mm of the initially augmented ridge width was measured for the test and control group, respectively. Together, these results clearly indicated that the early membrane exposure in lateral ridge augmentation procedure resulted in significantly lower ridge width gain probably due to a significant higher resorption of the augmented graft during the healing process.

Still, the ridge width gain in both groups was sufficient to allow for the successful placement of dental implants in all 14 subjects without any complication. The exposed matrix barrier degraded within 6–7 weeks or was covered by soft tissue without any further complications. This observed degradation time is markedly longer than that of collagen membrane, which is reported to be completely resorbed 1 to 2 weeks after exposure [18, 34]. The prolonged degradation time of matrix barrier seems to provide prolonged protecting of the underlying graft supporting the bone regeneration process. During this healing process, all exposures did resolve within 6–7 weeks and no membrane had to be extracted. During this period, the exposed bioresorbable matrix barrier became covered with keratinized tissue over time. The secondary healing in exposed area lead to a subsequent increase in the width of keratinized tissue superior to the band of keratinized tissue observed in the control group (Fig. 1a). This shows the epithelization nor the subsequent keratinization process was not altered by an inflammatory situation that could have been triggered by the presence of the matrix barrier or its degradation product. This demonstrated the good healing properties of this barrier membrane. However, the gain of keratinized tissue was not quantitatively measured; thus, this is a clinical observation rather than a documented outcome. The predictability of gaining both keratinized tissue and horizontal ridge dimension simultaneously needs further investigation to confirm this observation. The other main advantage using a bioresorbable matrix barrier over non-resorbable PTFE membrane in the GBR procedures was that all exposures did resolve within 6–7 weeks without any complications and without the need of second surgery to extract the barrier. This might be an important advantage in the

Table 3 Alveolar ridge width reduction

Groups	Grafted ridge width	Ridge width at the re-entry	Grafted ridge reduction (mm)
Exposed (test)	9.7 ± 0.9	5.0 ± 1.4	4.7 ± 1.4
Non-exposed (control)	9.1 ± 0.8	6.0 ± 1.1	3.1 ± 0.9
Fisher-Pitman	$p = 1.00$	$p = 0.260$	$p = 0.030$

The residual alveolar ridge width plus graft width was measured at the crestal level at the entry and re-entry procedure. In the test and control group, the mean of the grafted width was 9.7 and 9.1 mm, respectively. Graft reduction was 4.7 and 3.1 mm for the test and control group, respectively. The percentage of the graft reduction was calculated using the formula: ([Amount of graft reduction/Grafted alveolar bone width] × 100. p values for between-groups analysis are displayed

patient showing a thin biotype and in situations where primary closure is difficult to achieve in the GBR procedures.

The microbial contamination of the matrix barrier during exposure could be another important factor that might hamper bone formation within the underlying graft. This factor has not been investigated in the present study. However, it has been reported by other groups that the resorbable matrix barrier per se might be less prone to bacterial contamination and can be better cleaned using disinfectant agents such as chlorhexidine rinse than PTFE membranes [35]. Matrix membrane presents an outer and inner surface. The external surface is more occlusive (the pore sizes are bigger than those of internal surface) to allow gingival tissue penetration. The internal layer, smaller pores, prevents further penetration of the gingival tissue through the barrier, thus protecting new bone formation underneath the barrier. From clinical observation, the space between the two layers seemed already occupied by connective tissue protecting the inner layer and leaving only the outer layer of the matrix exposed to the oral cavity and subsequent degradation. Still, this clinical observation has to be confirmed in further studies.

The results from this study suggest that primary flap closure over the matrix barrier is preferable leading to better ridge width gain than when the matrix is left exposed or early exposures happen. However, exposures were not completely detrimental to the lateral ridge augmentation and sufficient ridge width gain could be achieved allowing for successful implant placement. In critical cases, where 1 or 2 mm less bone would affect the esthetic results, the matrix barrier should not be left exposed and due care should be taken to avoid any exposures during healing after primary closure was achieved.

Conclusions

Within the limits of this case-controlled study, it can be concluded that lateral ridge augmentation procedures in atrophic alveolar ridges using bioresorbable matrix barriers without achieving primary flap closure or in the case of early exposures can still lead to clinically satisfying ridge width gain that allows for the placement of dental implants. However, exposures seem to limit the ridge width gain. Therefore, in esthetic challenging situations, efforts should be made to achieve primary wound closure and to avoid subsequent membrane exposure.

Acknowledgements
We like to thank to Dr. Lorenz Uebersax for his help during the preparation of this article.

Authors' contributions
MAE and MEG have made substantial contributions in completing all the surgical parts and collecting all the parameters from the subjects. HG was involved in analyzing, interpreting, and supervising the study. DM revised it critically and helped in finalizing the manuscript and giving important intellectual content. All authors read and approved the final manuscript.

Competing interests
Authors Mehmet A Eskan, Marie-Eve Girouard, Dean Morton, and Henry Greenwell state that there are no competing interests.

Author details
[1]Sisli, Istanbul, Turkey. [2]Sherbrooke, Québec, Canada. [3]Department of Prosthodontics, Indiana University School of Dentistry, Indianapolis, IN 46202, USA. [4]Department of Oral Health and Rehabilitation, Division of Periodontics, University of Louisville School of Dentistry, Louisville, KY 40292, USA. [5]Clinic Eska, Terrace Fulya, Tesvikiye Mah., Hakki Yeten Cad, Sisli, Istanbul, Turkey.

References

1. Agarwal G, Thomas R, Mehta D. Postextraction maintenance of the alveolar ridge: rationale and review. Compend Contin Educ Dent. 2012;33:320–324, 326. quiz 327, 336.
2. Horvath A, Mardas N, Mezzomo LA, Needleman IG, Donos N. Alveolar ridge preservation. A systematic review. Clin Oral Investig. 2013;17:341–63.
3. Buser D, Dula K, Belser U, Hirt HP, Berthold H. Localized ridge augmentation using guided bone regeneration. 1. Surgical procedure in the maxilla. Int J Periodontics Restorative Dent. 1993;13:29–45.
4. Simion M, Jovanovic SA, Tinti C, Benfenati SP. Long-term evaluation of osseointegrated implants inserted at the time or after vertical ridge augmentation. A retrospective study on 123 implants with 1–5 year follow-up. Clin Oral Implants Res. 2001;12:35–45.
5. Benic GI, Bernasconi M, Jung RE, Hammerle CH. Clinical and radiographic intra-subject comparison of implants placed with or without guided bone regeneration: 15-year results. J Clin Periodontol. 2016. doi:10.1111/jcpe.12665.
6. Wang HL, Boyapati L. "PASS" principles for predictable bone regeneration. Implant Dent. 2006;15:8–17.
7. Al Salamah L, Babay N, Anil S, Al Rasheed A, Bukhary M. Guided bone regeneration using resorbable and non-resorbable membranes: a histological study in dogs. Odontostomatol Trop. 2012;35:43–50.
8. Simion M, Trisi P, Maglione M, Piattelli A. A preliminary report on a method for studying the permeability of expanded polytetrafluoroethylene membrane to bacteria in vitro: a scanning electron microscopic and histological study. J Periodontol. 1994;65:755–61.
9. Park SH, Wang HL. Clinical significance of incision location on guided bone regeneration: human study. J Periodontol. 2007;78:47–51.
10. Moses O, Pitaru S, Artzi Z, Nemcovsky CE. Healing of dehiscence-type defects in implants placed together with different barrier membranes: a comparative clinical study. Clin Oral Implants Res. 2005;16:210–9.
11. Deeb GR, Wilson GH, Carrico CK, Zafar U, Laskin DM, Deeb JG. Is the tunnel technique more effective than open augmentation with a titanium-reinforced polytetrafluoroethylene membrane for horizontal ridge augmentation? J Oral Maxillofac Surg. 2016;74:1752–6.
12. Magnusson I, Batich C, Collins BR. New attachment formation following controlled tissue regeneration using biodegradable membranes. J Periodontol. 1988;59:1–6.
13. Rachana C, Sridhar N, Rangan AV, Rajani V. Horizontal ridge augmentation using a combination approach. J Indian Soc Periodontol. 2012;16:446–50.
14. Kleinheinz J, Buchter A, Kruse-Losler B, Weingart D, Joos U. Incision design in implant dentistry based on vascularization of the mucosa. Clin Oral Implants Res. 2005;16:518–23.
15. Beitlitum I, Artzi Z, Nemcovsky CE. Clinical evaluation of particulate allogeneic with and without autogenous bone grafts and resorbable collagen membranes for bone augmentation of atrophic alveolar ridges. Clin Oral Implants Res. 2010;21:1242–50.
16. Jung RE, Halg GA, Thoma DS, Hammerle CH. A randomized, controlled clinical trial to evaluate a new membrane for guided bone regeneration around dental implants. Clin Oral Implants Res. 2009;20:162–8.
17. McAllister BS. Scalloped implant designs enhance interproximal bone levels. Int J Periodontics Restorative Dent. 2007;27:9–15.
18. Tal H, Kozlovsky A, Artzi Z, Nemcovsky CE, Moses O. Cross-linked and non-cross-linked collagen barrier membranes disintegrate following surgical exposure to the oral environment: a histological study in the cat. Clin Oral Implants Res. 2008;19:760–6.
19. Hugoson A, Ravald N, Fornell J, Johard G, Teiwik A, Gottlow J. Treatment of

class II furcation involvements in humans with bioresorbable and nonresorbable guided tissue regeneration barriers. A randomized multi-center study. J Periodontol. 1995;66:624–34.
20. Laurell L, Falk H, Fornell J, Johard G, Gottlow J. Clinical use of a bioresorbable matrix barrier in guided tissue regeneration therapy. Case series J Periodontol. 1994;65:967–75.
21. Lundgren AK, Sennerby L, Lundgren D, Taylor A, Gottlow J, Nyman S. Bone augmentation at titanium implants using autologous bone grafts and a bioresorbable barrier. An experimental study in the rabbit tibia. Clin Oral Implants Res. 1997;8:82–9.
22. Cortellini P, Tonetti MS, Lang NP, Suvan JE, Zucchelli G, Vangsted T, et al. The simplified papilla preservation flap in the regenerative treatment of deep intrabony defects: clinical outcomes and postoperative morbidity. J Periodontol. 2001;72:1702–12.
23. Stavropoulos A, Karring T. Long-term stability of periodontal conditions achieved following guided tissue regeneration with bioresorbable membranes: case series results after 6-7 years. J Clin Periodontol. 2004;31:939–44.
24. Falk H, Laurell L, Ravald N, Teiwik A, Persson R. Guided tissue regeneration therapy of 203 consecutively treated intrabony defects using a bioabsorbable matrix barrier. Clinical and radiographic findings. J Periodontol. 1997;68:571–81.
25. Eickholz P, Kim TS, Steinbrenner H, Dorfer C, Holle R. Guided tissue regeneration with bioabsorbable barriers: intrabony defects and class II furcations. J Periodontol. 2000;71:999–1008.
26. Christensen DK, Karoussis IK, Joss A, Hammerle CH, Lang NP. Simultaneous or staged installation with guided bone augmentation of transmucosal titanium implants. A 3-year prospective cohort study. Clin Oral Implants Res. 2003;14:680–6.
27. Eskan MA, Greenwell H, Hill M, Morton D, Vidal R, Shumway B, et al. Platelet-rich plasma-assisted guided bone regeneration for ridge augmentation: a randomized, controlled clinical trial. J Periodontol. 2014;85:661–8.
28. Lundgren D, Sennerby L, Falk H, Friberg B, Nyman S. The use of a new bioresorbable barrier for guided bone regeneration in connection with implant installation. Case Reports Clin Oral Implants Res. 1994;5:177–84.
29. Dan Lundgren TMaJG. The development of a bioresorbable barrier for guided tissue regeneration. The Journal of The SDA. 1994;86:741-756
30. Seol KY, Kim SG, Kim HK, Moon SY, Kim BO, Ahn JM, et al. Effects of decortication in the treatment of bone defect around particulate dentin-coated implants: an experimental pilot study. Oral Surg Oral Med Oral Pathol Oral Radiol Endod. 2009;108:529–36.
31. Fiorellini JP, Nevins ML. Localized ridge augmentation/preservation. A systematic review. Ann Periodontol. 2003;8:321–7.
32. Verardi S, Simion M. Management of the exposure of e-PTFE membranes in guided bone regeneration. Pract Proced Aesthet Dent. 2007;19:111–7.
33. Machtei EE. The effect of membrane exposure on the outcome of regenerative procedures in humans: a meta-analysis. J Periodontol. 2001;72:512–6.
34. Tal H, Kozlovsky A, Artzi Z, Nemcovsky CE, Moses O. Long-term bio-degradation of cross-linked and non-cross-linked collagen barriers in human guided bone regeneration. Clin Oral Implants Res. 2008;19:295–302.
35. Zucchelli G, Pollini F, Clauser C, De Sanctis M. The effect of chlorhexidine mouthrinses on early bacterial colonization of guided tissue regeneration membranes. An in vivo study. J Periodontol. 2000;71:263–71.

Zirconia implants and peek restorations for the replacement of upper molars

José María Parmigiani-Izquierdo[2], María Eugenia Cabaña-Muñoz[2], José Joaquín Merino[2] and Arturo Sánchez-Pérez[1,3*]

Abstract

Background: One of the disadvantages of the zirconia implants is the lack of elasticity, which is increased with the use of ceramic or zirconia crowns. The consequences that could result from this lack of elasticity have led to the search for new materials with improved mechanical properties.

Case presentation: A patient who is a 45-year-old woman, non-smoker and has no medical record of interest with a longitudinal fracture in the palatal root of molar tooth 1.7 and absence of tooth 1.6 was selected in order to receive a zirconia implant with a PEEK-based restoration and a composite coating. The following case report describes and analyses treatment with zirconia implants in molars following a flapless surgical technique. Zirconia implants are an alternative to titanium implants in patients with allergies or who are sensitive to metal alloys. However, one of the disadvantages that they have is their lack of elasticity, which increases with the use of ceramic or zirconia crowns. The consequences that can arise from this lack of elasticity have led to the search for new materials with better mechanical properties to cushion occlusal loads. PEEK-based restoration in implant prosthetics can compensate these occlusal forces, facilitating cushioning while chewing.

Conclusion: This procedure provides excellent elasticity and resembles natural tooth structure. This clinical case suggests that PEEK restorations can be used in zirconia implants in dentistry.

Keywords: Dental implants, Zirconia, Osseointegration, Ceramics, Polyether ketone, Elastic modudus

Background

In the field of implant dentistry, the most widely used implants over the past 40 years are those manufactured from titanium [1], which are still the most popular.

The recent demands for materials without metal alloys in dentistry, together with the increased sensitivity and allergies of some patients, have promoted the development of new materials.

An example of this is zirconia-based dental implants, known as zirconia or zirconium oxide implants. Its biocompatibility and its extraordinary mechanical properties make it suitable for numerous situations. Its main advantage lies in its elasticity which is greater than that of titanium and much greater than that of cortical bone. To avoid overload of the underlying bone from the direct transmission of biting impacts, several materials that can absorb part of this excess force have developed.

One of the prosthetic options lies in the combined use of PEEK restorations with composite coating on zirconia implants due to their physical and mechanical properties and their biocompatibility.

Case presentation

A patient who is a 45-year-old woman and non-smoker has no medical record of interest. The patient complained of pain in the right second upper molar. She said that she felt intense pain while chewing. The pain was accentuated with occlusion and while chewing, making normal functioning impossible. The patient mentioned the absence of piece 16, which had been extracted 8 years previously.

Clinical examination showed a longitudinal fracture in the palatal root of molar tooth 17, which was confirmed by a radiographic examination (Fig. 1), which was removed

* Correspondence: arturosa@um.es
[1]Periodontics Unit, Faculty of Medicine and Dentistry, University of Murcia (Spain), Murcia, Spain
[3]Clínica Odontologíca Universitaria, Hospital Morales Meseguer, 2ª planta, C/ Marqués de los Vélez s/n, Murcia 30008, Spain
Full list of author information is available at the end of the article

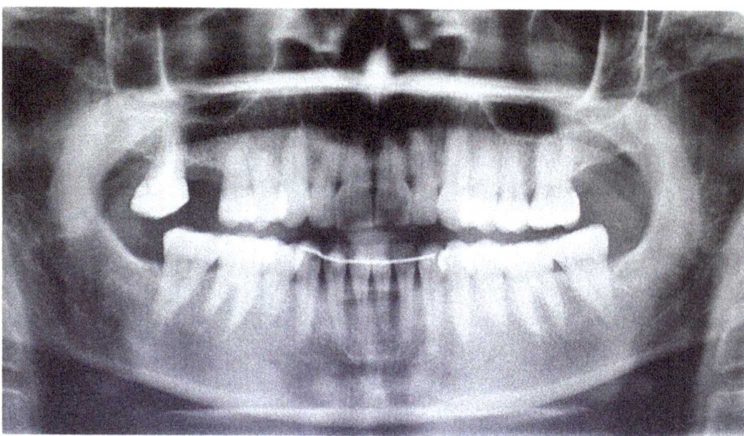

Fig. 1 Diagnostic radiographic exploration previous to treatment

during this appointment. Due to the absence of both molars, the patient expressed a desire to replace them with implants. She also worried about having metal in her mouth and insisted on an alternative material to titanium implants, as well as her intention to replace her molars with metal-free restorations. After 4 months of healing, we proposed as a treatment 2 white SKY (Bredent®) zirconia implants, (4.5 × 10 mm and 4.5 × 8 mm), with PEEK restorations and composite coating. The patient was informed about the intention to publish the results and agreed that the data from this study were public. The patient accepts the treatment and signs informed consent. The CIROM clinical committee has approved the oral surgery for Zirconia and PEEK implantation to the patient.

Initial exam

The edentulous crest showed an adequate amount of attached gingiva, thick enough to perform a flapless technique using a circular scalpel, [2] allowing the integrity of the peri-implant structures to be maintained, while diminishing post-operative pain [3].

Surgical technique

For the flapless technique, we made two circular punch incisions in the gums, with a circular scalpel. The mucous plug was withdrawn with a periosteotome while maintaining the integrity of the gum around the incisions. We continued with the drilling indicated by the manufacturer, to insert two white SKY (Bredent®) zirconia implants of 10 mm length × 4.5 mm diameter in positions 17 and 16 (8 mm length × 4 mm diameter) (Fig. 2).

Healing period

Fifteen days after surgery, the appearance of the soft tissue was excellent, with no signs of inflammation in the mucosa. The patient mentioned the absence of bleeding and pain during the post-operation period. At the same time, we made a clinical and radiological evaluation.

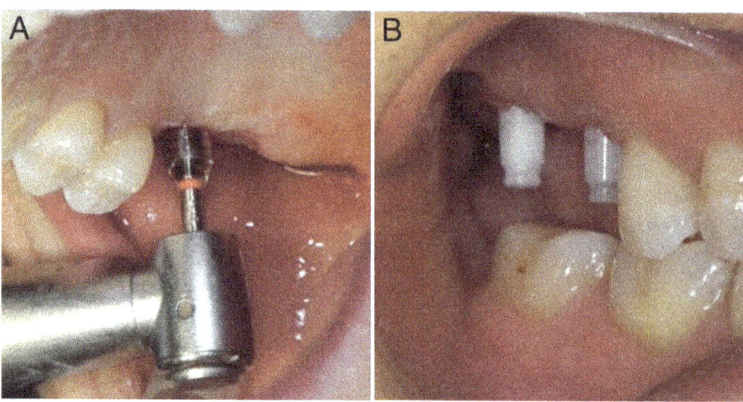

Fig. 2 Flapless surgical technique, atraumatic surgical procedure for zirconium implants using the circular scalpel (**a**)–sharp, clean cut without bleeding (**b**)

Three months after surgery, the stumps of the implants were carved to improve their parallelism with a special diamond drill (Kit Bredent®). Finally, we took impressions for the final restoration with polyether (Impregum, 3 M ESPE) without using retraction threads.

The final restorations were produced using CAD/CAM System Juvora® for the PEEK structure with composite coating (Anaxdent®). For cementation ionomer glass cement reinforced with resin was used (GC FujiCEM, GC Europe N.V.) (Figs. 3 and 4).

Tracking

A clinical and radiographic review carried out a year after the initial surgery showed the complete success of the procedure according to Albrektsson's criteria and the natural aspect of the soft tissue around the restorations (Fig. 5).

Discussion

Intraoral conditions (saliva pH, acidic drinks, bacterial plaque, etc.) interact with metals, increasing corrosion, a phenomenon that also affects titanium implants [4, 5]. Amongst other reasons, this is whereby patients increasingly request the use of materials free of metallic alloys. In response to this growing demand, zirconia implants are considered an alternative, due to their low reactivity [6].

In recent years, several implant manufacturers have investigated the behaviour of zirconia implants on hard and soft tissues. The characteristics of their biocompatibility, together with good osseointegration, make them clear candidates for clinical use in dentistry [7, 8]. One of the advantages of these implants is the absence of cracks (gap) between pillar and implant since they are made in a single block. (Bredent®, Straumman®) [9, 10]. However, this feature implies the need to carve the pillars to achieve proper parallelisation.

Several studies have shown that zirconia implants present a similar healing pattern to titanium implants, both as regards the healing time and marginal bone stability [11–13]. However, there is a controversy over the long-term stability of the bone-implant interface, which depends on several factors such as surface, composition and design of the implant. Other important factors to consider are the implant-stump-crown connection, as well as the composition of the restorative material and the occlusal load transmitted by the antagonist tooth.

In terms of the load-cushioning capacity of the prosthetic elements, the use of PEEK as a prosthetic structure on implants has increased in recent years [14]. PEEK is a high-density thermoplastic polymer with a linear aromatic semi-crystalline structure that has exceptional physical and chemical properties as regards toughness, hardness and elasticity. Also, its low molecular weight, combined with the absence of metal, allows its use as excellent biocompatible prosthetic denture material.

PEEK has a modulus of elasticity (E-modulus 4 GPa) great overdenture implants compared to other conventional materials such as titanium (E-module 110 GPa) or zirconium dioxide (E-modulus 210 GPa).

In addition, the bending resistance of metal-ceramic restorations stands at around 400 to 600 Mpa. [15], in contrast to new composite coatings that have a Vickers hardness of approximately 400 MPa and a bending capacity of 314 MPa. Conversely, zirconia is three times harder (1200 HV) and its resistance to bending is 1400 Mpa [16].

As a whole, all of these features mean that the use of materials of high rigidity will result in direct transmission of chewing forces to the zirconia implant. This potential overload could cause bone reabsorption around the implants [17]. Some authors claim that this relation only exists in cases accompanied by a previous inflammatory process (of infectious origin), [18] where bone loss would be accelerated.

To avoid exceeding the adaptive limits of the bone and maintain the proper stimulation of mechanical stress that will keep the bone vital [19], PEEK components seem a viable alternative to obtaining a similar modulus to that of cortical bone. In this way, bone could be stimulated, favouring remodelling without overload [20]. It would concentrate the load by absorbing and distributing the same [21]. Its capacity of load absorption has led

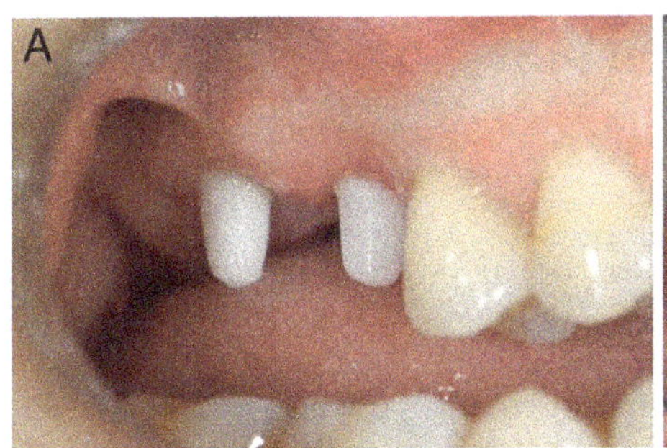

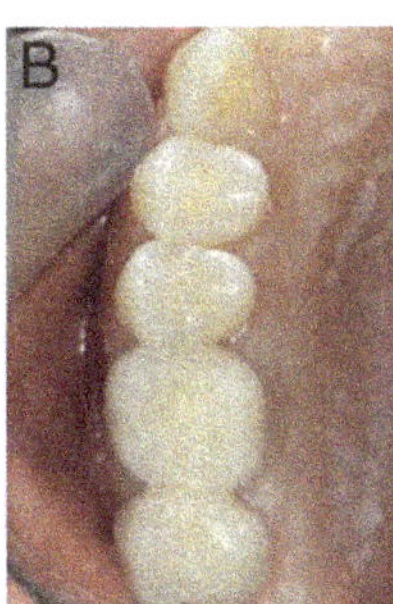

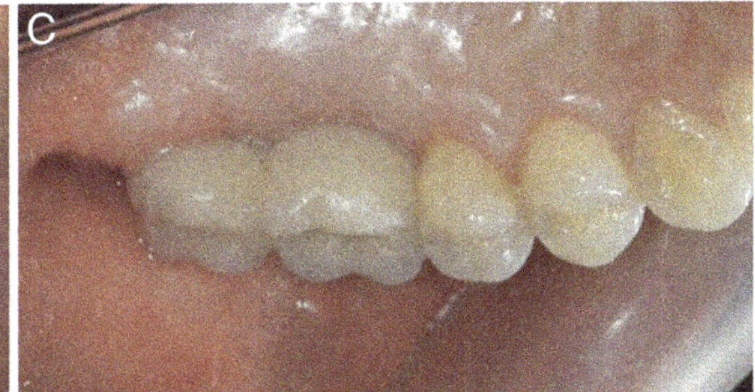

Fig. 3 Final restaurations: The parallelism of the implants is achieved by carving the non-submerged part **a** occlusal view and **b** lingual view

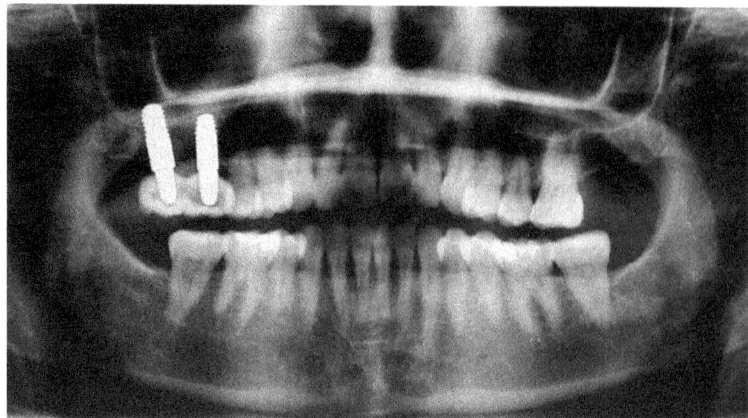

Fig. 4 Follow-up after 1 year, no radiographic sign was appreciating and the osseointegration was satisfactory

some authors to recommend its use in patients with severe bruxism [22].

Finite element analysis suggests that maximum contact pressure at the bone-titanium implant interface can be significantly reduced by using a PEEK crown rather than a ceramic crown [23].

In addition to PEEK, new coatings based on PMMA or composite materials (Anaxblent®Anaxdent®, Nexco®Ivoclar®, Solidex®Shofu®, Novo.lign®Bredent®, etc.) which incorporate ceramic fillings have been developed. Due to their molecular structure, these materials have excellent density and homogeneity [24]. The micro filling integrated into the polymer matrix increases abrasion resistance, at the same time as providing optimal elasticity which resembles the natural structure of a tooth. Although these restorations show good colour stability and a long-lasting shine, texture and brightness, they differ substantially from ceramic coatings which have excellent optical properties that enable them to achieve better long-term aesthetic results.

None of the authors have any competing interests in the manuscript. All authors have performed important contribution and have read and approved the final version to be published.

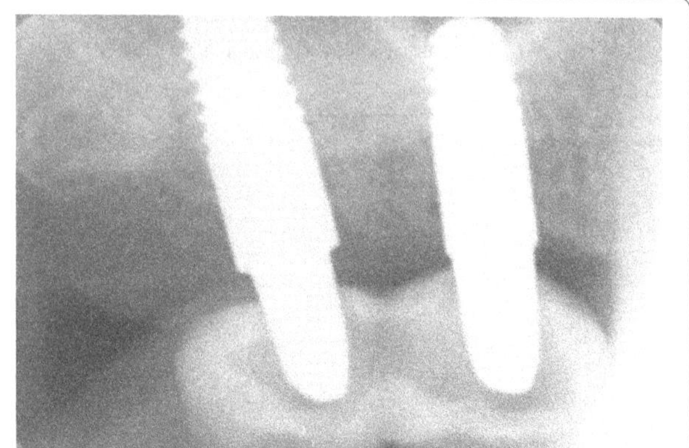

Fig. 5 Periapical X ray after 1 year of follow-up, the bone was stable and no sign of peri-implantitis was shown

Conclusions

Zirconia implants with PEEK restorations can be considered a good alternative for replacing natural teeth. Their biocompatibility and biostability make them a promising material for those patients who suffer from allergies and sensitivity to metal alloys.

PEEK restorations are a valid and alternative recommendation when using zirconia implants because of their cushioning effect and elastic modulus, which absorb occlusal forces and wear like a natural tooth, which could optimise and preserve osseointegration with time.

Within the limitations of this study, we recommend the combined use of zirconia implants, PEEK structures and PMMA coatings in patients with intolerance to or rejection of metal alloys.

Authors' contributions

SPA participated in its design and coordination, helped to draft the manuscript and is the corresponding author. PIJM performed the surgery and patient treatment. CMME participated in its design and coordination and helped to draft the manuscript. MJJ participated in its design and coordination and helped to draft the manuscript. All authors read and approved the final manuscript.

Competing interests

The authors Arturo Sánchez-Pérez, José María Parmigiani-Izquierdo, María Eugenia Cabaña-Muñoz, José Joaquín Merino certify that they have no affiliations with or involvement in any organization or entity with any financial interest (such as honoraria; educational grants; participation in speakers' bureaus; membership, employment, consultancies, stock ownership, or other equity interest; and expert testimony or patent-licensing arrangements) or non-financial interest (such as personal or professional relationships, affiliations, knowledge or beliefs) in the subject matter or materials discussed in this manuscript.

Author details

[1]Periodontics Unit, Faculty of Medicine and Dentistry, University of Murcia (Spain), Murcia, Spain. [2]Clínica CIROM, Murcia 30001, Spain. [3]Clínica Odontologíca Universitaria, Hospital Morales Meseguer, 2ª planta, C/ Marqués de los Vélez s/n, Murcia 30008, Spain.

References

1. Brånemark PI, Hansson BO, Adell R, Breine U, Lindström J, Hallén O, et al. Osseointegrated implants in the treatment of the edentulous jaw. Experience from a 10-year period. Scand j plast reconstr surg suppl. 1977;16:1–132.
2. Parmigiani-Izquierdo JM. TécnicaAtraumática en Implantología. Rev esp odontoestomatológica implant. 11:30–5.
3. Parmigiani-Izquierdo JM, Sánchez-Pérez A, Cabaña-Muñoz ME. A pilot study of postoperative pain felt after two implant surgery techniques: a randomized blinded prospective clinical study. Int j oral maxillofac implants. 2013;28:1305–10.
4. Sedarat C, Harmand MF, Naji A, Nowzari H. In vitro kinetic evaluation of titanium alloy biodegradation. J periodontal res. 2001;36:269–74.
5. Chaturvedi TP. An overview of the corrosion aspect of dental implants (titanium and its alloys). Indian j dent res off publ indian soc dent res. 2009;20:91–8.
6. Wenz HJ, Bartsch J, Wolfart S, Kern M. Osseointegration and clinical success of zirconia dental implants: a systematic review. Int j prosthodont. 2008;21:27–36.
7. Andreiotelli M, Wenz HJ, Kohal R-J. Are ceramic implants a viable alternative to titanium implants? A systematic literature review. Clin oral implants res. 2009;20 Suppl 4:32–47.
8. Stadlinger B, Hennig M, Eckelt U, Kuhlisch E, Mai R. Comparison of zirconia and titanium implants after a short healing period. A pilot study in minipigs. Int j oral maxillofac surg. 2010;39:585–92.
9. Gahlert M, Burtscher D, Pfundstein G, Grunert I, Kniha H, Roehling S. Dental zirconia implants up to 3 years in function: a retrospective clinical study and evaluation of prosthetic restorations and failures. Int j oral maxillofac implants. 2013;28:896–904.
10. Gahlert M, Kniha H, Weingart D, Schild S, Gellrich N-C, Bormann K-H. A prospective clinical study to evaluate the performance of zirconium dioxide dental implants in single-tooth gaps. Clin oral implants res. 1 de abril de 2015;
11. Gahlert M, Roehling S, Sprecher CM, Kniha H, Milz S, Bormann K. In vivo performance of zirconia and titanium implants: a histomorphometric study in mini pig maxillae. Clin oral implants res. 2012;23:281–6.
12. Bormann K-H, Gellrich N-C, Kniha H, Dard M, Wieland M, Gahlert M. Biomechanical evaluation of a microstructured zirconia implant by a removal torque comparison with a standard Ti-SLA implant. Clin oral implants res. 2012;23:1210–6.
13. Oliva J, Oliva X, Oliva JD. One-year follow-up of first consecutive 100 zirconia dental implants in humans: a comparison of 2 different rough surfaces. Int j oral maxillofac implants. 2007;22:430–5.
14. Siewert B, Parra M. Eine neue Werkstoffklasse in der Zahnmedizin: PEEK als Gerüstmaterial bei 12-gliedrigen implantatgetragenen Brücken. Z zahnärztl implant. 29:148–59.
15. Callís EM. Fundamentos de la estética bucal en el grupo anterior. Quintessence; 2001. 401 p.
16. Steger E. Sistema CAD/CAM Zirkonzahn. Quintessenza odontotec. 2013;10:70–82.
17. Berglundh T, Persson L, Klinge B. A systematic review of the incidence of biological and technical complications in implant dentistry reported in prospective longitudinal studies of at least 5 years. J clin periodontol. 2002; 29 Suppl 3:197-212-233.
18. Duyck J, Vandamme K. The effect of loading on peri-implant bone: a critical review of the literature. J oral rehabil. 2014;41(10):783–94.
19. Frost HM. Perspectives: bone's mechanical usage windows. Bone miner. 1992;19:257–71.
20. Huiskes R, Weinans H, van Rietbergen B. The relationship between stress shielding and bone resorption around total hip stems and the effects of flexible materials. Clin orthop. 1992;274:124–34.
21. Ponnappan RK, Serhan H, Zarda B, Patel R, Albert T, Vaccaro AR. Biomechanical evaluation and comparison of polyetheretherketone rod system to traditional titanium rod fixation. Spine j off j north am spine soc. 2009;9:263–7.
22. Schwitalla AD, Spintig T, Kallage I, Müller W-D. Flexural behavior of PEEK materials for dental application. Dent mater off publ acad dent mater. 2015;31:1377–84.
23. Schwitalla AD, Abou-Emara M, Spintig T, Lackmann J, Müller WD. Finite element analysis of the biomechanical effects of PEEK dental implants on the peri-implant bone. J biomech. 2015;48:1–7.
24. Rosentritt M, Preis V, Behr M, Sereno N, Kolbeck C. Shear bond strength between veneering composite and PEEK after different surface modifications. Clin oral investig. 2015;19:739–44.

Three-dimensional computer-guided implant placement in oligodontia

Marieke A. P. Filius[1], Joep Kraeima[1], Arjan Vissink[1], Krista I. Janssen[2], Gerry M. Raghoebar[1] and Anita Visser[1*]

Abstract

Background: The aim of computer-designed surgical templates is to attain higher precision and accuracy of implant placement, particularly for compromised cases.

Purpose: The purpose of this study is to show the benefit of a full three-dimensional virtual workflow to guide implant placement in oligodontia cases where treatment is challenging due compromised bone quantity and limited interdental spaces.

Patient and methods: A full, digitalized workflow was performed for implant placement in two oligodontia patients. Accuracy was assessed by calculating the coordinates of the entry point (shoulder) and apex (tip) as well as the angular deviation of the planned and actual implants.

Results: Implant placement could be well performed with the developed computer-designed templates in oligodontia. Mean shoulder deviation was 1.41 mm (SD 0.55), mean apical deviation was 1.20 mm (SD 0.54) and mean angular deviation was 5.27° (SD 2.51).

Conclusion: Application of computer-designed surgical templates, as described in this technical advanced article, aid in predictable implant placement in oligodontia where bone quantity is scarce and interdental spaces are limited.

Keywords: Oligodontia, Dental implants, Computer-guided implant dentistry, Guided surgery

Introduction

Oligodontia is the congenital absence of six or more permanent teeth, excluding third molars [1]. The need for oral rehabilitation in patients with oligodontia is high as they often suffer from functional and aesthetic problems due to a high number of missing teeth. Implant-based prosthodontics seem to be favourable to improve oral function and aesthetics in oligodontia [2].

Implant treatment in oligodontia is, in general, complex. The available bone volume is often limited for implant placement (e.g. above the mandibular nerve) due to jawbone underdevelopment in the area with the agenetic teeth as well as that the bone volume can be reduced due to physiological resorption of the alveolar process after a deciduous tooth without a successor has been lost. Moreover, the available interdental space and angulation of the neighbouring teeth are often unfavourable for implant placement in oligodontia cases.

Computer-designed surgical templates based on (cone beam) computer tomographic ((CB)CT) images have enabled higher precision and accuracy in implant planning [3]. Although this technique is promising, it has, as yet, not been tested in oligodontia. In this technical advanced article, we show the benefit of a full three-dimensional (3D) virtual workflow to guide implant placement in oligodontia, including an analysis of the accuracy of the actual implant placement in both cases.

Patient and methods

Implant planning and placement

Pre-implant procedure and 3D planning

A CBCT (ICat, Image Sciences International, Hatfield, UK; 576 slices, voxel size 0.3 mm, FOV: 11 × 16 cm) was made of two oligodontia patients (for patient details, see Figs. 1 and 2) for implant planning. Detailed patient

* Correspondence: a.visser@umcg.nl
[1]Department of Oral and Maxillofacial Surgery, University of Groningen and University Medical Center Groningen, PO Box 30.001, 9700 RB Groningen, The Netherlands
Full list of author information is available at the end of the article

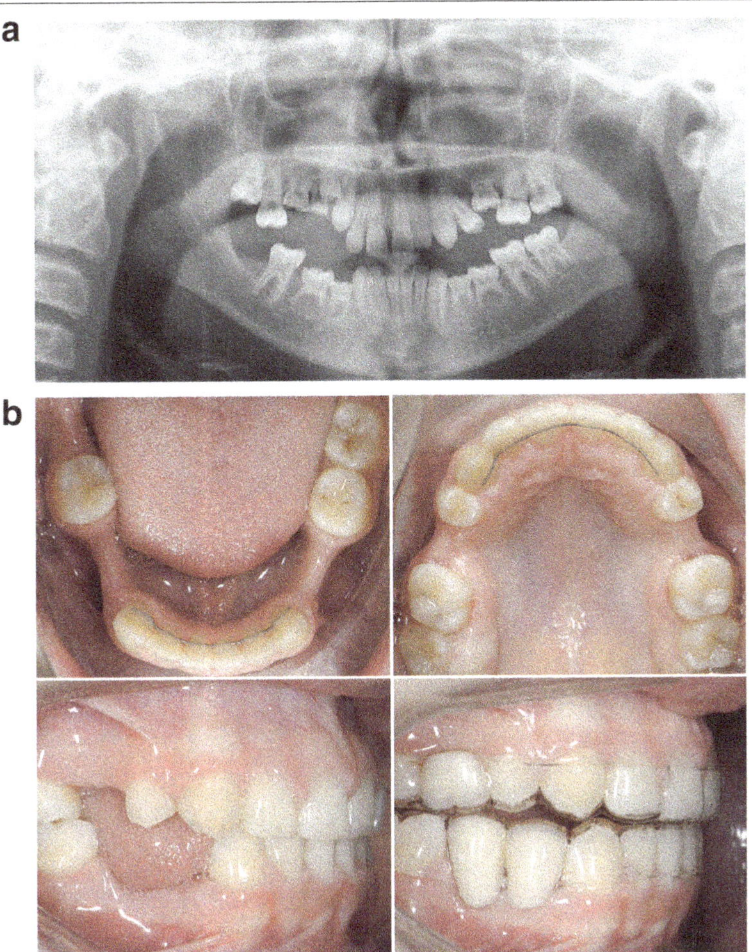

Fig. 1 **a** Patient 1—orthopantomogram (OPT) at age of 13. Situation before extraction of the ankylosed deciduous teeth 55, 54, 65, 74, 75, 84, and 85 and start of orthodontic treatment. Eleven permanent teeth (including 4 third molars) were congenitally missing. **b** Patient 1—post-orthodontic situation at age of 16. The top of the mandibular processus alveolaris is small (*upper*). The interdental space at location of the second premolars in the maxilla is 7 and 14 mm at location of the premolars in the mandible. Six dental implants were planned (locations 15, 25, 34, 35, 44 and 45). Implant placement (inclusive bone augmentation with the autogenous retromolar mandibular bone 3 months before implant placement at the place of the 25) was postponed until the age of 18. Essix retainers were used to safeguard the width of the diastemas

information was obtained with regard to the nerve position and bone quality and quantity. In addition, a digital intra-oral scan was made to get a detailed 3D image of the dentition (Chairside Oral Scanner: C.O.S., Lava™).

CBCT and intra-oral scanning data were combined using Simplant Pro (Dentsply, Hasselt, Belgium) in order to obtain a detailed 3D model of both patients (Fig. 3a, b) for virtual implant planning. The intra-oral scans, representing the dentition, were superimposed by a registration process, based on the contour of the corresponding dentition, onto the CBCTs. The intra-oral scan data was imported into the 3D virtual plan software as a *stl*-file. First, the objects representing the upper and lower dentition were globally positioned on the 3D data of the CBCT using manual translation functions. Next, exact positioning was determined using translation and rotation functions, starting in the mid-sagittal plane based on the contour of the model projected on the two-dimensional (2D) CT data. Refinements to the position were made while scrolling through the 2D CBCT data.

Virtual set-ups of the ultimate treatment goal were made for both patients with the virtual planning software Simplant Pro (Fig. 4a–c). Virtual teeth were aligned in the 3D virtual model. Based on the position of these teeth, the implants were planned in the optimal prosthodontic position; tooth size, optimal implant position, location of the mandibular nerve, bone quality and volume and antagonists were also accounted for. The planning was done by the technical physician (J.K.) for both cases, and the implant positions were checked and

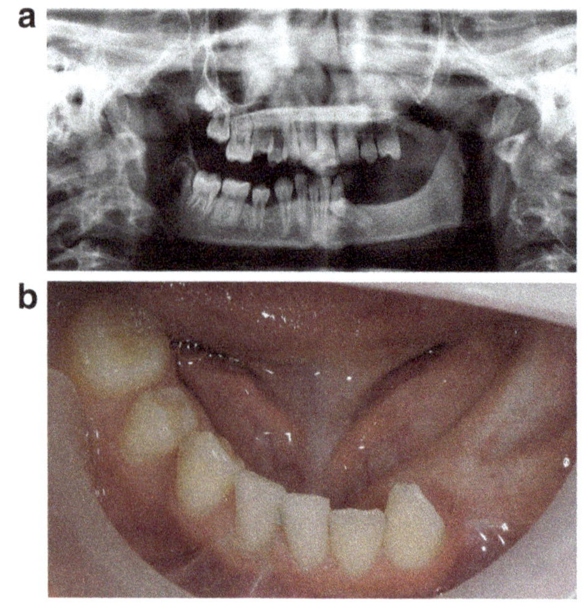

Fig. 2 a Patient 2—pre-implant orthopantomogram (OPG) at the age of 12. Situation before start of orthodontic and implant treatment. Eleven permanent teeth (including 2 third molars) were congenitally missing and the 34 is impacted. To erect the 34, orthodontic treatment was desired. Due to the lack of stable anchorages in the third quadrant, it was decided to place one implant at tooth region 35 for orthodontic anchorage and future prosthetics. Due to very limited bone height virtual implant planning was needed to avoid damage to the mandibular nerve. **b** Patient 2—mandible, pre implant intra-oral situation at the age of 12. The 34 is not visible in the oral cavity

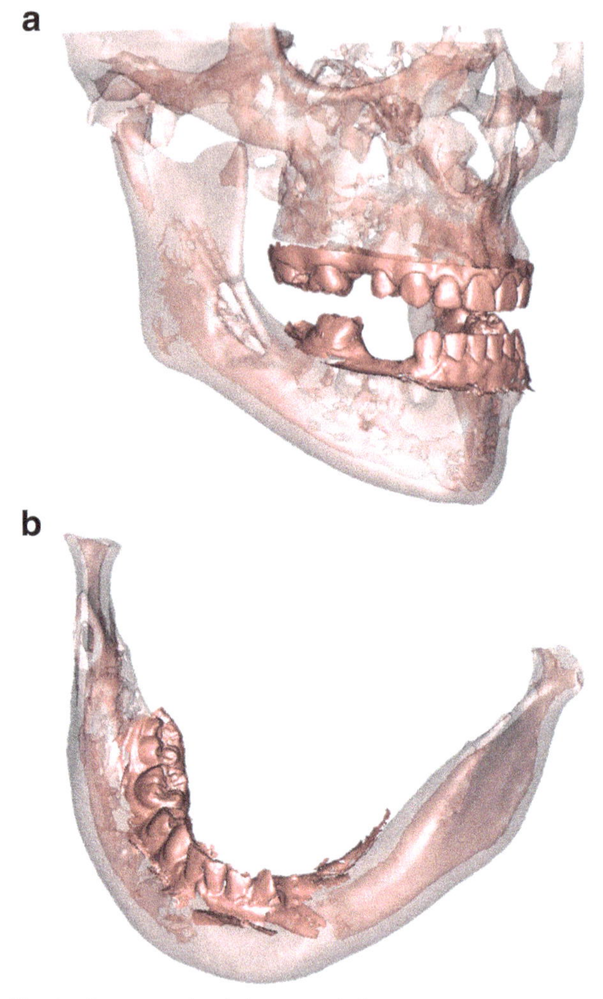

Fig. 3 a Patient 1—detailed 3D model of the combined data from the CBCT and intra-oral scan at age of 18. **b** Patient 2—detailed 3D model of the combined data from the CBCT and intra-oral scan at age of 12

optimized by the prosthodontist (M.F. and A.V.), orthodontist (K.J.) and surgeon (G.R.).

Fabricating 3D templates

Tooth-supported implant drilling templates were designed by the dental technician, based on the final virtual set-ups using the Geomagic Freeform software (3D Systems, Rock Hill, USA), and then fabricated out of polymethacrylate (Fig. 5a, b). The positioning of each implant was enabled with a 5-mm outer diameter metal drill sleeve (Nobel Guide, Nobel Biocare Holding AG, Zürich-Flughafen, Switzerland; Fig. 5a) as drill sleeves minimize deviation in drill position. The templates were checked for fit and stability in the intra-oral situation.

Implant placement

After raising a mucoperiostal flap, the dental implants were placed using the virtual developed tooth-supported drilling templates using metal inserts (Fig. 5c). It was checked whether no dehiscences of the implant surface were present.

Results

Clinical and radiographic assessments

The surgical guides fitted well and facilitated implant placement. All implants were placed in the native bone. No dehiscences of the implant surface occurred.

Post-operative orthopantomograms (OPT) of patients 1 and 2 are shown in Figs. 6 and 7. In patient 1, six implants were placed (NobelParallel Conical Connection implants, Nobel Biocare Holding AG, Zürich-Flughafen, Switzerland; Length 8.5 mm; diameter 3.25 mm). In patient 2, one implant (Straumann Standard Plus, Institut Straumann AG, Basel, Switzerland; Length 4.0 mm; diameter 4.1 mm) was placed at region 35. For patient 2, after osseointegration, the temporary prosthetic construction with a bracket to erupt the 34 was placed. Eruption of the 34 was already seen after 3 months of

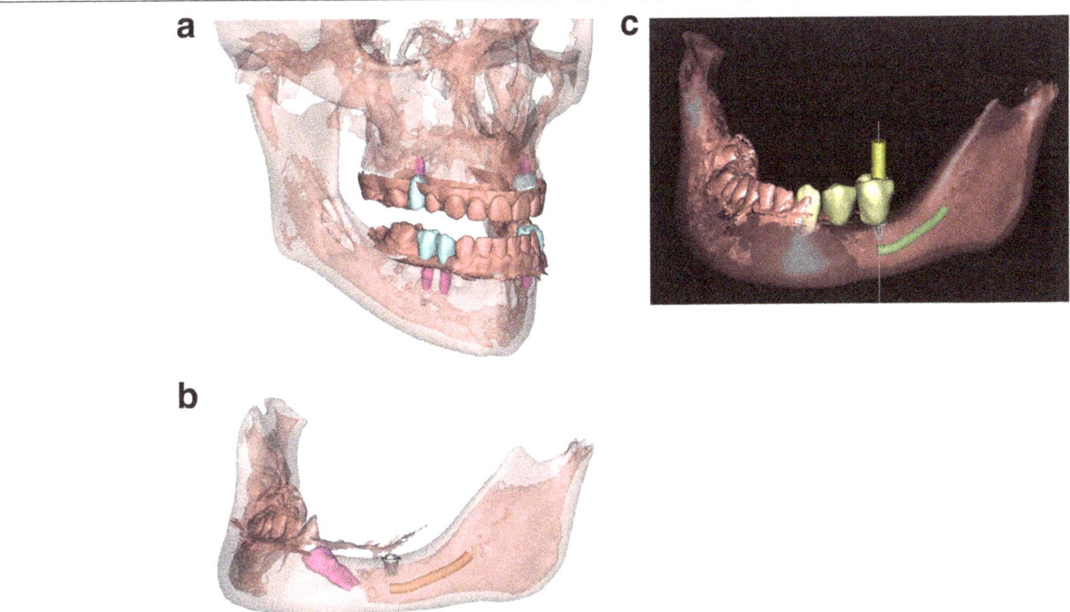

Fig. 4 a Patient 1—virtual set-up of the ultimate treatment goal. **b** Patient 2—virtual set-up of the ultimate implant position. One short dental implant was planned in region 35, based on the location of the mandibular nerve (*orange*), the impacted 34 (*pink*) and the bone quality and volume. **c** Patient 2—virtual set-up of the ultimate prosthetic treatment goal

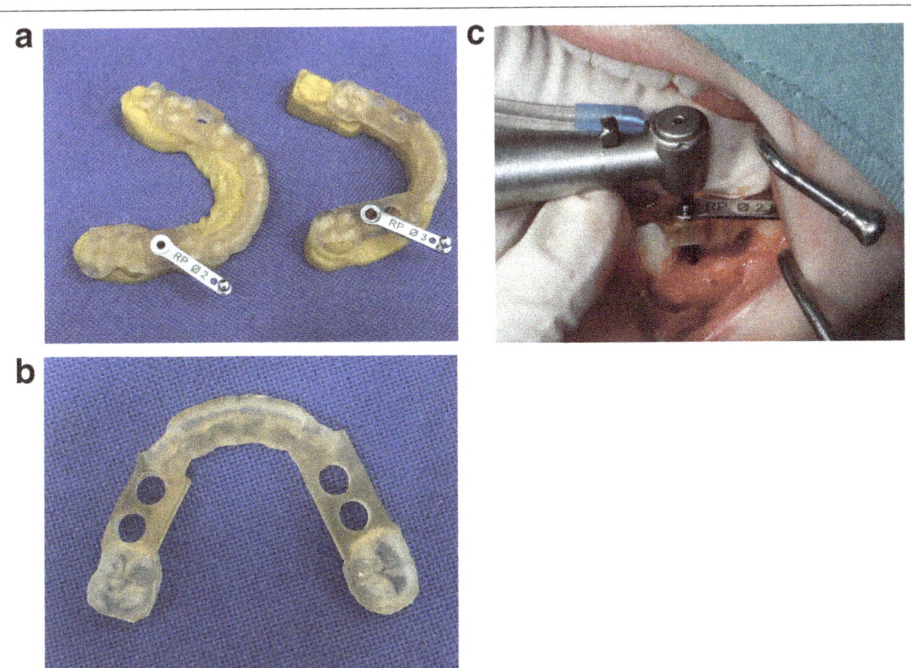

Fig. 5 a Drilling templates of patient 1. Printed model of the maxilla (*left*) and mandible (*right*) with drilling template and metal drilling inserts (Nobel biocare). **b** Drilling template for the mandible of patient 1. **c** Implant placement of patient 1. Dental implant placement in the mandible using the virtual developed tooth-supported templates and metal drilling inserts

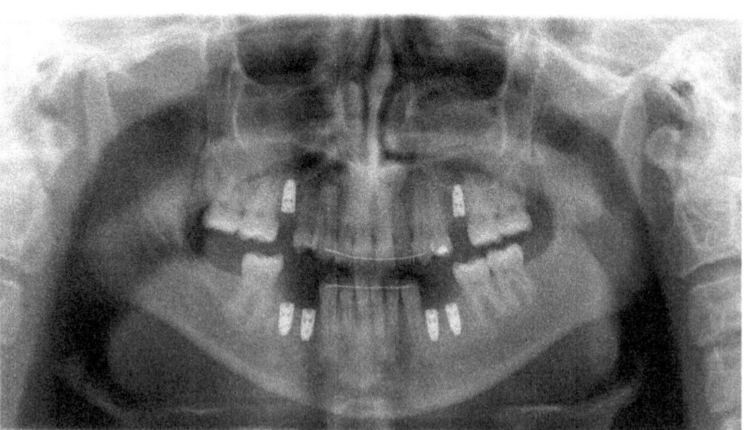

Fig. 6 Patient 1—post-operative orthopantomogram (OPT) at age of 18

orthodontic treatment (Figs. 7 and 8). Figure 9 shows the prosthodontic end result of patient 1.

Assessment of accuracy of implant placement

To assess the accuracy of the implant placement, post-operative CBCTs were made of both patients. 3D models of the postoperative result were obtained and superimposed on the data of the implant planning using a surface based alignment method (iterative closest point algorithm) and the same threshold value as used for the pre-operative scans. To deal with the scattering on the post-operative CBCT images in the implant regions, all implants were virtually matched with cylindrical shapes, positioned on the 2D CT data. These cylinders had the same dimensions as the implants and thus adequately represented the implants. The implant placement accuracy was calculated by comparing the pre- and post-implant placement coordinates of the entry point (shoulder), apex (tip) and angular deviation of the implants. Table 1 shows the accuracy data as Euclidian distances (ED) in millimetres (mm) of the entry point (shoulder) and apex (tip) of the implants as well as the degree of angular deviation of all implants ($n = 7$). Mean shoulder deviation was 1.41 mm (SD 0.55); mean apical deviation, 1.20 mm (SD 0.54); and mean angular deviation, 5.27° (SD 2.51). Figure 10 shows the actual differences in the planned and actual location of the implants of patient 1.

Discussion

This technical advanced article illustrated the benefit of a full three-dimensional virtual workflow to guide implant placement in oligodontia cases as well as that implants can be reliably placed at the planned positions with the technique proposed.

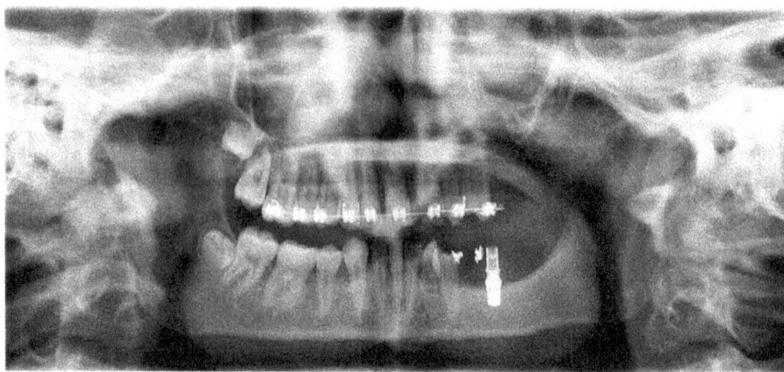

Fig. 7 Patient 2—post-operative orthopantomogram (OPT) at age of 13. Situation 10 months after implant placement. Three months after starting the orthodontic treatment, the 34 is already erected

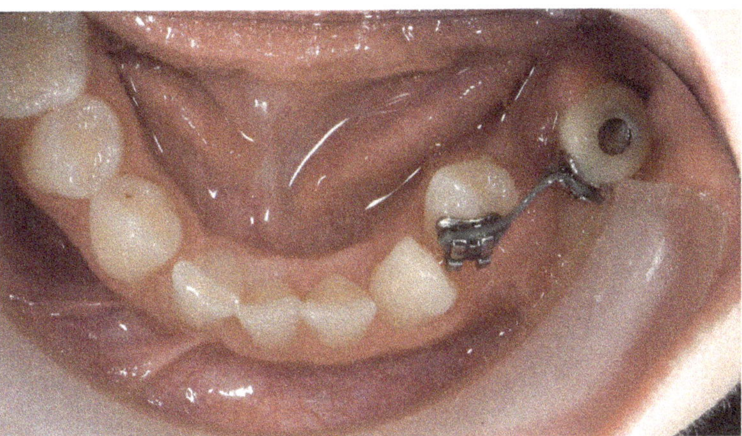

Fig. 8 Patient 2—intra-oral situation during orthodontic treatment at the age of 14. A temporary crown with bracket is fixed on the dental implant. Eight months after start of orthodontic treatment, the 34 is already close to the planned end position

The described full three-dimensional virtual workflow has several advantages. First, the surgeon is pre-operatively better informed about the requirements for the prosthodontic treatment with regard to the implant position. Second, the patient is pre-operatively better informed about the surgical procedure as well as the prosthodontic end result. The current costs are a limitation of this technique as fully digital planning is more expensive in comparison to a conventional approach. The expectation is that these costs will decrease with the time as this technique will be used more often in the future and probably the costs of the dental technician can also be reduced. At the moment, the extra costs for a full digital planning are reimbursed by Dutch health insurance companies. However, to the best of our knowledge, this (extra) reimbursement is not common in many other countries.

The difference in position between the virtually planned and actually placed implants, according to our workflow, resembles the deviation in implant placement for virtually planned and placed implants in non-oligodontia patients [3–6]. Schneider et al. [4] report in their systematic review a mean deviation of 1.07 mm (95% CI 0.76–1.22 mm) at the shoulder and 1.63 mm (95% CI 1.26–2 mm) at the apex as well as a mean angular deviation of 5.26° (95% CI 3.94–6.58°). More recent studies report similar results [3, 6]. Thus, the accuracy of virtual implant planning in oligodontia patients is comparable to that reported in non-oligodontia cases.

A variety of factors (i.e. technical, product, mechanical, procedure and environmental factors) can affect the accuracy of implant placement [7]. Commonly, implant placement accuracy is higher by experienced surgeons [8], but patient-related factors are often less easy to

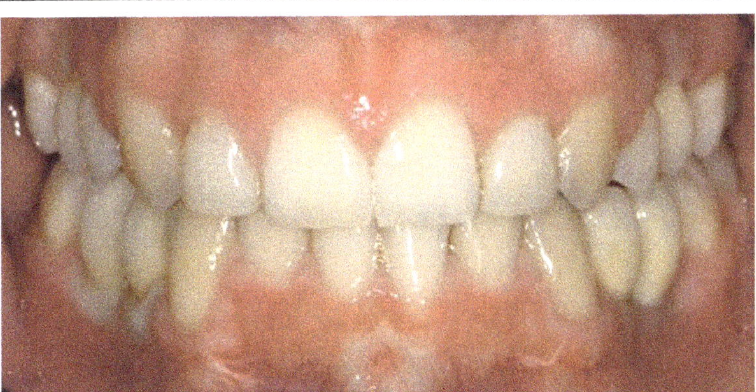

Fig. 9 Patient 1—prosthodontic end result 5 months after implant placement

Table 1 Accuracy data: Euclidian distances (ED, mm) of the apex (tip) and entry point (shoulder) and the degree (°) of angular deviation (axis) of the implants ($n = 7$)

Patient	Location implant (tooth nr)	Shoulder				Tip				Axis			
		X	*Y*	*Z*	ED (mm)	*X*	*Y*	*Z*	ED (mm)	*X*	*Y*	*Z*	(°)
1	15 planned	51.52	51.16	47.69		51.69	51.31	56.48		−0.02	−0.02	1.00	
	15 actual	52.85	51.82	48.89	1.91	52.57	50.64	57.60	1.58	0.03	0.13	−0.99	9.10
1	25 planned	90.72	51.04	48.83		90.43	49.74	57.52		0.03	0.15	−0.99	
	25 actual	91.42	50.29	51.04	2.43	90.88	49.60	59.78	2.31	0.06	0.08	−1.00	4.40
1	34 planned	89.21	47.78	16.06		88.12	45.53	24.49		0.12	0.26	−0.96	
	34 actual	88.39	47.86	16.15	0.82	87.90	45.96	24.57	0.49	0.06	0.22	−0.97	4.40
1	35 planned	91.44	51.17	27.24		91.90	53.25	18.72		0.05	0.24	−0.97	
	35 actual	91.02	51.17	26.14	1.18	91.44	54.07	18.00	1.18	−0.05	−0.34	−0.94	5.90
1	44 planned	58.46	48.01	14.10		58.28	46.58	22.77		0.02	0.16	−0.99	
	44 actual	58.34	49.51	13.77	1.54	57.88	46.98	22.02	0.94	0.05	0.29	−0.96	7.90
1	45 planned	55.98	54.54	15.58		55.52	52.54	24.13		0.05	0.23	−0.97	
	45 actual	55.44	54.48	15.03	0.78	54.95	52.78	23.41	0.95	0.06	0.24	−0.97	0.68
2	35 planned	129.71	50.02	66.16		129.68	50.06	71.34		0.01	−0.01	−1.00	
	35 actual	128.5	50.28	66.15	1.24	128.70	49.99	71.31	0.98	−0.04	0.06	−1.00	4.50
Mean					1.41				1.20				5.27
SD					0.55				0.54				2.54

control. Some progress has been made to control patient factors by using tooth-supported drilling templates, as demonstrated here; they enable a more precise transfer of the virtual implant planning to the surgical site than mucosa- or bone-supported templates [6, 9]. However, there is still a need to identify appropriate evaluation techniques and mechanisms capable of optimizing transfer precision and eliminating errors of three-dimensional planning and guiding systems for the partially dentate jaw [10]. Planning is complex, and high transfer precision is not always easy to accomplish, particularly in oligodontia cases with a large number of missing teeth. With the use of the described method, pre-operative implant planning is possible and placement is more predictable.

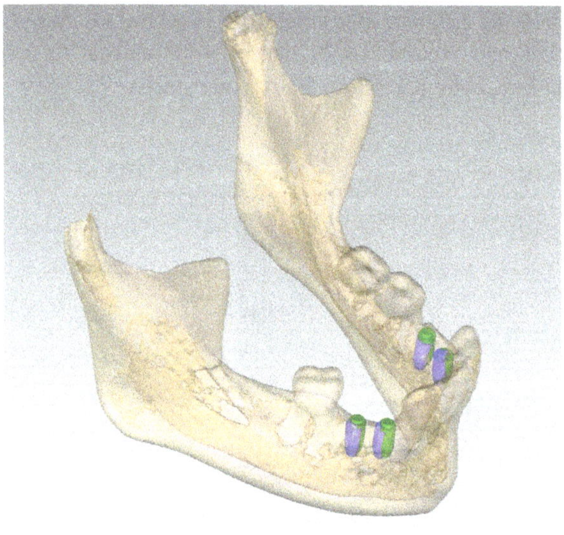

Fig. 10 Patient 1—post-operative evaluation of placement accuracy of the implants in the mandible. *Green* is the planned position; *blue* is the actual position

Conclusion

This technical advanced article introduces a fully digitalized workflow for implant planning in complex oligodontia cases. The application of computer-designed surgical templates enables predictable implant placement in oligodontia, where bone quantity and limited interdental spaces can be challenging for implant placement. The stepwise approach described in this technical advanced article provides the dentist and surgeon with a basis to plan and guide the preferred implant placement in oligodontia cases.

Abbreviations

(CB)CT: (Cone beam) computer tomography; 2D: Two-dimensional; 3D: Three-dimensional; ED: Euclidian distances; OPT: Orthopantomogram

Acknowledgements

The authors like to sincerely thank all co-workers from the Department of Orthodontics, University Center Groningen, The Netherlands, for the potent collaboration during the treatment process.

We also kindly thank native English speaker Jadzia Siemienski for critically reading our manuscript and making suggestions to improve the English.

Funding
This research did not receive any specific grant from funding agencies in the public, commercial or not-for-profit sectors.

Authors' contributions
MAPF and JK contributed to the 3D planning and in writing the manuscript. GMR carried out the implant placement and contributed in writing the manuscript. AVissink contributed in writing the manuscript and gave final approval for submission. KIJ performed the orthodontic treatment and contributed in writing the manuscript. AVisser performed the prosthodontic treatment and contributed in writing the manuscript. All authors read and approved the final manuscript.

Competing interests
Author Marieke Filius, Joep Kraeima, Arjan Vissink, Krista Janssen, Gerry Raghoebar and Anita Visser state that there are no conflicts of interest.

Author details
[1]Department of Oral and Maxillofacial Surgery, University of Groningen and University Medical Center Groningen, PO Box 30.001, 9700 RB Groningen, The Netherlands. [2]Department of Orthodontics, University of Groningen and University Medical Center Groningen, PO Box 30.001, 9700 RB Groningen, The Netherlands.

References
1. Schalk-van der Weide Y, Beemer FA, Faber JA, Bosman F. Symptomatology of patients with oligodontia. J Oral Rehabil. 1994;21:247–61.
2. Filius MA, Cune MS, Raghoebar GM, Vissink A, Visser A. Prosthetic treatment outcome in patients with severe hypodontia: a systematic review. J Oral Rehabil. 2016;43:373–87.
3. Shen P, Zhao J, Fan L, et al. Accuracy evaluation of computer-designed surgical guide template in oral implantology. J Craniomaxillofac Surg. 2015;43:2189–94.
4. Schneider D, Marquardt P, Zwahlen M, Jung RE. A systematic review on the accuracy and the clinical outcome of computer-guided template-based implant dentistry. Clin Oral Implants Res. 2009;20:73–86.
5. Van Assche N, van Steenberghe D, Guerrero ME, et al. Accuracy of implant placement based on pre-surgical planning of three-dimensional cone-beam images: a pilot study. J Clin Periodontol. 2007;34:816–21.
6. D'haese J, Van De Velde T, Komiyama A, Hultin M, De Bruyn H. Accuracy and complications using computer-designed stereolithographic surgical guides for oral rehabilitation by means of dental implants: a review of the literature. Clin Implant Dent Relat Res. 2012;14:321–35.
7. Yatzkair G, Cheng A, Brodie S, Raviv E, Boyan BD, Schwartz Z. Accuracy of computer-guided implantation in a human cadaver model. Clin Oral Implants Res. 2015;26:1143–9.
8. Rungcharassaeng K, Caruso JM, Kan JY, Schutyser F, Boumans T. Accuracy of computer-guided surgery: a comparison of operator experience. J Prosthet Dent. 2015;114:407–13.
9. Ozan O, Turkyilmaz I, Ersoy AE, McGlumphy EA, Rosenstiel SF. Clinical accuracy of 3 different types of computed tomography-derived stereolithographic surgical guides in implant placement. J Oral Maxillofac Surg. 2009;67:394–401.
10. Platzer S, Bertha G, Heschl A, Wegscheider WA, Lorenzoni M. Three-dimensional accuracy of guided implant placement: indirect assessment of clinical outcomes. Clin Implant Dent Relat Res. 2013;15:724–34.

24

Autogenous bone grafts in oral implantology—is it still a "gold standard"? A consecutive review of 279 patients with 456 clinical procedures

Andreas Sakkas[1*], Frank Wilde[1], Marcus Heufelder[1], Karsten Winter[2] and Alexander Schramm[1,3]

Abstract

Background: This study assessed the clinical outcomes of graft success rate and early implant survival rate after preprosthetic alveolar ridge reconstruction with autologous bone grafts.

Methods: A consecutive retrospective study was conducted on all patients who were treated at the military outpatient clinic of the Department of Oral and Plastic Maxillofacial Surgery at the military hospital in Ulm (Germany) in the years of 2009 until 2011 with autologous bone transplantation prior to secondary implant insertion. Intraoral donor sites (crista zygomatico-alveolaris, ramus mandible, symphysis mandible, and anterior sinus wall) and extraoral donor site (iliac crest) were used. A total of 279 patients underwent after a healing period of 3–5 months routinely computer tomography scans followed by virtual implant planning. The implants were inserted using guided oral implantation as described by Naziri et al. All records of all the consecutive patients were reviewed according to patient age, history of periodontitis, smoking status, jaw area and dental situation, augmentation method, intra- and postoperative surgical complications, and surgeon's qualifications. Evaluated was the augmentation surgical outcome regarding bone graft loss and early implant loss postoperatively at the time of prosthodontic restauration as well a follow-up period of 2 years after loading.

Results: A total of 279 patients underwent 456 autologous augmentation procedures in 546 edentulous areas. One hundred thirteen crista zygomatico-alveolaris grafts, 104 ramus mandible grafts, 11 symphysis grafts, 116 grafts from the anterior superior iliac crest, and 112 sinus lift augmentations with bone scrapes from the anterior facial wall had been performed. There was no drop out or loss of follow-up of any case that had been treated in our clinical center

(Continued on next page)

* Correspondence: ansakkas@yahoo.com
[1]Department of Oral and Plastic Maxillofacial Surgery, Military Hospital Ulm, Academic Hospital of the University of Ulm, Oberer Eselsberg 40, 89081 Ulm, Germany
Full list of author information is available at the end of the article

(Continued from previous page)

in this 3-year period. Four hundred thirty-six (95.6%) of the bone grafts healed successfully, and 20 grafts (4.4%) in 20 patients had been lost. Fourteen out of 20 patients with total graft failure were secondarily re-augmented, and six patients wished no further harvesting procedure. In the six patients, a partial graft resorption was detected at the time of implantation and additional simultaneous augmentation during implant insertion was necessary. No long-term nerve injury occurred. Five hundred twenty-five out of 546 initially planned implants in 259 patients could be inserted into successfully augmented areas, whereas 21 implants in 20 patients due to graft loss could not be inserted. A final rehabilitation as preplanned with dental implants was possible in 273 of the 279 patients. The early implant failure rate was 0.38% concerning two out of the 525 inserted implants which had to be removed before the prosthodontic restoration. Two implants after iliac crest augmentation were lost within a period of 2 years after loading, concerning a total implant survival rate after 2 years of occlusal loading rate of 99.6% after autologous bone augmentation prior to implant insertion.

Conclusions: This review demonstrates the predictability of autologous bone material in alveolar ridge reconstructions prior to implant insertion, independent from donor and recipient site including even autologous bone chips for sinus elevation. Due to the low harvesting morbidity of autologous bone grafts, the clinical results of our study indicate that autologous bone grafts still remain the "gold standard" in alveolar ridge augmentation prior to oral implantation.

Keywords: Autologous bone augmentation, Gold standard, Intraoral bone grafts, Complications, Dental implants, Donor site

Background

Oral implantation has a significant role in the rehabilitation of patients. Bone reconstruction techniques have been advanced in order to optimize the esthetic and functional outcome. However, the restoration of the oral function of atrophic alveolar crests still remains a challenge in oral implantology. Bone augmentation procedures are often indicated to allow implant placement in an optimal three-dimensional position to obtain long-term function and predictable esthetic outcome for prosthodontic restorations [1]. The extent of atrophy of the alveolar crest dictates whether the bone augmentation procedures may be performed simultaneously with the implant placement or as a separate procedure [2].

Among the different available augmentation materials, only autologous bone combines osteoconductive, osteoinductive, and osteogenic characteristics compared to bone substitute and composite materials [3]. Because of its properties and absence of immunological reactions, autologous bone grafts have been considered as the "gold standard" and most effective material in bone regeneration procedures [4–7]. Success rates exceeding 95% have been achieved, even when major augmentation procedures with autologous bone had to be carried out for severely resorbed jaws [8, 9]. However, limitations of autografts which include restricted donor sites and possible harvesting morbidity, reports of unpredictable resorption, and limited available bone volume had been reported for intraoral bone grafts [1, 9].

The most frequently applied bone augmentation techniques are staged guided bone regeneration procedures which include transplantation of an autologous bone block adding mechanical support to the covering soft tissues [10]. A number of different donor sites offering membranous or endochondral bone from regional or distant sites are available. The grafts differ considerably as far as embryology, histology, mechanical properties, and the volume that can be harvested are concerned. The choice of a specific donor site often is based on a number of different aspects like the expected donor site morbidity or bone resorption rate [8, 9]. Especially, sinus floor elevation is an established method of bone augmentation in the atrophic posterior maxilla [11].

Although the iliac crest is most often used in jaw reconstruction, a significant bone resorption has been mentioned [12]. This disadvantage, and the fact that dental implants do not always require a large amount of bone, has increased the use of autologous block bone grafts from intraoral sources [13]. Bone grafts from intraoral donor sites offer several benefits like surgical accessibility, proximity of donor and recipient sites, and less discomfort for the patient and less morbidity as compared with extraoral locations [14].

Intraoral harvesting has been reported to be associated with a relevant morbidity, and the significant graft resorption or their oral exposures are two of the most frequently reported complications [15]. The choice of the intraoral donor site is usually based on the amount, geometry, and type of bone required for alveolar reconstruction, and additionally, the incidence of intra- and postoperative complications should be considered [16, 17]. Six systematic literature reviews related to lateral atrophic ridges regenerated with intraoral bone block grafts have been reported and found evidence of bone gain and high implant success rates [18–22].

In the recent years, several alternatives have been investigated to supply the reported disadvantages of autologous bone. Allogenic grafts have been extensively used obtained from individuals from the same species but with different genetic load [23]. An allogenic graft is considered to be biocompatible with great applicability, exhibits good postoperative response without donor site morbidity, and is available in unlimited quantities [24, 25]. Furthermore, the anorganic bovine bone has received attention in the literature, since it yielded a long-term success in ridge augmentation technique. It is widely used for vertical and horizontal augmentation, sinus lift procedures, and socket treatment after tooth extraction [26]. While for sinus lift procedures bone substitutes have proven to achieve reliable results, we still lack clinical evidence that bone substitutes are equally reliable for horizontal and vertical augmentation of the dentoalveolar process.

In our military outpatient center exclusively, autologous bone transplantations harvested from different donor sites were used intraorally (crista zygomatico-alveolaris, ramus mandible, symphysis mandible, anterior sinus wall) and extraorally (iliac crest) to reconstruct severe horizontal and/or vertical alveolar ridge atrophy prior to implant placement. The aim of this study was to assess the clinical outcomes in terms of postoperative complications and harvesting morbidity, graft success rate, and implant survival rate, in a 2-year follow-up after alveolar ridge reconstructions with autologous bone grafts.

Methods

Patient selection

For this retrospective cohort study, we reviewed the records of all patients without exclusion criteria who were referred to the department of oral and plastic maxillofacial surgery at the military hospital of Ulm, Germany, between January 2009 and December 2011 for alveolar ridge augmentations prior to implant insertions using autologous bone grafts harvested from different donor sites and unilateral or bilateral sinus floor elevations with a lateral approach. There was no dropout or loss of follow-up of any patient that had been treated in our clinical center in this 3-year period (dropout rate = 0).

The files of 279 patients with a total of 456 augmentation procedures were reviewed.

At the first appointment for all included 279 patients, the medical and dental history as well as smoking habits was recorded using a standardized questionnaire.

During the initial clinical examination, the periodontal status was determined by means of a comprehensive periodontal assessment: lost teeth, teeth with bone loss over 5 mm, mobility grade, and periodontal pocket >4 mm were used to define a history of periodontal disease. Approximal Plaque Index (API) according to Lange and Sulcus Bleeding Index (SBI) according to Mühlemann and Son were also assessed at the first clinical examination [27, 28].

Occlusal and prosthodontic analyses were performed clinically as well as with the aid of dental casts.

The need for restorative treatment was also stated during this first appointment.

The preoperative radiological assessment included careful evaluation of the dental status and any pathologic conditions using panoramic X-rays and, potentially, computed tomography.

Indication for bone augmentation

Indication for the need for bone augmentation procedures was determined by means of the following parameters:

- Presence of severe alveolar ridge atrophy rated classes IV and V according to the Cawood and Howell classification [29]
- Residual maxillary bone less than 5 mm from the alveolar crest to the sinus floor

The indication for augmentation of the alveolar ridge defect was evaluated on the basis of a clinical examination with oral inspection and the use of dental casts and a radiological examination using panoramic radiographs to observe the height and width of the alveolar ridge and to identify structures of risk like the mandibular canal or the maxillary sinus. Three-dimensional radiographs had been used when clinical examination and two-dimensional radiographs were not sufficient to prove alveolar ridge dimensions. In 30.8% (83/279 patients), preoperative 3D CT examination had to be performed to assess the need and volume of bony reconstruction needed prior to implant insertion. All patients were informed in advance that bone grafting was necessary prior to implant placement because of the inadequate bone quality. Occlusal analysis was performed, diagnostic wax-ups were prepared on the articulated casts, and restorative treatment needs to be determined.

Surgical protocol

Bone block onlay graft procedures

A standardized two-stage surgical protocol was used, and all sites were treated in a similar fashion. In the first intervention, a bone block harvested from the donor site was fixed with osteosynthesis titanium screws to the recipient site as an onlay graft to achieve a horizontal and/or vertical enlargement of the alveolar ridge. Placement of the bone graft was always guided by an augmentation template as described by Schramm et al. [30–32]. In the second procedure, 3 to 5 months later, the screws were removed and the implants were placed using guided oral implantation as described by Naziri et al. The number of bone blocks and donor sites and the number of implants inserted in each augmented site were recorded. The choice of donor site, either left or right, was determined preoperatively based on defect morphology and recipient site location. Every bone harvesting procedure was performed using the same standardized surgical technique.

Intraoral autologous bone block grafts were harvested using piezoelectric surgery from the following donor sites:

- Lateral zygomatic buttress (crista zygomatico-alveolaris)
- Ramus mandible in the retromolar area
- Symphysis mandible

An oscillating saw and/or chisels were used for harvesting bone from the inner surface of the iliac crest (crista iliaca anterior superior).

The recipient site was dissected and pre-conditioned using a Safescraper device (C.G.M. S.p.A., Divisione Medicale META, Italy). The collected bone was preserved in a sterile environment until grafting. The block grafts were fixed with the aid of 1.0–2.0-mm diameter titanium osteosynthesis screws, and bone chips were packed around the bone blocks to fill gaps between the bone blocks and recipient buccal/labial wall. Any rough edges on the bone blocks were smoothed with a rotating burr and diamond burr. The entire graft was always covered by a collagen membrane (Bio-Gide, Geistlich Biomaterials, Wolhusen, Switzerland) and the periosteum was released to ensure a tension-free closure. The flap was closed with 3/0, 4/0, and 5/0 resorbable sutures.

Grafting from the iliac crest was always performed under general anesthesia in a two-team approach. The iliac crest was exposed and autogenous grafts from the anterosuperior inner edge of the iliac wing were harvested with an oscillating saw and/or a chisel, keeping a safe distance of around 2 cm from the anterosuperior iliac spine. After harvesting the bone grafts, the corticocancellous bone blocks were positioned by means of the technique described above.

The quantity of the bone needed for augmentation from the different donor sites was always depended on the size and form of the alveolar ridge defect and was evaluated always clinically before harvesting. The exact dimensional measurement of the bone blocks harvested and their radiological comparison in order to assess the resorption rate at the time of implantation was not investigated in this study. Each donor site provided a different bone quality according to the form and thickness.

Sinus lift procedures

Unilateral or bilateral sinus floor elevations in a two-stage procedure were also included in this study. The sinus augmentations were carried out with autogenous bone chips from the lateral sinus wall gained with a scraper device (C.G.M. S.p.A., Divisione Medicale META, Italy) as well as from the iliac crest, when the operation was combined with onlay grafts from the iliac crest.

Where the sinus lift procedures were concerned, the incision was made on the top of the alveolar ridge cutting the keratinized attached mucosa. A mucoperiosteal flap was raised, and the preparation started with the bone scraper (Safescraper; C.G.M. S.p.A., Divisione Medicale META, Italy). The bone from the anterior and lateral walls of the sinus was collected as part of the antrostomy. The preparation was concluded with the aid of a large round diamond bur to minimize the risk of Schneiderian membrane perforation. The Schneiderian membrane was carefully elevated using special mucosal sinus elevators until sufficient space for the impaction of bone material was created.

In addition to the bone already gained with the bone scraper device from the sinus wall during the antrostomy, bone was harvested with the same device from the maxillary buccal buttress, if more volume was needed. By taking this approach, the collection of enough bone for the augmentation of at least two implantation sites was feasible with a mean surgical time of 5 to 10 min for harvesting. In cases where an additional augmentation was performed with grafts from the iliac crest, the sinus lifting was performed with spongeous bone chips from the iliac crest instead of the bone gained locally with the bone scraper.

After impaction of the bone graft material in the sinus cavity, the bony sinus window was covered with a resorbable collagen membrane (Bio-Gide®, Geistlich Biomaterials, Baden-Baden, Germany). Finally, the mucoperiosteal flap was replaced and sutured without periosteal release if no additional bone block augmentation was performed at the same operation site.

Implant placement

After a healing period of 3 to 5 months, computed tomography scans were performed, followed by virtual implant planning using coDiagnostiX® software (Dental Wings GmbH, Chemnitz, Germany). After transfer of the planning into surgical guides, the augmented regions were re-opened, the screws which had been inserted during bone block augmentations were removed, and the implants were inserted using guided oral implantation as described by Naziri et al. [33]. All patients were recalled every 6 months for clinical and radiological examination within a period of 2 years after prosthodontic rehabilitation.

The implant success rate was clinically and radiographically evaluated over a follow-up period of 2 years after prosthesis loading according to the criteria of Buser et al. described below [34]:

- Implant in situ
- No permanent disorders such as pain and dysesthesia
- No peri-implant infection
- No implant mobility
- No persistent peri-apical radio-translucency

Data collection

The following data were collected from the patients' medical files regarding bone augmentation during the postoperative healing period until prosthetical rehabilitation:

- Medical history of patient
- Age of patient at the time of bone harvesting and augmentation
- History of periodontal disease
- Smoking habits
- Donor site
- Jaw area and dental situation of the recipient site
- Intraoperative complications
- Postoperative complications after augmentation
- Management of complications
- Bone graft stability and clinical resorption prior to implant placement
- Complications after implantation in a 2-year follow-up after prosthesis
- Experience of surgeon (resident or consultant)

Complications

Complications related to autologous bone augmentation and implant procedures were registered using the following definitions:

Intraoperative complications
- Intraoperative perforation of the Schneiderian membrane

Early postoperative complications
- Soft tissue dehiscency, when a separation of the suture line with or without exposure of the barrier membrane occurred
- Wound infection/inflammation characterized by pain, swelling, redness, fever and/or purulent discharge that required additional antibiotic treatment
- Bone graft exposure with or without screw mobilization
- Sensory disturbance if altered sensation at the neural supply area of alveolar inferior nerve, lingual nerve, and infraorbital nerve was recorded after surgery
- Symptoms of sinusitis after surgery on the posterior maxilla
- Secondary hemorrhage at the donor or recipient site

Late postoperative complications
- Surgical removal of the bone graft, defined as *bone graft failure*
- Early implant loss, when assessed before the placement of prosthetical restorations
- Late implant loss, when assessed within 2 years after prosthetical restorations
- Sensory disturbance, if altered sensation at the neural supply area of alveolar inferior nerve, lingual nerve, and infraorbital nerve was recorded at the time of reentry for dental implantation 4 to 5 months after bone augmentation.

Additional augmentation procedures with bone chips needed at the time of implant placement to obtain sufficient implant coverage as a result of partial graft resorption or inadequate primary augmentation were recorded. The dimensions of the bony defects and the quantitative success of the bone augmentation were not measured in this study. Due to the retrospective design of this study and the use of resorbable membranes and since all implants were inserted submerged, no reentry procedure was indicated to allow clinical evaluation of the augmented hard tissue volume. When re-augmentation procedures were needed by patients who suffered from a bone graft failure, the second procedures were not included in our statistical evaluation.

Classification of implant failure

Early and late implant loss was documented in this study, defining the clinical success of osseointegration. Early implant failures were assessed before the acquisition of osseointegration, i.e., before the placement of prosthodontic restorations. Early implant failure could occur from the time of placement, during the healing phase and before abutment connection. The implant inserted after re-augmentation was not included in the survival rate analysis. Late implant failures were documented within a period of up to 2 years after loading of the prosthodontic restorations. Implant and prosthodontic restoration design were not evaluated.

Result presentation

Demographic data and complication rates were presented descriptively. The results were additionally analyzed in percentage terms and presented in the form of tables and diagrams.

Results

Patient characteristics

Two hundred seventy-nine patients—250 men and 29 women—underwent 456 augmentation procedures involving autologous bone grafts prior to implant placement. The patients ranged in age from 18.5 to 71.5 years (average 43.1 years) at the moment of augmentation surgery.

Of those patients, 162 (58.1%) were younger than 40 years of age and 117 (41.9%) were older than 40 years of age. Caries or periodontitis was, in the majority of cases, the cause of primary tooth loss (89.9%, $n = 251$), followed by trauma in 20 (7.1%) of the cases, and agenesis in eight cases (3.0%).

Regarding the alveolar crest situation preoperatively, 163 defects were recorded as single-tooth gap, 119 as free-ending dental arch, and 79 as tooth gap involving more than one tooth. Edentulism was observed in 19 of the cases. Three hundred one bone harvesting procedures were performed for augmentation of the maxilla and 155 for the mandible.

One hundred ninety of 279 patients were operated in the maxilla, while 69 patients were augmented only in the maxilla, and 20 patients were treated in the maxilla and mandible.

Ninety-three (33.3%) of the patients were smokers and 186 were non-smokers.

With reference to the gingival/periodontal indices, 174 (62.3%) patients had an API score <20%, while 105 (37.7%) patients had an API score ≥20 and ≤30% prior to augmentation. The SBI showed a score of <20% in 213 (76.3%) patients and ≥20 and ≤30% in 66 (23.7%) patients. Patients with higher scores than 30% had not been treated since this was the prerequisite to implant treatment. As regards of SBI, 213 (76.3%) patients showed a score <20%, in contrast to 66 (23.7%) patients with SBI score 20–30%.

Patient characteristics are listed in Table 1.

Three hundred donor sites were necessary to perform the 456 augmentation procedures. One hundred thirteen bone grafts were harvested from the zygomatic buttress (crista zygomatico-alveolaris), 104 grafts from the mandibular ramus (retromolar area), 38 grafts from the iliac crest (spina iliaca anterior superior), 36 grafts from the lateral sinus wall, and 9 grafts from the mandibular symphysis.

A total of 112 sinus floor elevations were performed. In all of the cases, implants were inserted in a two-stage procedure. The donor site for harvesting the bone for the sinus elevations was in 76 procedures in the iliac crest area, and in 36 procedures, the bone was harvested with a bone scraper device from the lateral sinus wall at the site of sinus lifting.

Table 1 Patient characteristics at the time of augmentation

Patient characteristics	N (%)
Gender[a]	
Male	250 (89.6%)
Female	29 (10.4%)
Age[a]	
<40 years	162 (58.0%)
>40 years	117 (42.0%)
Smoking habits[a]	
Smokers	93 (33.3%)
Non-smokers	186 (66.6%)
API score[a]	
<20%	174 (62.3%)
≥20%	105 (37.6%)
SBI score[a]	
<20%	213 (76.3%)
≥20%	66 (23.6%)
Cause of tooth loss[a]	
Caries/periodontitis	251 (89.9%)
Trauma	20 (7.1%)
Hypodonty	8 (3.0%)
Augmentation site in the upper or lower jaw[a]	
Only maxilla	190 (68.1%)
Only mandible	69 (33.9%)
Both maxilla and mandible	20 (7.1%)
Dental situation[b]	
Tooth gap	99 (21.7%)
Single-tooth gap	163 (35.7%
Free-end dental arch	154 (33.7%)
Edentulous	40 (8.9%
Surgeon[c]	
Residents	223 (35.2%)
Senior consultants	410 (64.8%)

[a]N refers to the total number of the study patients ($N = 279$)
[b]N refers to the total number of the augmented areas ($N = 456$)
[c]N refers to the total number of the surgical approaches ($N = 633$)

The distribution and number of transplanted grafts are illustrated in Table 2 according to different donor sites and grafting methods.

Where the surgical experience of the surgeons is concerned, residents performed 223 (35.2%) procedures in total, whereas consultants performed 410 (64.8%) procedures.

Surgical outcome

Four hundred thirty-six of 456 augmentation procedures were performed successfully.

Table 2 Donor sites and numbers of bone grafts as well as distribution in patients in this study

Donor site	Bone grafts (*N*)/patients (*N*)
Lateral zygomatic buttress	113/112
Mandibular ramus (retromolar)	104/86
Mandibular symphysis	11/9
Iliac crest for alveolar ridge augmentation Iliac crest for sinus floor elevation	116/38 76/38
Bone chips harvested with a Safescraper device from the lateral sinus wall for sinus floor elevation	36/34
Total	456/279

Table 3 Intra- and postoperative complications after autologous bone harvesting

Postoperative complications	%/procedures (*N*)
At donor site[a]	
Wound infection	2.6% (8/300)
At recipient site[b]	
Soft tissue dehiscence	6.3% (24/378)
Wound infection	5.8% (22/378)
Graft exposure	5.5% (21/378)
Maxillary sinusitis	0.5% (2/378)
Hemorrhage	0.26% (1/378)
Nerve disturbance	
Temporary hypoesthesia mental nerve after grafting from ramus mandible	10.5% (11/104)
Temporary hypoesthesia lingual nerve after grafting from ramus mandible	2.8% (3/104)
Temporary hypoesthesia mental/lingual nerve after grafting from symphysis mandible	0%
Temporary hypoesthesia infraorbital nerve[c]	2.6% (6/225)
Sinus membrane perforation[c]	4.8% (11/225)

[a] *N* refers to the total number of donor sites ($N = 300$)
[b] *N* refers to the total number of recipient sites ($N = 378$)
[c] *N* refers to the total number of the surgical approaches in the maxilla ($N = 225$)

Seven of the 104 mandibular ramus grafts, two of the 113 zygomatic buttress grafts, and one of the 11 symphysis grafts were lost. Out of the 38 iliac crest procedures, there were eight regions with graft failures. In two sinus floor elevations after two-stage procedure, bone grafting failed. Twenty bone grafts failed in total (4.3%).

Fourteen of 20 patients with total graft failure were augmented secondarily. Three patients with retromolar graft loss were re-augmented with contra-lateral retromolar grafts. Two patients with loss of zygomatic buttress grafts underwent re-augmentation after graft harvesting from the contra-lateral site. One patient who lost a mandibular symphysis graft was re-augmented with a retromolar graft, and eight patients who lost their iliac crest grafts at the implant site were also re-augmented with bone blocks from the mandibular ramus. The healing period for all the re-augmented patients was uneventful, and implants could be inserted without any further complications after integration of the bone grafts.

Six of the 20 patients who suffered from a graft loss (four after retromolar bone grafts and two after sinus floor elevation) wished no further augmentation procedure and were treated with a conventional prosthetic restoration.

In six patients, a partial graft resorption was detected at the time of implantation and an additional simultaneous augmentation with bone chips harvested with the Safescraper device (C.G.M. S.p.A., Divisione Medicale META, Italy) was then necessary in order to ensure the osseointegration of the implants. Two out of these six cases had grafts from the crista zygomatico-alveolaris, two from the ramus mandible and two from the iliac crest.

Distribution of the harvesting methods, intra- and postoperative complications of the donor and recipient site, and bone graft survival related to the different autologous augmentation procedures are listed in Table 3 and presented in Figs. 1, 2, and 3.

Crista zygomatico-alveolaris

One hundred thirteen zygomatic bone grafts were harvested in 112 patients. Two out of the 112 patients were treated in two different alveolar sites while the rest of the patients in only one atrophic area for augmentation of the maxilla. Of the 113 onlay bone graft procedures, 93 (82.3%) were defined as completely successful, while 20 (17.7%) had adverse effects, such as soft tissue dehiscence, swelling, wound infection, or graft exposure. Of the total areas with complications, four were defined in the donor site and 20 in the recipient area. Two patients developed postoperative symptoms of maxillary sinusitis in combination with persistent fistula at the donor site. By these two patients, a perforation of the maxillary sinus membrane was noted intraoperatively. The frequency of complications was higher in recipient sites. Except for minor complications such as soft tissue dehiscence ($n = 8$), wound infection and abscess formation were observed in five augmented areas and bone graft exposures in seven of the 113 cases. In two cases (1.7%), the bone graft was totally exposed in combination with wound infection and discharge of pus. The surgical removal of the graft was then inevitable; these two patients wished no further bone grafting operation and were finally treated with a conventional bridge reconstruction. Totally, 134 implants had been inserted in 111 augmented sites. In two cases, two implants were inserted with simultaneous bone chip augmentation because of partial bone graft resorption. None of the inserted

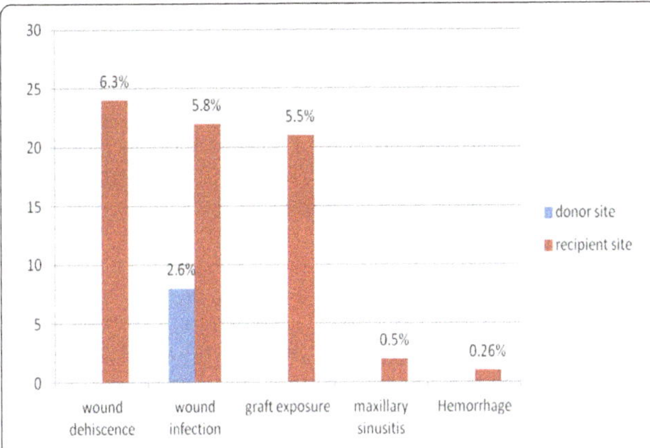

Fig. 1 Postoperative complications at the donor and recipient site, *N* refers to the total number of the donor sites (*N* = 300), *N* refers to the total number of the recipient sites (*N* = 378)

implants did fail due to lack of osseointegration at the time of prosthodontic restoration.

Ramus mandible (retromolar)

A total of 104 retromolar bone graft procedures in 86 patients were conducted. Twenty-two harvesting procedures were performed for augmentation of the maxilla and 82 for the mandible. Seven retromolar bone grafts (93.2%) in seven single-tooth gap dental regions by seven patients had been lost. Therefore, seven implants could not be inserted in augmented alveolar sites after graft failure. Three of the patients with total graft failure were secondarily augmented with retromolar grafts, harvested from the contra-lateral site, and all initially planned dental implants had been successfully inserted. The other four patients wished no further surgical procedure and were treated with a conventional prosthodontic restoration. A total of 155 implants had been inserted in 97 augmented sites. In 95 of the 97 cases, the implant insertions were uneventful; in two cases, the need of additional simultaneous bone chip augmentation due to partial graft resorption was essential. None of the inserted implants failed due to lack of osseointegration at the time of prosthodontic restoration.

Symphysis mandible

Eleven bone graft procedures harvesting from the mandibular symphysis were performed in nine patients. All procedures involving the mandible were done in the same surgical field for donor and recipient site. Two out of nine patients were treated in two different alveolar sites, while the rest of the patients in only one atrophied area. Of the 11 onlay bone grafts, 10 (90.9%) were defined as completely successful. In one patient, wound infection and abscess formation were developed and the bone graft had to be surgically removed. This patient after wound healing was re-augmented with a bone graft from the ramus mandible and could be successfully restored with an implant prosthesis as initially planned. A total of 10 dental implants were inserted in 10 augmented sites. None of the inserted implants failed due to lack of osseointegration at the time of prosthodontic restoration.

Iliac crest

Thirty-eight patients underwent a total of 116 augmentation procedures harvesting from the iliac crest. In 20 patients, a bone graft augmentation of the maxilla and the mandible in combination with bilateral sinus floor augmentations was performed. Eighteen patients had augmentations only in the maxilla, involving bone grafting and sinus lift elevations. Totally, 76 sinus lifts with bone material from the iliac crest had been performed. Eight grafts in eight patients developed wound infection combined with graft exposure, and the grafts were surgically removed. These patients were re-augmented with bone blocks from the mandibular ramus in the respective regions of bone loss. According to the donor site, one of 38 patients appeared with wound infection at the

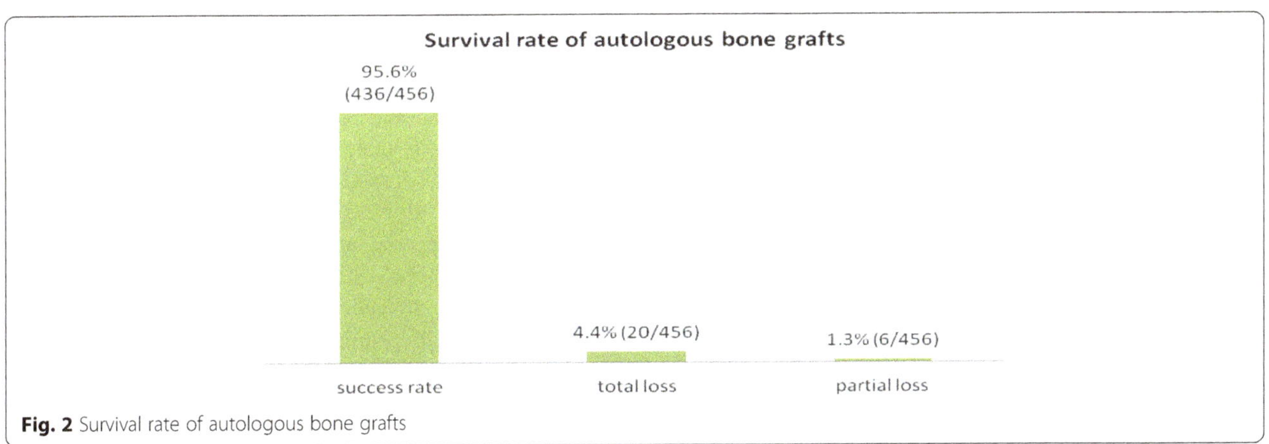

Fig. 2 Survival rate of autologous bone grafts

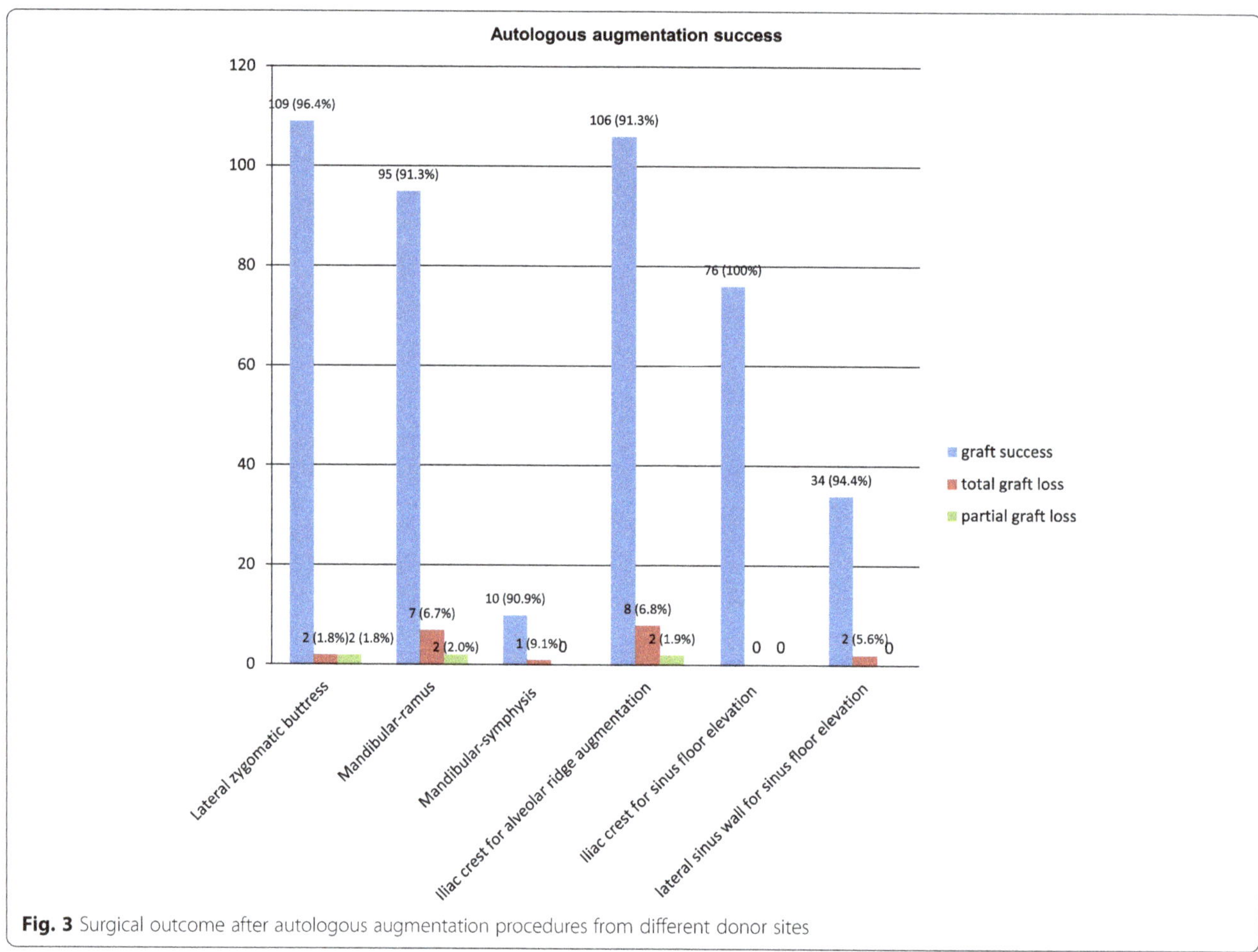

Fig. 3 Surgical outcome after autologous augmentation procedures from different donor sites

harvested iliac crest site. In the recipient sites occurred a higher complication rate. One case of soft tissue dehiscence, wound infection, and abscess formation was observed by six augmented areas and bone graft exposures in six of the cases. In addition, one patient showed a postoperative hemorrhage at the augmented area. A total of 187 implants had been inserted in 106 augmented areas. In two cases, two implants were inserted with simultaneous bone chip augmentation because of partial bone graft resorption. Two implants in two patients out of the 187 inserted implants were removed before the final prosthodontic restoration. One hundred eighty-five inserted implants showed regular osseointegration at the time of prosthodontic loading. Two implants were lost within 2 years after loading. These two implants concerned two patients after iliac crest graft augmentation and had to be removed due to development of peri-implantitis; the first 18 months and the second about 20 months after loading.

Sinus floor elevation

One hundred twelve sinus floor elevations had been performed in 72 patients to treat severely atrophic posterior maxilla using autogenous bone grafts. In 34 patients (36 sinus lifts), a sinus elevation was performed with bone material from the lateral sinus wall, while 38 patients (76 sinus lifts) underwent bone harvesting from the iliac crest. Of the 112 sinus floor elevations, 95 (84.8%) were uneventful, and 17 (15.2%) had adverse effects, such as swelling, wound infection with discharge of pus, or acute symptoms of sinusitis. Intraoperative complications in terms of perforation of the sinus membrane were observed in 9.8% ($n = 11$) of the cases and postoperative complications in 15.1% ($n = 17$). Four out of 11 patients (36.3%) with membrane perforation experienced postoperative complications accompanied by swelling and wound infections. Local wound dehiscence without fluctuance was developed 10–14 days after surgery in 11 of these cases. In four cases, abscess was developed postoperatively. Symptoms of acute sinusitis, such as nasal congestion, headache, diffuse pain on the operated facial site, and fever or redness, were diagnosed in two patients 1 week after sinus floor elevation. According to their medical history, none of those patients had pathological findings in the sinus in the past. Despite the appropriate treatment and antibiotic therapy, the graft resorption was extremely providing no sufficient bone for implant placement. These two patients refused any additional surgical treatment. No postoperative hypoesthesia in the area of the infraorbital nerve was reported. A total of 166 dental implants were placed with satisfactory primary stability in the augmented areas; among them, 16 implants were placed in a simultaneous one-stage procedure in 16 sinus lifts in 16 patients after harvesting intraoral bone. The rest 150 implants were inserted in a secondarily two-stage procedure. None of the implants were lost during the healing period, and all implants showed osseointegration at the time of implant exposure.

Nerve damage

No permanent damage to any trigeminal nerves was evident in any of our entire cohort. All cases of postoperative hypoesthesia of the mental, lingual, or infraorbital nerve were just a temporary nature. At the time of implant surgery, none of these patients reported any persisting neural disturbances (Fig. 4).

In eleven patients, hypoesthesia of the mental area was mentioned, and three of them also reported sensation disturbance in the tongue after the harvesting and transplanting of a bone block from the mandibular ramus. However, in all of these cases of neural dysfunction, the recipient site for the grafts was in the mandible, so that, it was not possible to evaluate whether the nerve disturbances were caused by the harvesting of the bone block, by the augmentation procedure due to manipulation of the mental nerve or even by the inferior alveolar nerve block. None of the patients mentioned any isolated hypoesthesia in the lingual area. Infraorbital nerve hypoesthesia was reported postoperatively by two patients after the harvesting of grafts from the zygomatic buttress. There was no incidence of nerve disturbances after bone harvesting from the mandibular symphysis or from the iliac crest, or after sinus lift procedures.

Perforation of the Schneiderian membrane

Sinus membrane perforation was observed intraoperatively in 11 of the 112 elevated sinuses (9.8%). After such perforations, postoperative complications accompanied by significant swelling and wound infection could be seen in four of these cases. Antibiotic treatment made the healing process absolutely effective, and dental implants could later be successfully inserted in all of these cases.

Postoperative complications

Wound infections were observed in 2.6% of the donor sites ($n = 8/300$) and in 5.8% of the recipient sites ($n = 22/378$), while soft tissue dehiscences such as incision line opening occurred in 6.3% of the recipient sites ($n = 24/378$). Graft exposure was diagnosed in 21 of the 378 recipient sites (5.5%), while maxillary sinusitis occurred in 0.5% of the cases ($n = 2/378$), and only one patient ($n = 1/378$; 0.26%) suffered from postoperative hemorrhage. A detailed list of the postoperative complications that occurred after bone augmentation is given in Table 3.

Complication management

Regarding intraoperative complications, all sinus membrane perforations were covered with a resorbable collagen membrane (Bio-Gide®, Geistlich Biomaterials, Baden-Baden, Germany) which applied as sealant to overlap the site of perforation prior to insertion of the graft material. These patients were advised to avoid

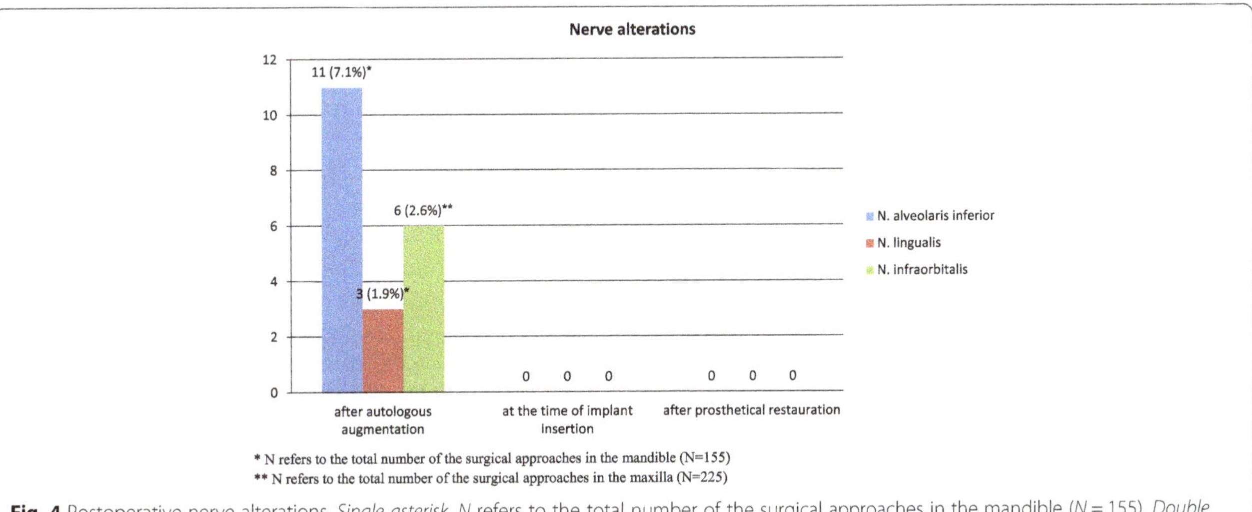

Fig. 4 Postoperative nerve alterations. *Single asterisk*, N refers to the total number of the surgical approaches in the mandible ($N = 155$). *Double asterisk*, N refers to the total number of the surgical approaches in the maxilla ($N = 225$)

physical stress, blowing their noses, or sneezing for a period of 3 weeks, and nose decongestant drops were prescribed.

Regarding postoperative swelling following the bone grafting procedure, most of the patients suffered a minimal facial deformity lasting not longer than 3–5 days. Swelling was so and otherwise an expected complication after surgery. At 2 weeks after the operation, none of the 179 patients reported persistent pain at the donor or recipient site.

Great importance was placed on the management of the postoperative complications. Minor effects such as soft tissue dehiscence with or without membrane exposure were treated conservatively with chlorhexidine mouth rinse (0.2%) and antibiotics either oral or intravenous (Augmentan®, GlaxoSmithKline Consumer Healthcare GmbH & Co. KG) achieving healing by secondary granulation. Patients with wound infection (n = ?) in the form of abscess formation had to be surgically drained, and systemic antibiotics were administered. In case of graft exposition without screw loosening (n = ?), the surgical field was revised, the bone block was refreshed with a diamond burr, and the flap was tensionlessly re-closed in combination parallel to antibiotic therapy. In case of graft exposure with screw mobility (n = ?), the bone grafts had been removed. All these patients were then scheduled to regular control appointments. Patients with symptoms of acute maxillary sinusitis after augmentation of the posterior maxilla (n = ?) were treated with antibiotic therapy and use of corticosteroid nasal spray for a period of 2 weeks.

Implant placement

The overall implant success rate was 99.2%. All implants, without exception, were placed with guided surgery after implant planning using the coDiagnostiX® software (Dental Wings GmbH, Chemnitz, Germany). Guided implant surgery was performed using insertion templates as described by Naziri et al. in all cases [34].

The average healing period until implant placement after bone harvesting was 4.53 months. Initially, 546 implants in 279 patients were planned. After the healing period, it was possible to place 525 implants in 436 successfully augmented areas in 259 patients. Three hundred implants were inserted in the maxilla and 225 in the mandible. The remaining 21 implants planned for 20 patients could not be placed. In six patients, an additional simultaneous augmentation with bone chips harvested with a bone scraper device was necessary to ensure that the entire implant shoulder was covered with bone. Two of these six patients had undergone augmentation with zygomatic buttress grafts, while two had received grafts from the mandibular ramus and two from the iliac crest.

A final rehabilitation with dental implants was possible in 97.9% of the patients (273 of 279). In the 14 patients who underwent re-augmentation due to primary graft failure, 15 implants could be successfully inserted later. The cases of implantation in a second time after re-augmentation were not included in our statistical evaluation. In the remaining six patients after graft failure, no re-augmentation was performed and no further implant treatment was desired.

Only two implants had to be removed from two patients before final prosthetic restoration due to lack of osseointegration, resulting in an early implant failure rate of 0.38%. These two implants were inserted in sites grafted with bone from the iliac crest. Both patients were smokers and had an SBI ≥ 20. The API of one of these two patients was also ≥20. With the exception of these two implants, all (523/525) were fully osseointegrated at the time of reentry for implant uncovery according to the Kerschbaum and Haastert criteria [35]. All of the implants were successful directly after prosthetic loading, based on the criteria of Buser et al. [34].

After prosthetic rehabilitation, all aspects of oral function were completely re-established in all patients. Two of 523 implants were lost within 2 years after prosthesis loading due to peri-implantitis. These data reveal a survival rate of 99.6% 2 years after prosthetic restoration.

The surgical outcome after augmentation and implantation procedures is presented in Fig. 5.

Discussion

Several grafting procedures have been described to create sufficient volume of bone for implant placement [8, 9]. Autologous bone grafts can be harvested by an intraoral approach (mandibular ramus, mandibular symphysis, zygomatic buttress) or from distant sites (iliac crest, calvaria, and etc.) [17, 36, 37]. However, bone harvesting potentially causes donor site morbidity which is a major issue for the patients who appreciate procedures that reduce morbidity [38]. In order to decrease surgery duration and donor site discomfort using autologous bone sources, bone substitutes from various bone origins such as allografts and xenografts for use in reconstructive implant surgery had been developed. The postulation that bone alternatives could successfully substitute the use of autologous bone and its osteoinductive, osteoconductive, and osteogenic properties is under consideration, and various studies have proven the benefits and appropriateness of its material for an ideal reconstruction of some selected atrophic ridges prior to implantation [19, 24].

The advantages of the use of autologous bone harvested for alveolar reconstruction must be carefully evaluated, while most of the studies have focused mainly on the reconstructive procedure at the recipient site or on the complications related to harvesting, and only a

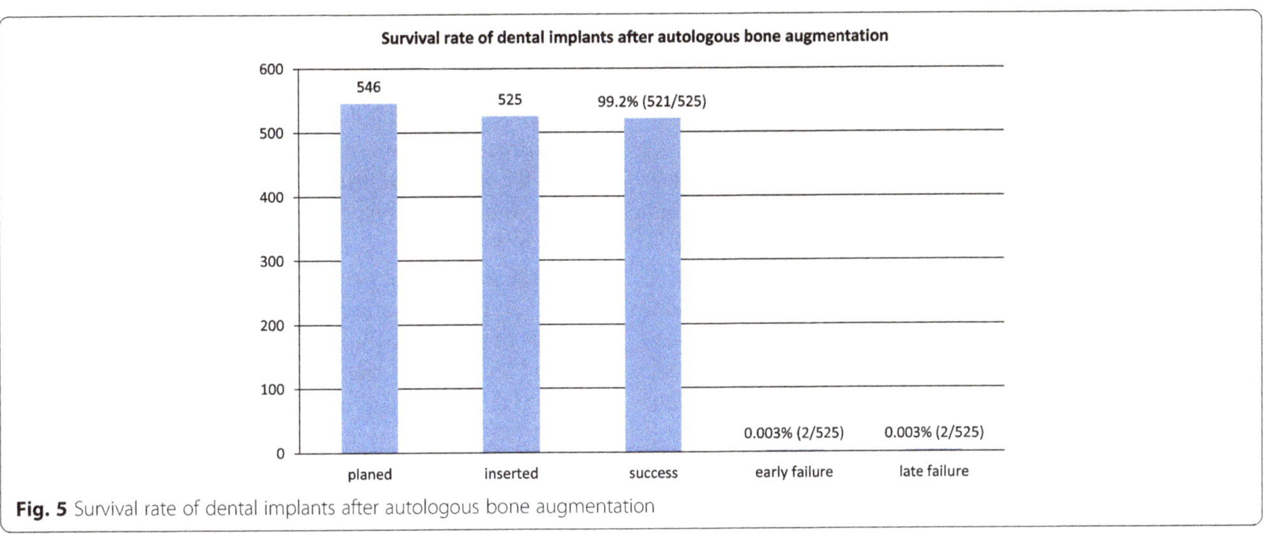

Fig. 5 Survival rate of dental implants after autologous bone augmentation

very limited number of studies have reported the final results of the augmentation procedure [39–41].

The present study aimed to evaluate the clinical outcome of augmentation and implant success rate after autologous bone harvesting from different donor sites and the following possibility and adequacy of implant insertion in grafted areas and on the potential risk factors for postoperative discomfort and graft or implant failure. In our patient study group, we evaluated the survival rate of grafts harvested from the mandibular ramus (retromolar region), symphysial region, alveolar zygomatic buttress, the anterior and lateral facial wall (sinus floor elevations), and the anterior superior iliac crest as well as the implant success rate in a period of 2 years after prosthodontic restauration.

Systematic reviews have failed to find evidence that one particular grafting technique is superior to others [10]. Intraoral bone grafts from the mandibular symphysis, mandibular ramus, and maxillary tuberosity provide a good treatment modality for ridge augmentation, and the amount of bone available for harvesting is sufficient for defects up to the width of three teeth [42]. Harvesting of retromolar and symphysis bone grafts are especially recommended in cases involving multiple tooth reconstruction in the mandible. The access to the symphysis has been described as being easier than that to the mandibular ramus [43]. Both techniques can be performed on an outpatient basis, while harvesting of bone from distant sites is associated with inpatient care and increased costs [44]. It is reported that both harvesting procedures are well accepted by the patients, but the ramus was preferred [9, 41, 45]. Both the harvesting and grafting procedures are usually performed in the same surgical field.

In our study, seven out of 104 retromolar grafts and one out of 11 symphysis grafts have been lost due to postoperative complications; this is in accordance with the study review of Nkenke and Neukam [9]. They demonstrated also the low graft failure rate and the well acceptance of these methods by the patients. The ramus should be considered the site of choice when block grafts are needed for horizontal or vertical augmentation or for unilateral sinus augmentation [39]. For bilateral sinus elevation or when a combination of sinus elevation and horizontal and/or vertical augmentation are needed, the symphysis or iliac crest should be evaluated as a possible donor site [46]. When distant donor sites have to be adopted, it can be assumed that the morbidity and complication rate arising from the iliac crest is low [9]. This is in accordance to our study results; only one patient mentioned postoperative discomfort on the recipient site and only eight out of 116 bone grafts had to be removed due to infection.

Postoperative morbidity after mandibular bone harvesting procedures was reported to be mainly related to temporary or permanent neural disturbances involving the inferior alveolar nerve and its branches [19]. In this study, only the incidence of the temporary hypoesthesia of the mandibular and lingual nerve after harvesting from the retromolar area could be detected. It was 10.4 and 2.8%, respectively, results that are suitable to the literature [9, 47]. No consistent nerve damage could be detected. All of them made a complete recovery over the short and medium term. The use of piezoelectric surgery may reduce the incidence of this complication offering a safer way of safely removing hard tissue without damaging soft tissue. However, it should not be forgotten that piezoelectric surgery has some critical disadvantages, including a longer operation time and heat generation during bone cutting [48]. Based on our study results, however, we can recommend this technique as a safe method to prevent nerve damage in autologous intraoral bone harvesting. More histological studies are needed to define the quality of the retromolar bone and its resorption in the follow-up evaluation. That could minimize the early resorption rate and optimize the surgical outcome.

Harvesting from the zygomatic buttress is a relative new method [49]. This technique is best suited for those situations where only moderate amounts of bone are needed, especially when implant surgery is undertaken in the maxilla in one to two dental regions. The convex cross-section of the bone graft is ideal for the reconstruction of alveolar projection loss in the anterior and posterior maxillary zone. The zygomatic buttress is a strong bony pillar providing pressure absorption and transduction in the facial skeleton. With the described technique, it is possible to harvest approximately 0.5 to 1 ml of bone without causing damage to surrounding tissues. Low morbidity in donor and recipient sites are mentioned. This donor site offers easy access with excellent visibility and yields good quality bone of correct morphology and has the great advantage that no muscles have to be detached, and the bony structure in this area is especially strong [17, 49]. This clinical experience of fewer difficulties in managing postoperative edema and pain following this method was also presented from Gellrich et al. [49]. Limiting factors are the mucous membrane of the adjacent maxillary sinus and the close relationship to the infraorbital foramen [50]. Further studies to the bone quality of this potential donor site in order to minimize the postoperative resorption rate are necessary.

Of the sinus floor elevations performed in this study, 84.8% were defined absolutely successful. Only two of our 72 patients having sinus lift operations could not finally be treated with dental implants. These results are comparable to other studies considering the sinus graft to be a safe treatment modality with few complications [6, 8, 51–53]. Raghoebar et al. reported incidences of sinus complication of less than 1% in 100 patients [54]. Perforation of the sinus membrane has often been reported as the most common intraoperative complication in case studies with a frequency between 10 and 30% [53, 55, 56]. In this study, this was observed in 9.8% of the cases. On the other side, Scarano et al. demonstrated a high number of successfully treated patients with implant survival rate of 98.0% 4 years after augmentation using biomaterials [57]. Garofalo supports maxillary sinus elevations with biomaterials as a safe oral surgery technique with rapid and optimal bone regeneration leading to anatomical and functional restoration [58]. It is still under discussion if the use of autologous bone is superior to bone substitutes in sinus floor elevation procedures [59].

A previous systematic review reported 5% soft tissue complications after augmentation of fenestration- and dehiscence-type bone defects using resorbable membranes [60]. Soft tissue dehiscences or infections in the early postoperative phase preceded 6.3% of the cases in our study. The increased risk of bone block resorption in case of dehiscence is well described, which underlines the importance of meticulous soft tissue handling and tension-free soft tissue closure [61]. Postoperative infection of the donor and the recipient site preceded 2.6 and 5.6% of our cases, respectively, which is in accordance with complication rates reported in previous studies [62, 63]. Ponte and Khoury reported five cases of graft exposure in 521 treated patients, which results in a complication rate of less than 1% [64]. In our study, graft exposure occurred in 5.5% of the cases. Reviewing the literature, Jensen and Terheyden reported a complication rate of close to 18% [10]. In particular, if a bone block was grafted for ridge augmentation, the complication rate was higher, reaching 29.8% [10].

The use of autologous bone in this study has shown excellent graft survival and success rate (95.6%). This is equal to the results from the studies on implants inserted in reconstructed sites [6, 8, 24]. The early implant survival rate of 99.7% found in the present material is very high comparable to that in the previous systematic reviews after staged horizontal ridge augmentation [9, 10, 22, 62, 65]. The implant survival rate of 99.2% within 2 years after prosthodontic restauration in this study is higher compared to that in studies of the international literature with implants placed in autologous grafted areas [9]. Even with complete resorption of the grafted bone, an implant survival rate can be reached [9, 66]. However, this high rate of implant survival reported in our cases has to be confirmed due to further studies with a longer time period of control after prosthodontic rehabilitation. There is evidence that ridge augmentation success rates were 92 to 100% for onlay bone grafts and implant survival rates were 90.4% for onlay grafts [20–22]. In our study, the graft total success was determined by 95.6%, proving the high effectiveness of autologous bone harvesting even using extraoral donor sites.

One of the most serious problems associated with the use of bone blocks could be their resorption at the recipient site. The literature shows variations of this resorption from 25 to 60% [9, 67]. A systemic review reported additional augmentation in 26.6% of cases using a particulate augmentation protocol and in 4.7% of the bone block cases [10]. Widmark et al. reported bone resorption after lateral bone block augmentation of up to 60% of the original bone graft volume at the time of implant abutment connection [68]. No radiological evaluation of the quantity and quality of the autologous bone harvested from different donor sites was carried out in this study. A lower percentage of 1.3% (6/436) of additional augmentation procedures at the time of implant placement was found in the present study and was not considered as primary complication [69]. The authors attributed the low graft resorption to the short healing period of 3 to 5 months, which has now proven to be sufficient for the revascularization of the graft and the secure insertion of dental implants as suggested in the past by various authors [70, 71]. Therefore, we suggest limiting the healing period after autologous bone grafting to a maximum of 3 to 6 months. This leads to earlier dental restorations compared to augmentations using bone substitutes, where the healing periods are often recommended up to 12 months. Strategies to minimize bone resorption after autologous grafting are discussed in the literature. However, further studies are necessary to identify factors influencing bone resorption [47, 72].

The results of the present study have to take into account the absence of a control group with patients undergoing bone augmentation procedures with bone substitutes (allogen, alloplastic, exogen). Without a comparative group of grafting surgeries using alternative bone material, only limited statements can be made.

However, the excellent surgical outcome of autologous surgical methods providing high survival rate of the grafts and inserted implants in our study proves for the first time the reliability and low comorbidity of autologous bone grafts in preprosthetic surgery for almost all kinds of intraoral and even for extraoral grafts from the iliac crest. Despite the study had a retrospective design, and the nature of a retrospective study inherently results in flaws, in this study there was no dropout of any patient operated in the years 2009–2011, and all patients operated with bone grafts prior to implant insertion in our department had been included in the study. This moreover reflects a prospective study design, which has never been reported in the literature before.

No evidence in the literature comparing surgical outcomes of autologous augmentations including postoperative morbidity from different donor sites, subject to graft and implant survival, has been reported. The relative short-term period of implant control after the prosthetic rehabilitation could be critical in order to define the implant success rate in augmented sites. Related to that, there was also no control group with implants placed in non-grafted areas that could facilitate the comparison of augmented and non-augmented areas. There was also no radiological evaluation of the graft resorption after harvesting; our findings were after clinical observation that could jeopardize the real dimensions of the graft at the time of implantation because of the missing comparison between pre- and post-augmentative situations. Future research could include control groups with large cohort size, long-term follow-up periods, and standardized criteria for defining bone graft and implant success or failure rate, in order to obtain rigorous evidence-based results. This will most likely only be achievable as single-arm multicenter studies.

Data on risk factors based on the original examination and documentation are difficult to assess the adverse effects of variable factors on the surgical prognosis because of the multifactorial genesis of surgical complications [73]. Factors such as gender, age, or smoking habit could be associated with postoperative complications after two-stage dentoalveolar reconstruction with autologous bone grafts. For example, a higher ratio of men compared to women (250 men to 29 women) was detected in this study. This can be logically explained due to the profession of the patients. The study was carried out in the military hospital of Ulm in Germany and the majority of the collective concerned male candidates. However, this inhomogeneity could significantly influence on the postoperative surgical outcome. It is a fact that conditions of the female nature, such as estrogen level alteration in postmenopausal women, may relate to bone graft resorption. To investigate the age-specific impact on the prognosis of these procedures, a prospective case control study in equal age and gender groups of patients is required. Possible risk factors for postoperative morbidity regarding complications at the donor and recipient sites after augmentation procedures with autologous bone grafts harvested from different donor sites were not analyzed in this study. An attempt to estimate the frequency with which postoperative complications occur in patients with different characteristics, such as age, gender, smoking habit, history of periodontitis, and more, in order to evaluate the influence of these factors on augmentation outcome and implant survival rate should be aimed in future studies.

Therefore, it has to be kept in mind that equal alternatives to autologous bone grafts in sinus floor augmentation are proven. It seems that the use of bone substitutes finally leads to implant survival rates that are comparable to those that can be achieved with implants placed in sinuses grafted with autologous bone [74]. In this respect, assessment of the defect should be carefully performed in order to provide the patient with the least invasive technique providing excellent long-term results. Our technique of using autologous bone scrapes from the anterior facial wall harvested during window preparation has proven to be equal to the use of bone substitutes. This technique combines augmentation with autologous material and the absence of comorbidity at the donor site. Surgeons therefore should consider using this technique in order to minimize the use of bone substitutes without additional harvesting morbidity.

Conclusions

The results of the clinical study proves the reliability and low comorbidity of autologous bone grafts in preprosthetic alveolar ridge reconstructions prior to implant insertion. The high graft success rate (95.6%) and the low early implant failure rate (0.38%) in a surveillance of all patients treated in three following years with this technique showing no exclusion and no dropout of any case for the first time proves that intraoral and extraoral autologous bone grafts could be further considered as the "gold standard" preprosthetic dentoalveolar reconstruction. This study demonstrates that the reconstruction of atrophic jaws with corticocancellous bone grafts from intraoral and extraoral donor sites is a predictable technique to facilitate dental rehabilitation of the atrophic ridge, associated with high bone survival rate and implant success. Although an increased number of bone substitutes exist, autologous bone has to be considered as the most effective material for two-stage preprosthodontic augmentation in oral implantation. Intraoral autologous grafts can serve as a reliable treatment option to reconstruct isolated defects for implant placement. Autologous onlay grafts from the ramus mandible, symphysis, and zygomatic buttress offer sufficient bone volume to reconstruct the atrophic jaw without any lasting harvesting morbidities. These sites are excellent treatment alternatives with high patient acceptance when reconstruction is necessary before implant insertion. Besides a successful reconstruction of the alveolar crest with correct selection of the donor site, patient acceptance of the procedure should be high, while the morbidity of the procedure should be minimal showing no persistent nerve damage, which was considered the main disadvantage of autologous bone grafts in the past. We cannot address the contribution of the use of piezoelectric surgery, grafting templates, and guided implant insertion to the reported results, but we could proof that with the described technique, predictable outcome lacking lasting morbidities can be achieved independently from surgical status such as residents, fellows, or consultants. Further studies should focus on long-term implant success rates in these patients. The influence of different patient characteristics as potential risk factors for postoperative morbidity may also be of interest for further investigations.

Acknowledgements

The authors thank the patients for their kindness to participate as study cases and the whole medical team at the Bundeswehrkrankenhaus Ulm.

Authors' contributions

AS participated in its design and coordination, carried out the data selection, and drafted the manuscript, and is the corresponding author. FW participated in its design and coordination and helped in drafting the manuscript. MH participated in its design and coordination and helped in drafting the manuscript. WK participated in the design of the study and performed the statistical analysis. AS contributed to the protocol preparation, preparation of the manuscript, and guidance of the study and was involved in drafting the manuscript and finalizing it for submission. All authors read and approved the final manuscript.

Competing interests

Andreas Sakkas, Frank Wilde, Marcus Heufelder, Karsten Winter, and Alexander Schramm declare that they have no competing interests.

Ethics approval and consent to participate

Patient recruitment and data collection for this study took place at the Department of Maxillofacial and Facial Plastic Surgery at the military/academic hospital of Ulm University, Germany. The research was conducted in full accordance with ethical principles, including the World Medical Association Declaration of Helsinki. The patients' data was referenced with the understanding and written consent of each patient, and the data was also anonymized and de-identified prior to analysis. Reporting was based on the recommendations of the "Strengthening the Reporting of Observational Studies in Epidemiology (STROBE)" initiative [75].

No research/experimentation was completed on humans and/or animals for these case reports.

All procedures performed in this study involving human participants were in accordance with the ethical standards of the institutional and/or national research committee and with the 1964 Helsinki Declaration and its later amendments or comparable ethical standards.

For this type of study, formal consent was not required.

Author details

[1]Department of Oral and Plastic Maxillofacial Surgery, Military Hospital Ulm, Academic Hospital of the University of Ulm, Oberer Eselsberg 40, 89081 Ulm, Germany. [2]Institute of Anatomy, Medical Faculty of Leipzig University, Leipzig, Germany. [3]Department of Oral and Plastic Maxillofacial Surgery, University Hospital Ulm, Ulm, Germany.

References

1. Jensen AT, Jensen SS, Worsaae N. Complications related to bone augmentation procedures of localized defects in the alveolar ridge. A retrospective clinical study. Oral Maxillofac Surg. 2016;20(2):115–22 [Epub ahead of print].
2. Buser D, Dula K, Hirt HP, Schenk RK. Lateral ridge augmentation using autografts and barrier membranes: clinical study with 40 partially edentulous patients. J Oral Maxillofac Surg. 1996;54:420–32.
3. Galindo-Moreno P, Avila G, Fernández-Barbero JE, Mesa F, O'Valle-Ravassa F, Wang HL. Clinical and histologic comparison of two different composite grafts for sinus augmentation: a pilot clinical trial. Clin Oral Implants Res. 2008;19:755–9.
4. Chiapasco M, Zaniboni M, Rimondini L. Autogenous onlay bone grafts vs. alveolar distraction osteogenesis for the correction of vertically deficient edentulous ridges: a 2–4-year prospective study on humans. Clin Oral Implants Res. 2007;18:432–40.
5. Moses O, Nemcovsky CE, Langer Y, Tal H. Severely resorbed mandible treated with iliac crest autogenous bone graft and dental implants: 17-year follow-up. Int J Oral Maxillofac Implants. 2007;22:1017–21.
6. Zizelmann C, Schoen R, Metzger MC, Schmelzeisen R, Schramm A, Dott B, Bormann KH, Gellrich N-C. Bone formation after sinus augmentation with engineered bone. Clin Oral Implants Res. 2007;18(1):69–73.
7. Sbordone C, Toti P, Guidetti F, Califano L, Pannone G, Sbordone L. Volumetric changes after sinus augmentation using blocks of autogenous iliac bone or freeze-dried allogeneic bone. A non-randomized study. J Craniomaxillofac Surg. 2014;42:113–8.
8. Stricker A, Schramm A, Marukawa E, Lauer G, Schmelzeisen R. Distraction osteogenesis and tissue engineering-new options for enhancing the implant site. Int J Periodontics Restorative Dent. 2003;23(3):297–302.
9. Nkenke E, Neukam FW. Autogenous bone harvesting and grafting in advanced jaw resorption: morbidity, resorption and implant survival. Eur J Oral Implantol. 2014;7:203–17.
10. Jensen SS, Terheyden H. Bone augmentation procedures in localized defects in the alveolar ridge: clinical results with different bone grafts and bone-substitute materials. Int J Oral Maxillofac Implants. 2009;24:218–36.

11. Del Fabbro M, Corbella S, Weinstein T, Ceresoli V, Taschieri S. Implant survival rates after osteotome-mediated maxillary sinus augmentation: a systematic review. Clin Implant Dent Relat Res. 2012;14:159–68.
12. Schwartz-Arad D, Dori S. Intraoral autogenous onlay block bone grafting for implant dentistry. Refuat Hapeh Vehashinayim. 2002;19:35–9. 77.
13. Misch CM. Ridge augmentation using mandibular ramus bone grafts for the placement of dental implants: presentation of a technique. Pract Periodontics Aesthet Dent. 1996;8:127–35.
14. Altiparmak N, Soydan SS, Uckan S. The effect of conventional surgery and piezoelectric surgery bone harvesting techniques on the donor site morbidity of the mandibular ramus and symphysis. Int J Oral Maxillofac Surg. 2015;44:1131–7.
15. Proussaefs P, Lozada J. The use of intraorally harvested autogenous block grafts for vertical alveolar ridge augmentation: a human study. Int J Periodontics Restorative Dent. 2005;25:351–63.
16. Fakhry A. The mandibular retromolar area as a donor site in maxillofacial bone grafting: surgical notes. Int J Periodontics Restorative Dent. 2011;31:275–83.
17. Sakkas A, Schramm A, Karsten W, Gellrich NC, Wilde F. A clinical study of the outcomes and complications associated with zygomatic buttress block bone graft for limited preimplant augmentation procedures. J Craniomaxillofac Surg. 2016;44(3):249–56.
18. Fiorellini JP, Nevins ML. Localized ridge augmentation/preservation. A systematic review. Ann Periodontol. 2003;8:321–7.
19. Chiapasco M, Zaniboni M, Boisco M. Augmentation procedures for the rehabilitation of deficient edentulous ridges with oral implants. Clin Oral Implants Res. 2006;17:136–59.
20. Esposito M, Grusovin MG, Felice P, Karatzopoulos G, Worthington HV, Coulthard P. The efficacy of horizontal and vertical bone augmentation procedures for dental implants—a Cochrane systematic review. Eur J Oral Implantol. 2009;2:167–84.
21. Clementini M, Morlupi A, Agrestini C, Ottria L. Success rate of dental implants inserted in autologous bone graft regenerated areas: a systematic review. Oral Implantol. 2011;4:3–10.
22. Kuchler U, von Arx T. Horizontal ridge augmentation in conjunction with or prior to implant placement in the anterior maxilla: a systematic review. Int J Oral Maxillofac Implants. 2014;29:14–24.
23. Leonetti JA, Koup R. Localized maxillary ridge augmentation with a block allograft for dental implant placement: case reports. Implant Dent. 2003;12:217–26.
24. Aghaloo TL, Moy PK. Which hard tissue augmentation techniques are the most successful in furnishing bony support for implant placement? Int J Oral Maxillofac Implants. 2007;22:49–70.
25. Margonar R, dos Santos PL, Queiroz TP, Marcantonio E. Rehabilitation of atrophic maxilla using the combination of autogenous and allogeneic bone grafts followed by protocol-type prosthesis. J Craniofac Surg. 2010;21:1894–6.
26. Fugazzotto PA. GBR using bovine bone matrix and resorbable and nonresorbable membranes. Part 2: clinical results. Int J Periodontics Restorative Dent. 2003;23:599–605.
27. Lange DE, Plagmann HC, Eenboom A, Promesberger A. Clinical methods for the objective evaluation of oral hygiene. Dtsch Zahnarztl Z. 1977;32:44–7.
28. Mühlemann HR, Son S. Gingival sulcus bleeding—a leading symptom in initial gingivitis. Helv Odontol Acta. 1971;15:107–13.
29. Cawood JI, Howell RA. A classification of the edentulous jaws. Int J Oral Maxillofac Surg. 1988;17:232–6.
30. Schramm A, Schön R, Rücker M, Barth E-L, Zizelmann C, Gellrich N-C. Computer assisted oral and maxillofacial reconstruction. Int J Comp Techn. 2006;14(1):71–7.
31. Schramm A, Gellrich N-C, Schmelzeisen R. Navigational surgery of the facial skeleton. New York: Springer Berlin Heidelberg; 2007 (ISBN-13 987-3-540-22357-3).
32. Schramm A, Gellrich N.C. Intraoperative Navigation und computerassistierte Chirurgie. In: Schwenzer N und Ehrenfeld M. Zahn-Mund-Kieferheilkunde, Mund-Kiefer-Gesichtschirurgie. 4. Auflage, (ed. Thieme). Stuttgart New York, 2010;479–499.
33. Naziri E, Schramm A, Wilde F. Accuracy of computer-assisted implant placement with insertion templates. GMS Interdiscip Plast Reconstr Surg DGPW. 2016; May 13; 5Doc15. eCollection 2016.
34. Buser D, Weber HP, Lang NP. Tissue integration of non-submerged implants. 1-year results of a prospective study with 100 ITI hollow-cylinder and hollow-screw implants. Clin Oral Implants Res. 1990;1:33–40.
35. Kerschbaum T, Haastert B. Statistische Verweildaueranalysen in der Implantologie. Implantologie. 1995;2:101–11.
36. Sittitavornwong S, Gutta R. Bone graft harvesting from regional sites. Oral Maxillofac Surg Clin North Am. 2010;22:317–30.
37. Myeroff C, Archdeacon M. Autogenous bone graft: donor sites and techniques. J Bone Joint Surg Am. 2011;7:2227–36.
38. Nkenke E, Eitner S, Radespiel-Tröger M, Vairaktaris E, Neukam FW, Fenner M. Patient-centred outcomes comparing transmucosal implant placement with an open approach in the maxilla: a prospective, non-randomized pilot study. Clin Oral Implants Res. 2007;18:197–203.
39. von Arx T, Buser D. Horizontal ridge augmentation using autogenous block grafts and the guided bone regeneration technique with collagen membranes: a clinical study with 42 patients. Clin Oral Implants Res. 2006;17:359–66.
40. Levin L, Nitzan D, Schwartz-Arad D. Success of dental implants placed in intraoral block bone grafts. J Periodontol. 2007;78:18–21.
41. Andersson L. Patient self-evaluation of intra-oral bone grafting treatment to the maxillary frontal region. Dent Traumatol. 2008;24:164–9.
42. Sant'Ana E. Short-term survival of osseointegrated implants installed in alveolar ridge reconstructed with autogenous graft (Thesis submitted to obtain PhD). Bauru School of Dentistry, São Paulo University, 1997.
43. Misch CM. Comparison of intraoral donor sites for onlay grafting prior to implant placement. Int J Oral Maxillofac Implants. 1997;12:767–76.
44. Sàndor GK, Nish IA, Carmichael RP. Comparison of conventional surgery with motorized trephine in bone harvest from the anterior iliac crest. Oral Surg Oral Med Oral Pathol Oral Radiol Endod. 2003;95:150–5.
45. Raghoebar GM, Meijndert L, Kalk WW, Vissink A. Morbidity of mandibular bone harvesting: a comparative study. Int J Oral Maxillofac Implants. 2007;22:359–65.
46. Cordaro L, Torsello F, Accorsi Ribeiro C, Liberatore M, Mirisola Di Torresanto V. Inlay-onlay grafting for three-dimensional reconstruction of the posterior atrophic maxilla with mandibular bone. Int J Oral Maxillofac Surg. 2010;39:350–7.
47. Cordaro L, Torsello F, Miuccio MT, di Torresanto VM, Eliopoulos D. Mandibular bone harvesting for alveolar reconstruction and implant placement: subjective and objective cross-sectional evaluation of donor and recipient site up to 4 years. Clin Oral Implants Res. 2011;22:1320–6.
48. Stelzle F, Frenkel C, Riemann M, Knipfer C, Stockmann P, Nkenke E. The effect of load on heat production, thermal effects and expenditure of time during implant site preparation—an experimental ex vivo comparison between piezosurgery and conventional drilling. Clin Oral Implants Res. 2014;25:e140–8.
49. Gellrich N-C, Held U, Schön R, Pailing T, Schramm A, Bormann K. Alveolar zygomatic buttress: a new donor site for limited preimplant augmentation procedures. J Oral Maxillofac Surg. 2007;65:275–80.
50. Verdugo F, Castillo A, Moragues MD, Pontón J. Bone microbial contamination influences autogenous grafting in sinus augmentation. J Periodontol. 2009;80:1355–64.
51. Wiltfang J, Schultze-Mosgau S, Merten HA, Kessler P, Ludwig A, Engelke W. Endoscopic and ultrasonographic evaluation of the maxillary sinus after combined sinus floor augmentation and implant insertion. Oral Surg Oral Med Oral Pathol Oral Radiol Endod. 2000;89:288–91.
52. Barone A, Santini S, Sbordone L, Crespi R, Covani U. A clinical study of the outcomes and complications associated with maxillary sinus augmentation. Int J Oral Maxillofac Implants. 2006;21:81–5.
53. Felice P, Pistilli R, Piattelli M, Soardi E, Barausse C, Esposito M. 1-stage versus 2-stage lateral sinus lift procedures: 1-year post-loading results of a multicentre randomised controlled trial. Eur J Oral Implantol. 2014;7:65–75.
54. Raghoebar GM, Meijer HJ, Telleman G, Vissink A. Maxillary sinus floor augmentation surgery with autogenous bone grafts as ceiling: a pilot study and test of principle. Clin Implant Dent Relat Res. 2013;15:550–7.
55. Scabbia A, Cho KS, Sigurdsson TJ, Kim CK, Trombelli L. Cigarette smoking negatively affects healing response following flap debridement surgery. J Periodontol. 2001;72:43–9.
56. Sakkas A, Konstantinidis I, Winter K, Schramm A, Wilde F. Effect of Schneiderian membrane perforation on sinus lift graft outcome using two different donor sites: a retrospective study of 105 maxillary sinus elevation procedures. GMS Interdiscip Plast Reconstr Surg DGPW. 2016; Mar 2;5: Doc11. doi: 10.3205/iprs000090. eCollection 2016.
57. Scarano A, Degidi M, Iezzi G, Pecora G, Piattelli M, Orsini G, Caputi S, Perrotti V, Mangano C, Piattelli A. Maxillary sinus augmentation with different biomaterials: a comparative histologic and histomorphometric study in man. Implant Dent. 2006;15(2):197–207.

58. Garofalo GS. Autogenous, allogenetic and xenogenetic grafts for maxillary sinus elevation: literature review, current status and prospects. Minerva Stomatol. 2007;56(7–8):373–92.
59. Del Fabbro M, Testori T, Francetti L, Weinstein R. Systematic review of survival rates for implants placed in the grafted maxillary sinus. Int J Periodontics Restorative Dent. 2004;24:565–77.
60. Chiapasco M, Zaniboni M. Clinical outcomes of GBR procedures to correct peri-implant dehiscences and fenestrations: a systematic review. Clin Oral Implants Res. 2009;20:113–23.
61. Felice P, Pellegrino G, Checchi L, Pistilli R, Esposito M. Vertical augmentation with interpositional blocks of anorganic bovine bone vs. 7-mm-long implants in posterior mandibles: 1-year results of a randomized clinical trial. Clin Oral Implants Res. 2010;21:1394–403.
62. Felice P, Marchetti C, Piattelli A, Pellegrino G, Checchi V, Worthington H, Esposito M. Vertical ridge augmentation of the atrophic posterior mandible with interpositional block grafts: bone from the iliac crest versus bovine anorganic bone. Eur J Oral Implantol. 2008;1:183–98.
63. Laino L, Iezzi G, Piattelli A, Lo Muzio L, Cicciù M. Vertical ridge augmentation of the atrophic posterior mandible with sandwich technique: bone block from the chin area versus corticocancellous bone block allograft—clinical and histological prospective randomized controlled study. Biomed Res Int. 2014;982104. doi: 10.1155/2014/982104.
64. Ponte A, Khoury F. The tunnel technique in bone grafting procedures: a clinical study (Abstract). Int J Oral Maxillofac Implants. 2004;19:766.
65. Pommer B, Frantal S, Willer J, Posch M, Watzek G, Tepper G. Impact of dental implant length on early failure rates: a meta-analysis of observational studies. J Clin Periodontol. 2011;38:856–63.
66. Chiapasco M, Casentini P, Zaniboni M, Corsi E. Evaluation of peri-implant bone resorption around Straumann Bone Level implants placed in areas reconstructed with autogenous vertical onlay bone grafts. Clin Oral Implants Res. 2012;23:1012–21.
67. Sclar AG. Strategies for management of single-tooth extraction sites in aesthetic implant therapy. J Oral Maxillofac Surg. 2004;62:90–105.
68. Widmark G, Andersson B, Ivanoff CJ. Mandibular bone graft in the anterior maxilla for single-tooth implants. Presentation of surgical method. Int J Oral Maxillofac Surg. 1997;26:106–9.
69. Laviv A, Jensen OT, Tarazi E, Casap N. Alveolar sandwich osteotomy in resorbed alveolar ridge for dental implants: a 4-year prospective study. J Oral Maxillofac Surg. 2014;72:292–303.
70. Heberer S, Rühe B, Krekeler L, Schink T, Nelson JJ, Nelson K. A prospective randomized split-mouth study comparing iliac onlay grafts in atrophied edentulous patients: covered with periosteum or a bioresorbable membrane. Clin Oral Implants Res. 2009;20:319–26.
71. Semper W, Kraft S, Mehrhof J, Nelson K. Impact of abutment rotation and angulation on marginal fit: theoretical considerations. Int J Oral Maxillofac Implants. 2010;25:752–8.
72. Wiltfang J, Jätschmann N, Hedderich J, Neukam FW, Schlegel KA, Gierloff M. Effect of deproteinized bovine bone matrix coverage on the resorption of iliac cortico-spongeous bone grafts—a prospective study of two cohorts. Clin Oral Implants Res. 2014;25:e127–32.
73. Chrcanovic BR, Albrektsson T, Wennerberg A. Smoking and dental implants: a systematic review and meta-analysis. J Dent. 2015;43:487–98.
74. Nkenke E, Stelzle F. Clinical outcomes of sinus floor augmentation for implant placement using autogenous bone or bone substitutes: a systematic review. Clin Oral Implants Res. 2009;20:124–33.
75. Vandenbroucke JP, von Elm E, Altman DG, Gøtzsche PC, Mulrow CD, Pocock SJ, Poole C, Schlesselman JJ, Egger M. STROBE Initiative. Strengthening the Reporting of Observational Studies in Epidemiology (STROBE): explanation and elaboration. Int J Surg. 2014;12:1500–24.

Retrospective cohort study of rough-surface titanium implants with at least 25 years' function

Tadashi Horikawa[1†], Tetsurou Odatsu[2*†], Takatoshi Itoh[1], Yoshiki Soejima[1], Hutoshi Morinaga[1], Naruyoshi Abe[1], Naoyuki Tsuchiya[1], Toshikazu Iijima[1] and Takashi Sawase[1,2]

Abstract

Background: The longitudinal clinical outcomes over decades contribute to know potential factors leading to implant failure or complications and help in the decision of treatment alternatives.

Methods: The cases of all patients who received dental implants treated with titanium plasma-sprayed surfaces and whose prostheses were set in the period 1984–1990 at seven private practices were retrospectively analyzed. The cumulative survival rate, the cumulative incidence of peri-implantitis, and the complication-free prosthesis rate were calculated with Kaplan-Meier survival curves, and the factors' influence on implant survival rate and the incidence of peri-implantitis were determined by a single factor in univariate analyses and multivariate analyses.

Results: A total of 223 implants and 106 prostheses were applied to 92 patients, and approx. 62% of the implants and patients dropped out over the 25 years following their treatment. The cumulative survival rates of the implants at 10, 15, and 25 years were 97.4, 95.4, and 89.8%, respectively. A significant difference was observed in the implant position. The cumulative incidences of peri-implantitis at 10, 15, and 25 years were 15.3, 21.0, and 27.9%, respectively. Significant differences were observed in the gender, implant type, and width of keratinized mucosa around the implant. The cumulative survival rates of mechanical complication-free prostheses at 10, 15, and 25 years were 74.9, 68.8, and 56.4%, respectively. The difference in the type of prosthesis resulted in significant differences.

Conclusions: The high rate of dropout during follow-up indicates the difficulty of determining long-term (> 25 years) prognoses. The gender, location, and width of keratinized mucosa affected the development of peri-implantitis, resulting in late failures. Implant-supported overdentures were frequently repaired. Tooth implant-supported prostheses are not recommended for long-term survival.

Keywords: Dental implants, Implant-supported prosthesis, Long-term survival, Titanium plasma-sprayed surface

Background

Dental implant treatment based on the concept of osseointegration [1] is now a widely accepted restorative treatment for fully and partially edentulous patients. In the earliest days of the use of osseointegrated implants, two different topographies were applied on the implant surfaces: a machined minimally rough titanium surface such as the Brånemark system and a rough microporous titanium plasma-sprayed surface such as the ITI system [2]. In clinical studies, the long-term (i.e., up to 20 years) survival rate of Brånemark-system implants was in the range of 80–99% [3–5] and that with ITI-system implants was 88–96% [6, 7].

Despite the high survival rates, implant-supported restorations are still subject to biological and mechanical complications. The focus in dental implant treatments has shifted from implant survival to (1) implant success, (2) peri-implant infection, and (3) long-term outcomes of prostheses. Since the increasing human life expectancy and most of the patients who undergo implant treatment are middle-aged (approx. 40–60 years old) [8, 9], the

* Correspondence: odatsu@nagasaki-u.ac.jp
†Equal contributors
[2]Department of Applied Prosthodontics, Graduate School of Biomedical Sciences, Nagasaki University, 1-7-1 Sakamoto, Nagasaki 852-8588, Japan
Full list of author information is available at the end of the article

Table 1 Age and gender distributions (n = 92)

Age/gender	Male	Female	Total
20–29	3	1	4
30–39	2	7	9
40–49	8	14	22
50–59	8	18	26
60–69	15	13	28
70–79	2	1	3
Total	38	54	92

determination of these longitudinal clinical outcomes over decades will contribute to the evaluation of treatment alternatives.

The aim of this retrospective study was not only to evaluate the long-term outcomes of solid-screw implants with a titanium plasma-sprayed (TPS) surface but also to assess the survival rates associated with the biological and mechanical complications.

Methods

Study design

This retrospective observational study was approved by the ethical committee of Nagasaki University (No. 1512). The cases of all of the patients who underwent dental implant treatment with a TPS-surfaced solid-screw implant and whose prosthesis was set in the years 1984–1990 at seven private practices were analyzed. All inserted implants were either a TPS-type (TPS-type, Institute Straumann, Basel, Switzerland) implant or a BONEFIT 45° shoulder-type (S-type, Institute Straumann) implant. We identified a total of 223 implants inserted into 92 patients.

Medical record assessment

Medical records were reviewed, and the patient-related parameters of age, gender, smoking habit, the date of

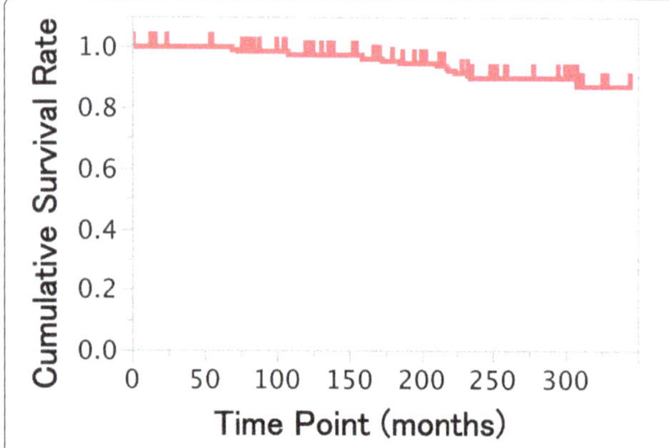

Fig. 1 Kaplan-Meier cumulative survival rate at 10, 15, and 25 years after the prosthesis setting

Table 2 Distribution of implants in situ (n = 223)

Position	1	2	3	4	5	6	7	Total
Maxilla	0	0	2	6	6	8	2	24
Mandible	7	32	8	30	20	59	43	199

implant surgery, and the date of the prosthesis setting were collected. The information of implant (length, diameter, type), site of implantation, width of keratinized mucosa, and additional pre- and/or post-implant surgery (i.e., bone augmentation, soft tissue management) was also collected. The types of prostheses were classified into implant-supported fixed prostheses, tooth implant-supported fixed prostheses, and implant-supported overdentures.

The endpoint of this study was set at December 31, 2015. Episodes of implant failure, biological complication (i.e., peri-implantitis with suppuration), and mechanical complications (i.e., component or laboratory-fabricated suprastructure's failure) were recorded.

Statistical analysis

JMP Pro software (ver. 11.2.0, SAS, Cary, NC, USA) was used for the statistical data analyses. The cumulative implant survival rate, the cumulative incidence of peri-implantitis, and the cumulative "complication-free" survival rate of implant-supported restorations were analyzed using the Kaplan-Meier survival estimator method. The cumulative "mechanical complication-free" survival rate of implant-supported restorations was estimated by a restoration-based analysis. The influence of the following variables on the implant survival rate and the incidence of peri-implantitis were determined by a single factor in univariate analyses (Kaplan-Meier) and multivariate analyses (Cox proportional hazards regression analysis): patient gender, smoking habit, implant type (S-type or TPS-type), implant position (three categories: maxilla, anterior mandible, posterior mandible), presence of additional soft tissue management (i.e., free-gingival graft, vestibular extension, and frenectomy), and the width of keratinized mucosa around implant (> 2 mm). The influence of patient gender and type of prosthesis on the complication-free survival rate of implant-supported restorations was

Table 3 Distribution of implants by diameter and location (n = 223)

Dia. (mm)	Maxilla anterior	Maxilla posterior	Mandible anterior	Mandible posterior	Total
3.5	1	2	15	14	32
4.0	0	0	13	17	30
4.1	1	20	19	118	158
4.8	0	0	0	3	3
Total	2	22	47	152	223

Table 4 Distribution of implants by length and location ($n = 223$)

Dia. (mm)	Maxilla anterior	Maxilla posterior	Mandible anterior	Mandible posterior	Total
8	0	8	3	8	19
10	0	5	9	73	87
11	1	0	1	6	8
12	1	9	7	44	61
14	0	0	13	13	26
17	0	0	11	7	18
20	0	0	3	1	4
Total	2	22	47	152	223

determined. The results were considered statistically significant at $p < 0.05$.

Results

Patient cohort

A total of 92 patients (38 men, 54 women; mean age 54.3 years, range 20–78) received implant-supported prostheses (at the seven private practices) between 1984 and 1990. The distribution of patients by age and gender is presented in Table 1. Fifty-seven patients (140 implants) were considered dropouts due to the fact that no data were obtained at the endpoint, but 25 years had passed since the prosthetic treatment delivery of one dropout patient (with four implants). The Kaplan-Meier estimate shows the censorings (Fig. 1), and they present unbiased throughout the observation period. The drop-out reasons for 42 patients were illness, moved away, and not showing up for check-ups; another 15 patients had passed away before the present analysis.

Implant diameter, length, and location

A total of 223 implants were placed in 15 fully edentulous patients and 77 partially edentulous patients. The distributions of implants by diameter, length, and location are presented in Tables 2, 3, and 4. Twenty-four implants were placed in the maxilla (10.8%), and 199 implants were placed in the mandible (89.2%). Only two implants were applied to the maxillary anterior region, whereas 152 implants (68.2%) were applied to the mandibular posterior region (Tables 2 and 3). Regarding the sizes of the implants, 4.1-mm dia. and 10-mm length were the most frequently used implant dimensions (70.9 and 39%, respectively).

Additional surgery

Four implants of one patient were inserted into the reconstructed mandible with iliac bone, due to an ameloblastoma. Additional soft tissue managements were applied to 96 implants. Free gingival graft was used for 86 implants, and frenectomy and vestibular extension were applied to 15 and 13 implants, respectively.

Cumulative survival rate and biological complications

Sixteen implants were lost during the observation period. The Kaplan-Meier cumulative survival rates were 97.4, 95.4, and 89.8% at 10, 15, and 25 years after the prosthesis setting, respectively (Fig. 1). After stepwise backward selection, implant position in the mandibular vs. the maxilla showed the significant difference in the cumulative survival rate (Table 5, Fig. 2c). The gender, implant type, additional soft tissue management, and width of keratinized mucosa did not provide significant differences with respect to the survival of the evaluated implants in this study (Fig. 2a, b, d, and e). The reasons for late failure were peri-implant infection (14 implants) and unknown (two implants).

A total of 48 implants were eventually accompanied by a peri-implant infection: the cumulative incidence of peri-implantitis was 9.5, 15.3, 21.0, and 27.9% at 5, 10, 15, and 25 years after the prosthesis delivery, respectively (Fig. 3). After stepwise backward selection, the gender, implant type, and width of keratinized mucosa showed the significant difference in the cumulative survival rate (Table 6, Fig. 4a, b, and e). The difference in implant position and additional soft tissue management did not result in significant differences with respect to the cumulative incidence of peri-implantitis (Fig. 4c, d).

Table 5 Cox regression analyses for implant survival

	Hazard ratio	95% confidence interval	p value
Gender (male)	1.99	0.538~8.201	0.3018
Implant type (TPS)	2.86	0.579~13.626	0.1897
Implant position (maxilla to mandibular/anterior)	40.09	4.062~994.751	0.0012
Implant position (maxilla to mandibular/posterior)	18.69	3.127~155.409	0.0013
Implant position (mandibular/anterior to mandibular/posterior)	0.47	0.022~3.912	0.5024
Additional soft tissue management (yes)	1.64	0.290~12.695	0.5808
Width of keratinized mucosa (> 2 mm)	0.78	0.166~3.294	0.7365

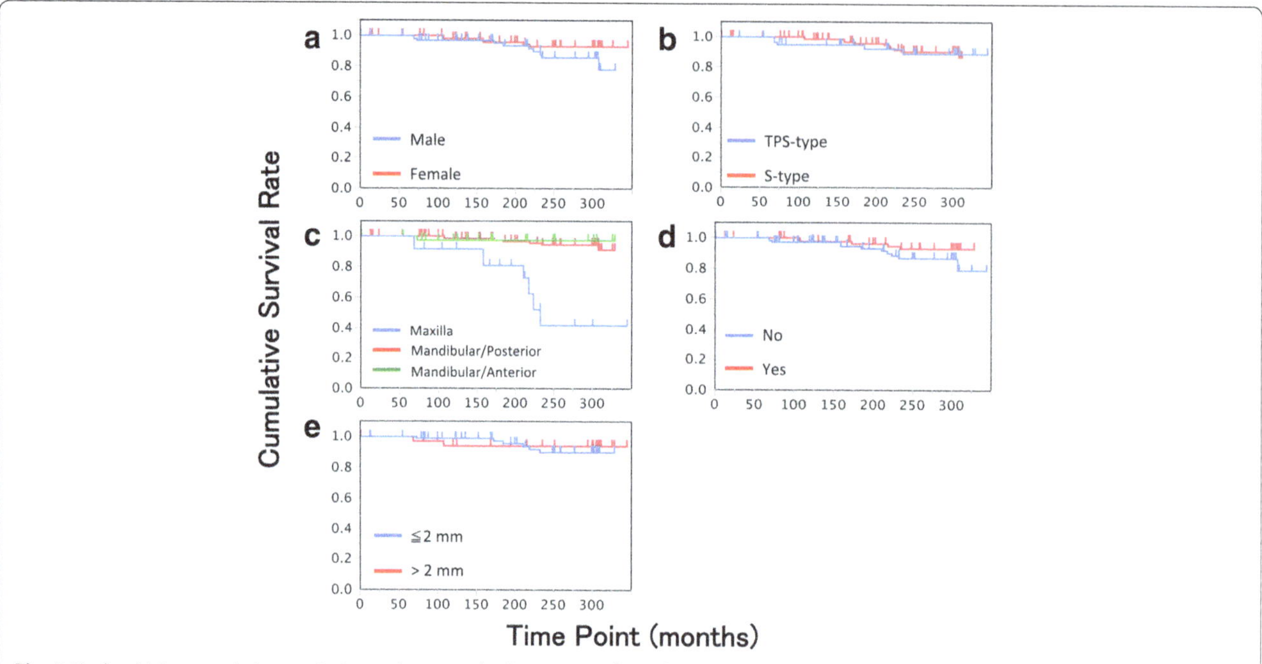

Fig. 2 Kaplan-Meier cumulative survival rates by **a** gender ($p = 0.1049$), **b** implant type ($p = 0.6259$), **c** implant position ($p < 0.0001$), **d** presence of additional soft tissue management ($p = 0.1149$), and **e** width of keratinized mucosa around implant ($p = 0.7132$). Log rank test was used for assessing statistical significance

Cumulative survival rate of mechanical complication-free prostheses

A total of 106 prostheses were applied to 92 patients. Nine prostheses were single crowns, 17 prostheses were implant-supported overdentures, and the other 80 prostheses were multiunit fixed partial dentures. Thirty-seven of the multiunit fixed partial dentures were splinted with natural teeth as an abutment (i.e., tooth implant-supported fixed prostheses). With respect to the materials of the occlusal surface, 21 of the fixed prostheses were veneered with porcelain, and the other 68 were made from dental alloys (Au-Pt or Au-Ag-Pd alloys).

The Kaplan-Meier cumulative survival rate of mechanical complication-free prostheses was 74.9, 68.8, and 56.4% at 10, 15, and 25 years (Fig. 5). The gender difference did not result in a significant difference with respect to the rate of mechanical complication-free prosthesis, but the difference in the type of prosthesis did (Table 7, Fig. 6a, b). For 11 of the 37 tooth implant-supported prostheses, the abutment teeth were extracted due to caries, periodontitis, or root fracture during the observation period. Regarding the implant-supported overdentures, the following mechanical complications were observed: the total number of relinings was 22 times; that of artificial tooth replacement was 17; attachment replacements were performed 15 times; bar

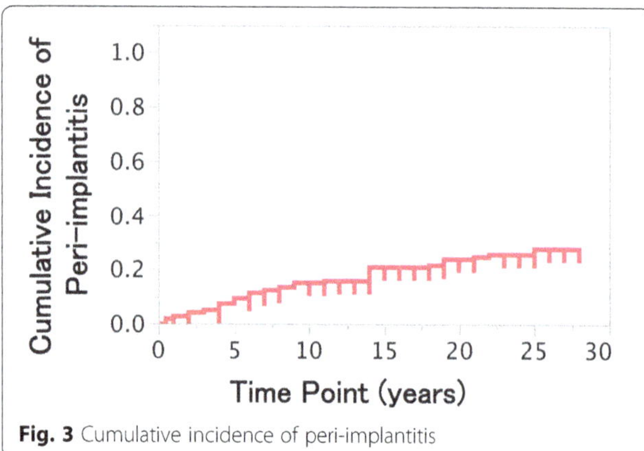

Fig. 3 Cumulative incidence of peri-implantitis

Table 6 Cox regression analyses for cumulative incidence of peri-implantitis

	Hazard ratio	95% confidence interval	*p* value
Gender (male)	2.38	1.138~5.362	0.0208
Implant type (TPS)	4.35	1.897~9.941	0.0006
Implant position (maxilla to mandibular/anterior)	6.08	1.384~24.436	0.0188
Implant position (maxilla to mandibular/posterior)	3.45	0.903~11.111	0.0679
Implant position (mandibular/anterior to mandibular/posterior)	0.57	0.207~1.442	0.2370
Additional soft tissue management (yes)	1.18	0.535~2.714	0.6826
Width of keratinized mucosa (> 2 mm)	0.24	0.094~0.559	0.0006

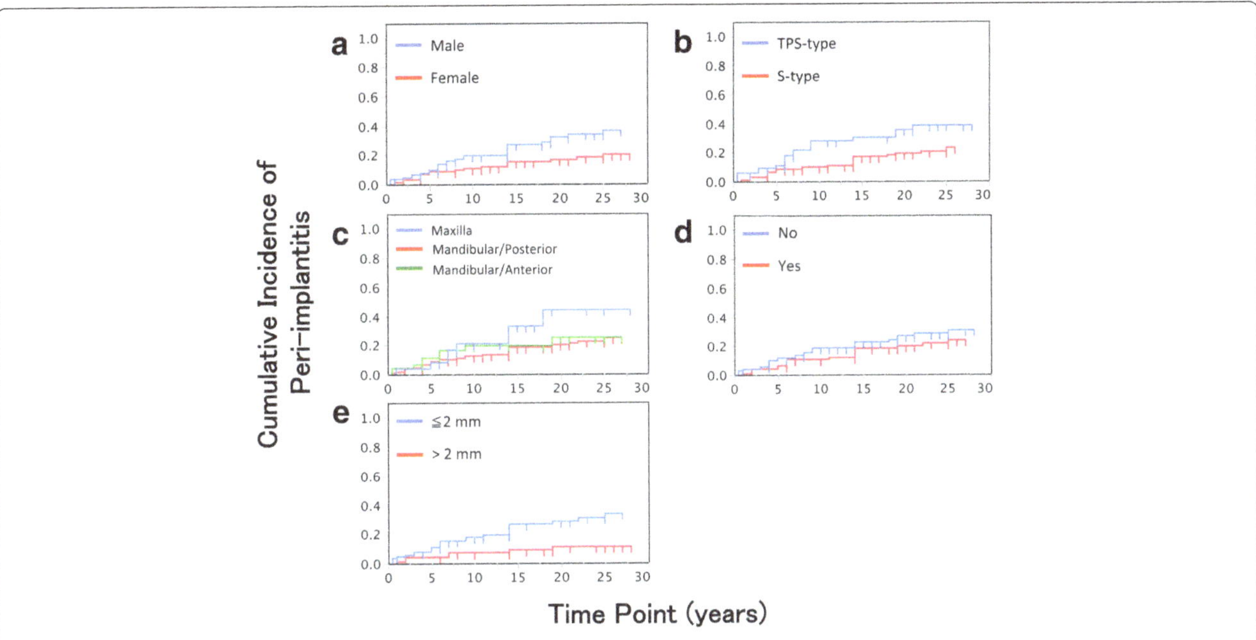

Fig. 4 Cumulative incidence of peri-implantitis by **a** gender (p = 0.0221), **b** implant type (p = 0.0128), **c** implant position (p = 0.2470), **d** presence of additional soft tissue management (p = 0.2488), and **e** width of keratinized mucosa around implant (p = 0.0045). Log rank test was used for assessing statistical significance

fractures were observed in three cases, and screw loosening occurred twice.

Discussion

Although all implants used in this study were withdrawn from the market about 20 years before, the longitudinal clinical outcomes over decades will help to better understand potential factors leading to implant failure or complications and assess the safe and predictable use of dental implant. Our analyses revealed a 25-year cumulative survival rate of 89.8% after the prosthesis setting, which seems comparable to the result of a recent study [7]. Although approx. 62% of the patients and implants in our original cohort dropped out during the follow-up period, according to Table 1, a majority of patients who underwent implant treatment were middle- and old-aged (82.6% of the patients were 40–69 years old) and thus some of the patients could not continue maintenance for varying reasons over a 25-year follow-up. The other 38% of the patients are healthy and likely to visit their dentists for maintenance, and they were included in the 25-year cumulative survival rate [7]. Therefore, the true long-term survival rate might have been lower than we reported herein due to bias from the patients who dropped out.

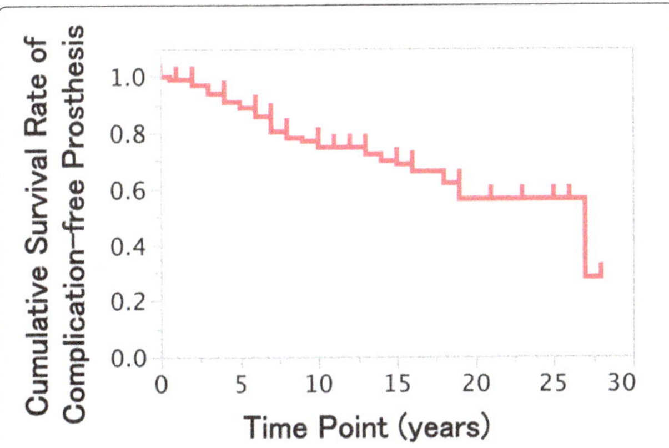

Fig. 5 Kaplan-Meier cumulative survival rate of complication-free prostheses at 10, 15, and 25 years after the prosthesis setting

In addition, only four implants of one patient were inserted into a re-constructed site from the iliac bone; no other bone augmentation procedure such as bone graft, guided bone regeneration (GBR), and sinus floor elevation were conducted. The principle of guided tissue regeneration (GTR) was introduced in 1982 [10], and GBR was introduced in 1988 [11]. The technique of sinus floor elevation was initially introduced in 1980 [12]. These complex augmentation procedures had not been common at that time [2], especially in private practices in Japan, and thus, they were not used for any of the patients in the present study. There is thus some degree of bias regarding the numbers of implant and the lengths of the implants according to the implant position. The number of implants applied to the maxilla anterior region was only two, since getting the esthetic result with implant prostheses was uncertain in those days. And the number of implants under 10 mm long was greater at posterior sites compared to anterior sites due to the sinus and inferior alveolar nerve.

Table 7 Cox regression analyses for cumulative survival rate of complication-free prostheses

	Hazard ratio	95% confidence interval	*p* value
Gender (male)	1.82	0.946~3.487	0.0725
Type of prostheses (implant-supported fixed prostheses to implant-supported overdenture)	0.04	0.013~0.108	< .0001
Type of prostheses (implant-supported fixed prostheses to tooth implant-supported fixed prostheses)	0.13	0.047~0.316	< .0001
Type of prostheses (tooth implant-supported fixed prostheses to implant-supported over denture)	0.31	0.148~0.654	0.0026

Peri-implantitis is the major reason for late failure [13, 14]. The consensus report of the Sixth European Workshop on Periodontology described peri-implant mucositis in approx. 80% of subjects restored with implant, and peri-implantitis in 28–56% of subjects [15]. In the present study, the cumulative incidence of peri-implantitis was 9.5, 15.3, 21.0, and 27.9% at 5, 10, 15, and 25 years after the prosthesis setting, respectively. Derks and Tomasi reported a positive relationship between the incidence of peri-implantitis and the mean function time by performing a meta-regression analysis of a systematic review [16], whereas the current cumulative result shown in Fig. 3 may represent the time course of the peri-implantitis incidence. Interestingly, the incidence of the peri-implantitis increased gradually with time; the rate of increase was approx. 1–1.5% per year.

Many potential factors associated with the incidence of peri-implantitis were reported [17, 18]. In the present study, the gender, implant type, and width of keratinized mucosa were identified as risk factors. Regarding gender, Koldsland et al. also reported a male population with overt peri-implantitis [19], whereas Attard and Zarb reported that women experienced more peri-implant bone loss than men [20]. Other studies and reviews reported that gender had no effect on peri-implantitis [21, 22]. Some other gender-related factors might affect the results.

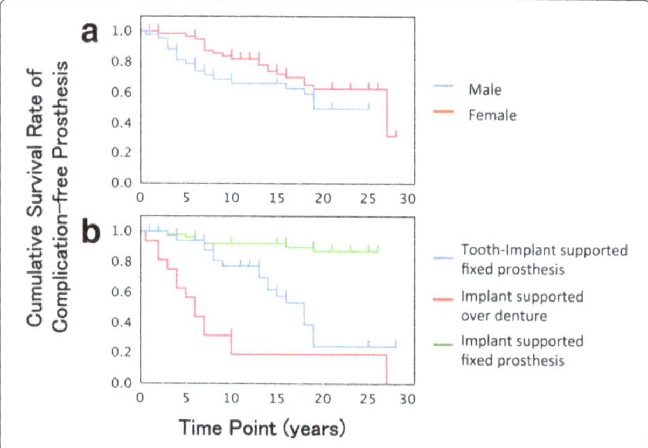

Fig. 6 Cumulative survival rate of complication-free prostheses by **a** gender ($p = 0.1220$) and **b** type of prostheses ($p < 0.0001$). Log rank test was used for assessing statistical significance

Regarding implant type, a difference between the S-types and the TPS-types is whether the existence of an abutment connection or not. The TPS-types are one-piece implants, and the S-types are two-piece but one-stage implants. Duda et al. reported that one-piece implants showed more marginal bone loss than two-piece implants [23]. In addition, a TPS surface is classified as "rough" surface when the surface roughness is more than 2 μm (Sa > 2 μm) [24]. Teughels et al. reported that a transmucosal implant surface with higher surface roughness facilitates biofilm formation [25] and thus TPS-type implants showed a higher incidence of peri-implantitis compared to the S-type.

Regarding the width of keratinized mucosa, many studies and a review have indicated that the presence of a sufficient width of keratinized mucosa is necessary for maintaining healthy peri-implants [26–29]. In the present study, when 2 mm of keratinized mucosa was used as the adequate width, the *p* value was 0.053 (data not shown). This also showed the tendency of the availability of keratinized mucosa around implants, and it may indicate that at least 2 mm of keratinized mucosa is preferable for the long-term success and survival of implants.

Our analysis showed that 16 of 223 implants were lost during the observation period. Among the six factors examined, only the implant position affected the cumulative implant survival rate and the main reason for implant failure was peri-implantitis (14/16 failed implants). However, the implant position did not affect the incidence of peri-implantitis. Compared to the mandible, the bone quality of the maxilla is lower [30] and the loading force is tilted to the implant axis. These factors might have acted as an exacerbating factor of peri-implantitis, resulting in the lower survival rate of the implants in the maxilla compared to the mandible.

Prosthetic complications occur due to the accumulation of mechanical damage to the implant, implant components, and supra-structures, resulting in the need for repairs and reconstructions of the implant prostheses, which may require time-consuming procedures and additional financial resources. The present investigation was a retrospective and multicenter study, and there were many differences in design patterns, materials, connections, and the attachment of supra-structures. It was therefore difficult to subdivide and review the factors that may affect the prosthetic survival rate, and only gender and type of prosthesis could be analyzed in this study.

The implant-supported fixed prostheses showed the highest complication-free survival rate in our study. It was reported that the veneering material's chipping/ fracture is the most common type of prosthetic complication for fixed prostheses [31, 32]. Pjetursson et al. reported that veneer fracture was observed in 13.5% of fixed prostheses after at least 5-year functioning [33]. In the present study, approx. 76% of the fixed prostheses were not veneered (metal occlusal surface), resulting in the lower complication rate after 25 years of functioning.

We also observed that the tooth-implant-supported prostheses had a lower complication-free rate than implant-supported fixed prostheses due to caries, periodontitis, or the root fracture of abutment teeth. Lang et al. reported that the survival rates of tooth implant-supported fixed partial dentures were 94.1% after 5 years and 77.8% after 10 years of functioning [31], and these results were almost the same as ours (93.9% after 5 years' and 77.2% after 10 years' functioning). Taking our results and those of Lang et al. into account, it appears that prosthetic complications of tooth implant-supported prostheses start arising after 7 years post-setting and then increase with time.

The implant-supported overdentures showed the lowest complication-free rate among the three implant types in the present study, due to the wear or fracture of artificial teeth, attachment fracture, and relines. Compared to another retrospective study of conventional complete dentures (without implant support) [34], our complication-free rate was higher and there was a difference in terms of the incidence of artificial tooth problems. That study showed a < 10% of incidence of artificial tooth problems during the first 5 years post-setting. The rigid support provided by an implant might have enhanced the loss, wear, and fracture of artificial teeth in our patients.

Conclusions

In conclusion, our analyses revealed a cumulative survival rate of 89.8% of TPS-surface implants with at least 25 years of functioning. The survival rate of maxillary positioned implants was significantly lower than that of mandibulary positioned implants. The patient gender, implant location, and width of keratinized mucosa affected the rate of peri-implantitis, resulting in late failure. Implant-supported overdentures were frequently repaired compared to the fixed prostheses due to the wear or fracture of artificial teeth, attachment fracture, and relines. Tooth implant-supported prostheses were not beneficial for long term owing to the troubles of abutment tooth.

Authors' contributions
TH, TO, and TS initiated and designed the retrospective study and drafted the manuscript including the preparation of figures and tables. TH, TAI, YS, HM, NA, NT, and TOI reviewed the medical records and collected the data. All authors revised the manuscript and approved the final manuscript.

Competing interests
Tadashi Horikawa, Tetsurou Odatsu, Takatoshi Itoh, Yoshiki Soejima, Hutoshi Morinaga, Naruyoshi Abe, Naoyuki Tsuchiya, Toshikazu Iijima, and Takashi Sawase declare that they have no competing interests.

Author details
[1]Kyushu Implant Research Group, 4-14 Kokaihonmachi, Chuo-ku, Kumamoto 860-0851, Japan. [2]Department of Applied Prosthodontics, Graduate School of Biomedical Sciences, Nagasaki University, 1-7-1 Sakamoto, Nagasaki 852-8588, Japan.

References

1. Brånemark PI, Adell R, Breine U, Hansson BO, Lindström J, Ohlsson A. Intra-osseous anchorage of dental prostheses. I. Experimental studies. Scand J Plast Reconstr Surg. 1969;3:81–100.
2. Buser D, Sennerby L, De Bruyn H. Modern implant dentistry based on osseointegration: 50 years of progress, current trends and open questions. Periodontol. 2017;73:7–21.
3. Ekelund JA, Lindquist LW, Carlsson GE, Jemt T. Implant treatment in the edentulous mandible: a prospective study on Brånemark system implants over more than 20 years. Int J Prosthodont. 2003;16:602–8.
4. Lekholm U, Gröndahl K, Jemt T. Outcome of oral implant treatment in partially edentulous jaws followed 20 years in clinical function. Clin Implant Dent Relat Res. 2006;8:178–86.
5. Astrand P, Ahlqvist J, Gunne J, Nilson H. Implant treatment of patients with edentulous jaws: a 20-year follow-up. Clin Implant Dent Relat Res. 2008;10:207–17.
6. Chappuis V, Buser R, Brägger U, Bornstein MM, Salvi GE, Buser D. Long-term outcomes of dental implants with a titanium plasma-sprayed surface: a 20-year prospective case series study in partially edentulous patients. Clin Implant Dent Relat Res. 2013;15:780–90.
7. Becker ST, Beck-Broichsitter BE, Rossmann CM, Behrens E, Jochens A, Wiltfang J. Long-term survival of Straumann dental implants with TPS surfaces: a retrospective study with a follow-up of 12 to 23 years. Clin Implant Dent Relat Res. 2016;18:480–8.
8. Buser D, Mericske-Stern R, Bernard JP, Behneke A, Behneke N, Hirt HP, Belser UC, Lang NP. Long-term evaluation of non-submerged ITI implants. Part 1: 8-year life table analysis of a prospective multi-center study with 2359 implants. Clin Oral Implants Res. 1997;8:161–72.
9. Lekholm U, Gunne J, Henry P, Higuchi K, Lindén U, Bergström C, van Steenberghe D. Survival of the Brånemark implant in partially edentulous jaws: a 10-year prospective multicenter study. Int J Oral Maxillofac Implants. 1999;14:639–45.
10. Nyman S, Lindhe J, Karring T, Rylander H. New attachment following surgical treatment of human periodontal disease. J Clin Periodontol. 1982;9:290–6.
11. Dahlin C, Linde A, Gottlow J, Nyman S. Healing of bone defects by guided tissue regeneration. Plast Reconstr Surg. 1988;81:672–6.
12. Boyne PJ, James RA. Grafting of the maxillary sinus floor with autogenous marrow and bone. J Oral Surg. 1980;38:613–6.
13. Hellem S, Karlsson U, Almfeldt I, Brunell G, Hamp SE, Astrand P. Nonsubmerged implants in the treatment of the edentulous lower jaw: a 5-year prospective longitudinal study of ITI hollow screws. Clin Implant Dent Relat Res. 2001;3:20–9.
14. Roos-Jansåker AM, Lindahl C, Renvert H, Renvert S. Nine- to fourteen-year follow-up of implant treatment. Part II: presence of peri-implant lesions. J Clin Periodontol. 2006;33:290–5.
15. Lindhe J, Meyle J, Group D European Workshop on Periodontology. Peri-implant diseases: Consensus Report of the Sixth European Workshop on Periodontology. J Clin Periodontol. 2008;35(Suppl 8):282–5.

16. Derks J, Tomasi C. Peri-implant health and disease. A systematic review of current epidemiology. J Clin Periodontol. 2015;42(Suppl 16):S158–71.
17. Sgolastra F, Petrucci A, Severino M, Gatto R, Monaco A. Periodontitis, implant loss and peri-implantitis. A meta-analysis. Clin Oral Implants Res. 2015;26:e8–16.
18. Stacchi C, Berton F, Perinetti G, Frassetto A, Lombardi T, Khoury A, Andolsek F, Di Lenarda R. Risk factors for peri-implantitis: effect of history of periodontal disease and smoking habits. A systematic review and meta-analysis. J Oral Maxillofac Res. 2016;7:e3.
19. Koldsland OC, Scheie AA, Aass AM. The association between selected risk indicators and severity of peri-implantitis using mixed model analyses. J Clin Periodontol. 2011;38:285–92.
20. Attard NJ, Zarb GA. Long-term treatment outcomes in edentulous patients with implant-fixed prostheses: the Toronto study. Int J Prosthodont. 2004;17:417–24.
21. Geckili O, Mumcu E, Bilhan H. The effect of maximum bite force, implant number, and attachment type on marginal bone loss around implants supporting mandibular overdentures: a retrospective study. Clin Implant Dent Relat Res. 2012;14(Suppl 1):e91–7.
22. Renvert S, Aghazadeh A, Hallström H, Persson GR. Factors related to peri-implantitis — a retrospective study. Clin Oral Implants Res. 2014;25:522–9.
23. Duda M, Matalon S, Lewinstein I, Harel N, Block J, Ormianer Z. One piece immediately loading implants versus 1 piece or 2 pieces delayed: 3 years outcome. Implant Dent. 2016;25:109–13.
24. Wennerberg A, Albrektsson T. Effects of titanium surface topography on bone integration: a systematic review. Clin Oral Implants Res. 2009; 20(Suppl 4):172–84.
25. Teughels W, Van Assche N, Sliepen I, Quirynen M. Effect of material characteristics and/or surface topography on biofilm development. Clin Oral Implants Res. 2006;17(Suppl 2):68–81.
26. Brito C, Tenenbaum HC, Wong BK, Schmitt C, Nogueira-Filho G. Is keratinized mucosa indispensable to maintain peri-implant health? A systematic review of the literature. J Biomed Mater Res B Appl Biomater. 2014;102:643–50.
27. Ferreira CF, Buttendorf AR, de Souza JG, Dalago H, Guenther SF, Bianchini MA. Prevalence of peri-implant diseases: analyses of associated factors. Eur J Prosthodont Restor Dent. 2015;23:199–206.
28. Ladwein C, Schmelzeisen R, Nelson K, Fluegge TV, Fretwurst T. Is the presence of keratinized mucosa associated with periimplant tissue health? A clinical cross-sectional analysis. Int J Implant Dent. 2015;1(1):11.
29. Canullo L, Peñarrocha-Oltra D, Covani U, Botticelli D, Serino G, Penarrocha M. Clinical and microbiological findings in patients with peri-implantitis: a cross-sectional study. Clin Oral Implants Res. 2016;27:376–82.
30. Ko YC, Huang HL, Shen YW, Cai JY, Fuh LJ, Hsu JT. Variations in crestal cortical bone thickness at dental implant sites in different regions of the jawbone. Clin Implant Dent Relat Res. 2017; doi: 10.1111/cid.12468.
31. Lang NP, Pjetursson BE, Tan K, Brägger U, Egger M, Zwahlen M. A systematic review of the survival and complication rates of fixed partial dentures (FPDs) after an observation period of at least 5 years. II. Combined tooth implant-supported FPDs. Clin Oral Implants Res. 2004;15:643–53.
32. Aglietta M, Siciliano VI, Zwahlen M, Brägger U, Pjetursson BE, Lang NP, Salvi GE. A systematic review of the survival and complication rates of implant supported fixed dental prostheses with cantilever extensions after an observation period of at least 5 years. Clin Oral Implants Res. 2009;20:441–51.
33. Pjetursson BE, Thoma D, Jung R, Zwahlen M, Zembic A. A systematic review of the survival and complication rates of implant-supported fixed dental prostheses (FDPs) after a mean observation period of at least 5 years. Clin Oral Implants Res. 2012;23(Suppl 6):22–38.
34. Dorner S, Zeman F, Koller M, Lang R, Handel G, Behr M. Clinical performance of complete dentures: a retrospective study. Int J Prosthodont. 2010;23:410–7.

Permissions

All chapters in this book were first published in IJID, by Springer; hereby published with permission under the Creative Commons Attribution License or equivalent. Every chapter published in this book has been scrutinized by our experts. Their significance has been extensively debated. The topics covered herein carry significant findings which will fuel the growth of the discipline. They may even be implemented as practical applications or may be referred to as a beginning point for another development.

The contributors of this book come from diverse backgrounds, making this book a truly international effort. This book will bring forth new frontiers with its revolutionizing research information and detailed analysis of the nascent developments around the world.

We would like to thank all the contributing authors for lending their expertise to make the book truly unique. They have played a crucial role in the development of this book. Without their invaluable contributions this book wouldn't have been possible. They have made vital efforts to compile up to date information on the varied aspects of this subject to make this book a valuable addition to the collection of many professionals and students.

This book was conceptualized with the vision of imparting up-to-date information and advanced data in this field. To ensure the same, a matchless editorial board was set up. Every individual on the board went through rigorous rounds of assessment to prove their worth. After which they invested a large part of their time researching and compiling the most relevant data for our readers.

The editorial board has been involved in producing this book since its inception. They have spent rigorous hours researching and exploring the diverse topics which have resulted in the successful publishing of this book. They have passed on their knowledge of decades through this book. To expedite this challenging task, the publisher supported the team at every step. A small team of assistant editors was also appointed to further simplify the editing procedure and attain best results for the readers.

Apart from the editorial board, the designing team has also invested a significant amount of their time in understanding the subject and creating the most relevant covers. They scrutinized every image to scout for the most suitable representation of the subject and create an appropriate cover for the book.

The publishing team has been an ardent support to the editorial, designing and production team. Their endless efforts to recruit the best for this project, has resulted in the accomplishment of this book. They are a veteran in the field of academics and their pool of knowledge is as vast as their experience in printing. Their expertise and guidance has proved useful at every step. Their uncompromising quality standards have made this book an exceptional effort. Their encouragement from time to time has been an inspiration for everyone.

The publisher and the editorial board hope that this book will prove to be a valuable piece of knowledge for researchers, students, practitioners and scholars across the globe.

List of Contributors

Josipa Radic, Bernd Stadlinger, Martin Rücker and Barbara Giacomelli-Hiestand
Clinic of Cranio-Maxillofacial and Oral Surgery, Centre of Dental Medicine, University of Zurich, Plattenstrasse 11, 8032 Zurich, Switzerland

Raphael Patcas
Clinic for Orthodontics and Paediatric Dentistry, Centre of Dental Medicine, University of Zurich, Plattenstrasse 11, 8032 Zurich, Switzerland

Arturo Sánchez-Pérez
Periodontics Unit, Faculty of Medicine and Dentistry, University of Murcia (Spain), Murcia, Spain
Clínica Odontologíca Universitaria, Hospital Morales Meseguer, 2ª planta, C/ Marqués de los Vélez s/n, Murcia 30008, Spain

José María Parmigiani-Izquierdo, María Eugenia Cabaña-Muñoz and José Joaquín Merino
Clínica CIROM, Murcia 30001, Spain

Naoki Tanabe
Department of Applied Mathematics and Informatics, Nihon University School of Dentistry, Tokyo 101-8310, Japan

Tetsurou Odatsu
Department of Applied Prosthodontics, Graduate School of Biomedical Sciences, Nagasaki University, 1-7-1 Sakamoto, Nagasaki 852-8588, Japan

Andreas Sakkas, Frank Wilde and Marcus Heufelder
Department of Oral and Plastic Maxillofacial Surgery, Military Hospital Ulm, Academic Hospital of the University of Ulm, Oberer Eselsberg 40, 89081 Ulm, Germany

Karsten Winter
Institute of Anatomy, Medical Faculty of Leipzig University, Leipzig, Germany

Alexander Schramm
Department of Oral and Plastic Maxillofacial Surgery, Military Hospital Ulm, Academic Hospital of the University of Ulm, Oberer Eselsberg 40, 89081 Ulm, Germany
Department of Oral and Plastic Maxillofacial Surgery, University Hospital Ulm, Ulm, Germany

Marieke A. P. Filius, Joep Kraeima, Arjan Vissink, Gerry M. Raghoebar and Anita Visser
Department of Oral and Maxillofacial Surgery, University of Groningen and University Medical Center Groningen, 9700 RB Groningen, The Netherlands

Krista I. Janssen
Department of Orthodontics, University of Groningen and University Medical Center Groningen, 9700 RB Groningen, The Netherlands

K. Sagheb, E. Schiegnitz, M. Moergel, B. Al-Nawas and W. Wagner
Department of Oral and Maxillofacial Surgery, Plastic Surgery, University Medical Centre of the Johannes Gutenberg-University Mainz, Mainz, Germany

C. Walter
Department of Oral and Maxillofacial Surgery, Plastic Surgery, University Medical Centre of the Johannes Gutenberg-University Mainz, Mainz, Germany
Mediplus, Oral and Maxillofacial Surgery, Private Praxis, Mainz, Germany

Cagasan Pirpir, Onur Yilmaz, Celal Candirli and Emre Balaban
Faculty of Dentistry, Department of Oral and Maxillofacial Surgery, Karadeniz
Technical University, Trabzon, Turkey

Waldemar Reich, Christian Heinzelmann, Bilal Al-Nawas and Alexander Walter Eckert
Department of Oral and Plastic Maxillofacial Surgery, Martin Luther University Halle-Wittenberg, Ernst-Grube Str. 40, 06120 Halle (Saale), Germany

Ramona Schweyen and Jeremias Hey
University School of Dental Medicine, Department of Prosthetic Dentistry, Martin Luther University Halle-Wittenberg, Magdeburger Straße 16, 06112 Halle (Saale), Germany

Lamiaa Said Elfadaly, Lamiaa Sayed Khairallah and Mona Atteya Al Agroudy
Fixed Prosthodontics, Cairo University, Giza, Egypt

B. Beger, M. Morlock, E. Schiegnitz and B. Al-Nawas
Department of Maxillofacial Surgery, University Medical Center of the Johannes Gutenberg-University Mainz, Augustusplatz 2, 55131 Mainz, Germany

H. Goetz
Biomaterials in Medicine (BioAPP), University Medical Center of the Johannes Gutenberg-University Mainz, Mainz, Germany

Ashish Kakar, Bappanadu H. Sripathi Rao and Shashikanth Hegde
Yenepoya University Dental College, University Road, Mangalore 575018, India

Nikhil Deshpande
Dental Foundations and Research Centre, Malad, Mumbai 400064, India

Heiner Nagursky and Annette Lindner
Department of Oral and Maxillofacial Surgery, Center for Dental Medicine, Medical Center—University of Freiburg, Hugstetter Str. 55, 79106 Freiburg, Germany

Aditya Patney and Harsh Mahajan
Mahajan Imaging Center, K-18 Hauz Khas Enclave, New Delhi 110016, India

Tibebu Tsegga and Thomas Wright
Department of Oral & Maxillofacial Surgery, San Antonio Military Medical Center, 3551 Roger Brooke Dr., Ft. Sam Houston 78234, TX, USA
Department of Oral & Maxilofacial Surgery, Wilford Hall Ambulatory Surgical Center, 2200 Bergquist Dr, Suite 1, Lackland AFB, TX 78236, USA

Dawlat Mostafa and Moustafa Aboushelib
Dental Biomaterials, Faculty of Dentistry, Alexandria University, Champolion St., Azarita, Alexandria, Egypt

Mehmet A. Eskan
Sisli, Istanbul, Turkey
Clinic Eska, Terrace Fulya, Tesvikiye Mah., Hakki Yeten Cad, Sisli, Istanbul, Turkey

Marie-Eve Girouard
Sherbrooke, Québec, Canada

Dean Morton
Department of Prosthodontics, Indiana University School of Dentistry, Indianapolis, IN 46202, USA

Henry Greenwell
Department of Oral Health and Rehabilitation, Division of Periodontics, University of Louisville School of Dentistry, Louisville, KY 40292, USA

Yusuke Zushi, Kazuki Takaoka, Joji Tamaoka, Miho Ueta, Kazuma Noguchi and Hiromitsu Kishimoto
Department of Oral and Maxillofacial Surgery, Hyogo College of Medicine, 1-1 Mukogawa-cho, Nishinomiya, Hyogo 663-8501, Japan

E. A. J. M. Schulten
Department of Oral and Maxillofacial Surgery/ Oral Pathology, VU University Medical Center/ Academic Centre for Dentistry Amsterdam (ACTA), 1007 MB Amsterdam, The Netherlands

N. Bravenboer
Department of Clinical Chemistry, VU University Medical Center, Amsterdam, The Netherlands

J. W. F. H. Frenken
Department of Oral and Maxillofacial Surgery, St. Antonius Hospital, Nieuwegein, The Netherlands

C. M. ten Bruggenkate
Department of Oral and Maxillofacial Surgery/ Oral Pathology, VU University Medical Center/ Academic Centre for Dentistry Amsterdam (ACTA), 1007 MB Amsterdam, The Netherlands
Department of Oral and Maxillofacial Surgery, Alrijne Hospital, Leiderdorp, The Netherlands

W. F. Bouwman
Department of Oral and Maxillofacial Surgery/ Oral Pathology, VU University Medical Center/ Academic Centre for Dentistry Amsterdam (ACTA), 1007 MB Amsterdam, The Netherlands
Department of Oral and Maxillofacial Surgery, The Tergooi Hospital, Blaricum, The Netherlands

Juliana Marulanda, Sharifa Alebrahim and Jocelyne Sheila Feine
Faculty of Dentistry, McGill University, Montreal, Quebec, Canada

Jagjit Singh Dhaliwal
Faculty of Dentistry, McGill University, Montreal, Quebec, Canada
PAPRSB, Institute of Health Sciences, Universiti Brunei Darussalam, Jalan Tungku Link, Gadong BE1410, Brunei Darussalam

Jingjing Li
Faculty of Medicine, McGill University, Montreal, Quebec, Canada

Monzur Murshed
Faculty of Dentistry, McGill University, Montreal, Quebec, Canada
Faculty of Medicine, McGill University, Montreal, Quebec, Canada
Shriners Hospital for Children, Montreal, Quebec H4A 0A9, Canada

Hiroko Ishii, Akemi Tetsumura, Yoshikazu Nomura, Shin Nakamura and Tohru Kurabayashi
Department of Oral and Maxillofacial Radiology, Graduate School of Medical and Dental Sciences, Tokyo Medical and Dental University, 1-5-45, Yushima, Bunkyo-ku, Tokyo, Japan

Masako Akiyama
URA, Research Administration Division, Tokyo Medical and Dental University, 1-5-45, Yushima, Bunkyo-ku, Tokyo, Japan

Sotirios Konstantinos Saridakis and Wilfried Wagner
Department of Oral and Maxillofacial Surgery - Plastic Surgery, University Medical Center, Johannes Gutenberg University of Mainz, Augustusplatz 2, 55131 Mainz, Germany

Robert Noelken
Department of Oral and Maxillofacial Surgery - Plastic Surgery, University Medical Center, Johannes Gutenberg University of Mainz, Augustusplatz 2, 55131 Mainz, Germany
Private Practice for Oral Surgery, Lindau/Lake Constance, Germany

Puria Parvini
Department of Oral Surgery and Implantology, Carolinum, Johann Wolfgang Goethe-University, Frankfurt, Germany

Frank Schwarz
Department of Oral Surgery and Implantology, Carolinum, Johann Wolfgang Goethe-University, Frankfurt, Germany
Department of Oral Surgery, Universitätsklinikum Düsseldorf, Düsseldorf, Germany

Robert Sader
Department for Oral, Cranio-Maxillofacial and Facial Plastic Surgery, Medical Center of the Goethe University Frankfurt, Frankfurt, Germany

Didem Sahin and Jürgen Becker
Department of Oral Surgery, Universitätsklinikum Düsseldorf, Düsseldorf, Germany

Dimitrios Apostolakis and Georgios Kourakis
Private Practice, Dental Radiology in Crete, Plateia 1866, No 39, 73100 Chania, Crete, Greece

Mai Ahmed Yousry El-Sheikh, Tamer Mohamed Nasr Mostafa and Mohamed Maamoun El-Sheikh
Prosthodontic Department, Faculty of Dentistry, Tanta University, Elgeish St., Tanta, Egypt

Eijiro Sakamoto, Rie Kido and Jun-ichi Kido
Department of Periodontology and Endodontology, Institute of Biomedical Sciences, Tokushima University Graduate School, 3-18-15 Kuramoto, Tokushima 770-8504, Japan

Yoritoki Tomotake and Yoshihito Naitou
Oral Implant Center, Tokushima University Hospital, Tokushima, Japan

Yuichi Ishida
Department of Oral and Maxillofacial Prosthodontics, Institute of Biomedical Sciences, Tokushima University Graduate School, Tokushima, Japan

E. Schiegnitz, K. Sagheb, A. Pabst and B. Al-Nawas
Department of Oral and Maxillofacial Surgery, Plastic Surgery, University Medical Centre of the Johannes Gutenberg-University, Augustusplatz 2, 55131 Mainz, Germany

P. W. Kämmerer
Department of Oral and Maxillofacial Surgery, Plastic Surgery, University of Rostock, Rostock, Germany

A. J. Wendt
Department of Prosthodontics, University of Hamburg-Eppendorf, Hamburg, Germany

M. O. Klein
Department of Oral and Maxillofacial Surgery, Plastic Surgery, University Medical Centre of the Johannes Gutenberg-University, Augustusplatz 2, 55131 Mainz, Germany
Oral and Maxillofacial Surgery, Private Praxis, Düsseldorf, Germany

Shinya Nakabayashi and Yoshiyuki Hagiwara
Implant Dentistry, Nihon University School of Dentistry Dental Hospital, Tokyo 101-8310, Japan

Atsushi Kamimoto and Keisuke Seki
Implant Dentistry, Nihon University School of Dentistry Dental Hospital, Tokyo 101-8310, Japan
Department of Comprehensive Dentistry and Clinical Education, Nihon University School of Dentistry, 1-8-13 Kanda-Surugadai, Chiyoda-ku, Tokyo 101-8310, Japan

Daniel Wiedemeier
Statistical Services, Centre of Dental Medicine, University of Zurich, Plattenstrasse 11, 8032 Zurich, Switzerland

Tadashi Horikawa, Takatoshi Itoh, Yoshiki Soejima, Hutoshi Morinaga, Naruyoshi Abe, Naoyuki Tsuchiya and Toshikazu Iijima
Kyushu Implant Research Group, 4-14 Kokaihonmachi, Chuo-ku, Kumamoto 860-0851, Japan

Takashi Sawase
Kyushu Implant Research Group, 4-14 Kokaihonmachi, Chuo-ku, Kumamoto 860-0851, Japan
Department of Applied Prosthodontics, Graduate School of Biomedical Sciences, Nagasaki University, 1-7-1 Sakamoto, Nagasaki 852-8588, Japan

Index

www.ingramcontent.com/pod-product-compliance
Lightning Source LLC
Chambersburg PA
CBHW082034190326
41458CB00010B/3363

* 9 7 8 1 6 3 9 2 7 0 5 2 1 *